Fibroblast Activation Protein Imaging

Editors

RODNEY J. HICKS
FREDERIK L. GIESEL
KEN HERRMANN

PET CLINICS

www.pet.theclinics.com

Consulting Editor
ABASS ALAVI

July 2023 • Volume 18 • Number 3

ELSEVIER

1600 John F. Kennedy Boulevard • Suite 1800 • Philadelphia, Pennsylvania, 19103-2899

http://www.pet.theclinics.com

PET CLINICS Volume 18, Number 3
July 2023 ISSN 1556-8598, ISBN-13: 978-0-323-93895-2

Editor: John Vassallo (j.vassallo@elsevier.com)
Developmental Editor: Karen Justine S. Dino

PET Clinics (ISSN 1556-8598) is published quarterly by Elsevier Inc., 360 Park Avenue South, New York, NY 10010-1710. Months of issue are January, April, July, and October. Periodicals postage paid at New York, NY, and additional mailing offices. Subscription prices per year are $275.00 (US individuals), $500.00 (US institutions), $100.00 (US students), $304.00 (Canadian individuals), $563.00 (Canadian institutions), $100.00 (Canadian students), $297.00 (foreign individuals), $563.00 (foreign institutions), and $140.00 (foreign students). To receive student and resident rate, orders must be accompanied by name of affiliated institution, date of term, and the signature of program/residency coordinator on institution letterhead. Orders will be billed at individual rate until proof of status is received. Foreign air speed delivery is included in all Clinics subscription prices. All prices are subject to change without notice. POSTMASTER: Send address changes to PET Clinics, Elsevier Health Sciences Division, Subscription Customer Service, 3251 Riverport Lane, Maryland Heights, MO 63043. **Customer Service: 1-800-654-2452 (U.S. and Canada); 314-447-8871 (outside U.S. and Canada). Fax: 314-447-8029. E-mail: journalscustomerservice-usa@elsevier.com (for print support); journalsonlinesupport-usa@elsevier.com (for online support).**

Reprints. For copies of 100 or more of articles in this publication, please contact the Commercial Reprints Department, Elsevier Inc., 360 Park Avenue South, New York, NY 10010-1710. Tel.: 212-633-3874; Fax: 212-633-3820; E-mail: reprints@elsevier.com.

PET Clinics is covered in MEDLINE/PubMed (Index Medicus).

Contributors

CONSULTING EDITOR

ABASS ALAVI, MD, MD (Hon), PhD (Hon), DSc (Hon)
Professor of Radiology and Neurology, Director of Research Education, Division of

Nuclear Medicine, Department of Radiology, Hospital of the University of Pennsylvania, Perelman School of Medicine, University of Pennsylvania, Philadelphia, Pennsylvania, USA

EDITORS

RODNEY J. HICKS, MB, BS, MD, FRACP
Department of Medicine, St Vincent's Medical School, The University of Melbourne, Australia; The Department of Medicine, Central Clinical School, The Alfred Hospital, Monash University, Melbourne, Australia

FREDERIK L. GIESEL, MD, MBA
Department of Nuclear Medicine, Medical Faculty and University Hospital Duesseldorf, Heinrich-Heine-University Duesseldorf,

Duesseldorf, Germany; Department of Nuclear Medicine, Heidelberg University Hospital, Heidelberg, Germany; Institute for Radiation Sciences, Osaka University, Osaka, Japan

KEN HERRMANN, MD, MBA
Professor, German Cancer Consortium (DKTK), Partner Site University Hospital Essen, Department of Nuclear Medicine, West German Cancer Center, University Hospital Essen, Essen, Germany

AUTHORS

JOHN W. BABICH, PhD
Ratio Therapeutics, Inc, Boston, Massachusetts, USA

SEBASTIAN BAUER, MD
Professor, Department of Medical Oncology, West German Cancer Center, University Hospital Essen, Hufelandstr, Germany; German Cancer Consortium (DKTK), Partner Site University Hospital Essen, Essen, Germany

FRANK M. BENGEL, MD, FAHA
Department of Nuclear Medicine, Hannover Medical School, Hannover, Germany

HAOJUN CHEN, MD, PhD
Department of Nuclear Medicine and Minnan PET Center, Xiamen Cancer Center, The First Affiliated Hospital of Xiamen University, School of Medicine, Xiamen University, Xiamen, China

PHYLLIS F. CHEUNG, PhD
Bridge Institute of Experimental Tumor Therapy, West German Cancer Center, University Hospital Essen, Essen, Germany; Division of Solid Tumor Translational Oncology, German Cancer Consortium (DKTK, Partner Site Essen), German Cancer Research Center, DKFZ, Heidelberg, Germany

KATHARINA DENDL, Can.Med
Department of Nuclear Medicine, University Hospital Heidelberg, Heidelberg, Germany; Department of Nuclear Medicine, University Hospital Duesseldorf, Duesseldorf, Germany

JOHANNA DIEKMANN, MD
Department of Nuclear Medicine, Hannover Medical School, Hannover, Germany

STEPHEN G. DIMAGNO, PhD
Ratio Therapeutics, Inc, Boston, Massachusetts, USA

GIANPAOLO DI SANTO, MD
Department of Nuclear Medicine, Medical University of Innsbruck, Innsbruck, Austria

SJOERD ELIAS, MD, PhD
Department of Epidemiology, Julius Center for Health Sciences and Primary Care, University Medical Center Utrecht, Utrecht University, Utrecht, the Netherlands

AARON S. ENKE, BS
Senior Director, Clinical Development, Clovis Oncology, Boulder, Colorado, USA

WOLFGANG P. FENDLER, MD
Professor, German Cancer Consortium (DKTK), Partner Site University Hospital Essen, Department of Nuclear Medicine, West German Cancer Center, University Hospital Essen, Essen, Germany

FREDERIK L. GIESEL, MD, MBA
Department of Nuclear Medicine, Medical Faculty and University Hospital Duesseldorf, Heinrich-Heine-University Duesseldorf, Duesseldorf, Germany; Department of Nuclear Medicine, Heidelberg University Hospital, Heidelberg, Germany; Institute for Radiation Sciences, Osaka University, Osaka, Japan

UWE HABERKORN, MD
Department of Nuclear Medicine, Heidelberg University Hospital, Heidelberg, Germany

RAINER HAMACHER, MD
Department of Medical Oncology, West German Cancer Center, University Hospital Essen, Hufelandstr, Germany; German Cancer Consortium (DKTK), Partner Site University Hospital Essen, Essen, Germany

KEN HERRMANN, MD, MBA
Professor, German Cancer Consortium (DKTK), Partner Site University Hospital Essen, Department of Nuclear Medicine, West German Cancer Center, University Hospital Essen, Essen, Germany

JESSICA D. JENSEN, MPH
Executive Vice President, Clinical Development, Point Biopharma, Indianapolis, Indiana, USA

KAZUKO KANEDA-NAKASHIMA, PhD
Division of Radiation Science, Institute for Radiation Sciences, Osaka University, MS-CORE, Forefront Research Center, Graduate School of Science, Osaka University, Osaka, Japan

YUICHIRO KADONAGA, PhD, MS-CORE
Forefront Research Center, Graduate School of Science, Osaka University, Department of Nuclear Medicine and Tracer Kinetics, Graduate School of Medicine, Osaka University, Osaka, Japan

LUKAS KESSLER, MD
Department of Nuclear Medicine, West German Cancer Center, University Hospital Essen, University of Duisburg-Essen, German Cancer Consortium (DKTK), Partner Site University Hospital Essen, German Cancer Research Center (DKFZ), Essen, Germany

STEFAN A. KOERBER, MD, PD
Department of Radiation Oncology and Radiation Therapy, Heidelberg University Hospital, Clinical Cooperation Unit Radiation Oncology, German Cancer Research Center, Heidelberg, Germany; Department of Radiation Oncology and Radiation Therapy, Barmherzige Brueder Hospital Regensburgh, Regensburg, Germany

ONNO KRANENBURG, PhD
Division of Imaging and Cancer, Laboratory Translational Oncology, University Medical Center Utrecht, Utrecht University, Utrecht, the Netherlands

CLEMENS KRATOCHWIL, MD
Department of Nuclear Medicine, Heidelberg University Hospital, Heidelberg, Germany

KATHARINA LÜCKERATH, PhD
Preclinical Theranostics, Department of Nuclear Medicine, University of Duisburg-Essen, German Cancer Consortium (DKTK), University Hospital Essen, Essen, Germany

MARNIX LAM, MD, PhD
Department of Radiology and Nuclear Medicine, University Medical Center Utrecht, Utrecht University, Utrecht, the Netherlands

HELENA LANZAFAME, MD
German Cancer Consortium (DKTK), Partner
Site University Hospital Essen, Department of
Nuclear Medicine, West German Cancer Center,
University Hospital Essen, Essen, Germany

QIN LIN, MD, PhD
Department of Radiation Oncology, Xiamen
Cancer Center, Xiamen Key Laboratory of
Radiation Oncology, The First Affiliated
Hospital of Xiamen University, School of
Medicine, Xiamen University, Xiamen, China

ILEKTRA A. MAVROEIDI, MD
Department of Medical Oncology, West
German Cancer Center, University Hospital
Essen, Hufelandstr, Germany; German Cancer
Consortium (DKTK), Partner Site University
Hospital Essen, Essen, Germany

CHRISTINE E. MONA, PhD
Ahmanson Translational Theranostic Division,
Department of Molecular and Medical
Pharmacology, University of California, Los
Angeles, Los Angeles, California, USA

YURIKO MORI, MD
Department of Nuclear Medicine, Medical
Faculty and University Hospital Duesseldorf,
Heinrich-Heine-University Duesseldorf,
Duesseldorf, Germany

SHERLY MOSESSIAN, PhD
Chief Scientific Officer, Sofie Biosciences Inc,
Dulles, Virginia, USA

EMIL NOVRUZOV, MD
Department of Nuclear Medicine, Medical
Faculty, Heinrich-Heine-University, University
Hospital Dusseldorf, Dusseldorf, Germany

FUAD NOVRUZOV, MD
Department of Nuclear Medicine, Azerbaijan
National Centre of Oncology, Baku, Azerbaijan

KIM M. PABST, MD
German Cancer Consortium (DKTK), Partner
Site University Hospital Essen, Department of
Nuclear Medicine, West German Cancer
Center, University Hospital Essen, Essen,
Germany

YIZHEN PANG, MD
Department of Nuclear Medicine and Minnan
PET Center, School of Medicine, Department
of Radiation Oncology, Xiamen Cancer Center,
Xiamen Key Laboratory of Radiation Oncology,
The First Affiliated Hospital of Xiamen
University, School of Medicine, Xiamen
University, Xiamen, China

MANUEL RÖHRICH, PhD, MD, (German PD)
Department of Nuclear Medicine, University
Hospital Heidelberg, Heidelberg, Germany

HANS-ULRICH SCHILDHAUS, MD
Professor, German Cancer Consortium
(DKTK), Partner Site University Hospital Essen,
Institute of Pathology, West German Cancer
Center, University Hospital Essen, Essen,
Germany

YOSHIFUMI SHIRAKAMI, PhD
Division of Radiation Science, Institute for
Radiation Sciences, Osaka University, MS-
CORE, Forefront Research Center, Graduate
School of Science, Osaka University, Osaka,
Japan

JENS T. SIVEKE, MD
Professor, Department of Medical Oncology,
West German Cancer Center, University
Hospital Essen, Hufelandstr, Germany;
German Cancer Consortium (DKTK), Partner
Site University Hospital Essen, Bridge Institute
of Experimental Tumor Therapy, West German
Cancer Center, University Hospital Essen,
Essen, Germany; Division of Solid Tumor
Translational Oncology, German Cancer
Consortium (DKTK), Partner Site Essen) and
German Cancer Research Center, DKFZ,
Heidelberg, Germany

ESTHER STRATING, MD
Division of Imaging and Cancer, Laboratory
Translational Oncology, University Medical
Center Utrecht, Utrecht University, Utrecht, the
Netherlands

LONG SUN, MD, PhD
Department of Nuclear Medicine and Minnan
PET Center, Xiamen Cancer Center, The First
Affiliated Hospital of Xiamen University,
School of Medicine, Xiamen University,
Xiamen, China

ANNA SVIRIDENKO, MD
Department of Nuclear Medicine, Medical
University of Innsbruck, Innsbruck, Austria

MARIJA TRAJKOVIC-ARSIC, PhD
Division of Solid Tumor Translational
Oncology, DKTK and German Cancer
Research Center (DKFZ) Partner Side
Essen; Bridge Institute of Experimental
Tumor Therapy, West German Cancer
Center, University Hospital Essen, Essen,
Germany

ANNE VAN DE LOO, BSC
Division of Imaging and Cancer, Laboratory
Translational Oncology, University Medical
Center Utrecht, Utrecht University, Utrecht, the
Netherlands

IRENE VIRGOLINI, MD
Department of Nuclear Medicine, Medical
University of Innsbruck, Innsbruck, Austria

TADASHI WATABE, MD, PhD
Assistant Professor, Department of Nuclear
Medicine and Tracer Kinetics, Graduate
School of Medicine, Institute for Radiation
Sciences, Osaka University, Osaka, Japan;
Department of Nuclear Medicine, Osaka
University, Suita, Japan

HUA WU, MD, PhD
Department of Nuclear Medicine and Minnan
PET Center, Xiamen Cancer Center, The First
Affiliated Hospital of Xiamen University,
School of Medicine, Xiamen University,
Xiamen, China

LIANG ZHAO, MD
Department of Nuclear Medicine and
Minnan PET Center, School of Medicine,
Department of Radiation Oncology, Xiamen
Cancer Center, Xiamen Key Laboratory of
Radiation Oncology, The First Affiliated
Hospital of Xiamen University, School
of Medicine, Xiamen University, Xiamen,
China

Contents

Fibroblast activation protein-α (FAP) has attracted increasing attention as a selective marker of cancer-associated fibroblasts (CAFs) and more broadly, of activated fibroblasts in tissues undergoing remodeling of their ECM due to chronic inflammation, fibrosis, or wound healing. Since FAP is critical to the initiation of metastatic growth, its expression will serve as a molecular marker to detect tumors at an earlier stage of development compared to currently available methods. The design of high affinity small molecule FAP inhibitor will allow for noninvasive imaging of activated fibroblast in cancer patients. Small molecule inhibitors of FAP are being developed for targeted radiotherapy of tumors.

Radiolabeled fibroblast activation protein inhibitor (FAPI) has been introduced as a promising PET tracer for imaging of pancreatic cancer. To date, FAPI PET/computed tomography (CT) has generally but not universally yielded higher radiotracer uptake and tumor-to-background contrast than ^{18}F-fluorodeoxyglucose PET/CT in primary tumors, involved lymph nodes, and visceral metastases. It may also be useful for the evaluation of the tumor response to chemotherapy. However, increased FAPI uptake may be observed in benign conditions, including pancreatitis, pancreatic tuberculosis, IgG4-related disease, and serous cystadenoma, and therefore, clinical, radiological, and pathological correlations are required.

Hepatocellular carcinoma (HCC) is the most common primary liver malignancy with worldwide high incidence and mortality. In more than 90% of cases, HCC arise from a cirrhotic liver that is mostly induced by viral diseases and especially in developed countries alcoholic steatohepatitis and non-alcoholic steatohepatitis. In contrast, cholangiocellular carcinoma (CCC) is a very rare cancer entity with a high mortality due to insidious onset. The only curative option for both cancer entities is a timely and definitive surgical therapy, which mandates an accurate early diagnosis. To this end, [18F]FDG PET/CT scan could demonstrate only little benefit, as there is an unmet clinical need for an alternative, pan-cancer agent for initial diagnostic work-up of CCC or evaluation of Milan criteria for HCC patients.

^{68}Ga-fibroblast activation protein inhibitor (FAPI)-PET is highly promising for head and neck cancers including oral squamous cell carcinomas, hypopharynx carcinomas, adenoid cystic carcinomas, thyroid cancer, and cervical cancer of unknown primary. For oral squamous cell carcinomas, hypopharynx carcinomas, and adenoid cystic carcinomas, ^{68}Ga-FAPI-PET has high potential for the assessment of primary tumors with impact on radiotherapy planning. ^{68}Ga-FAPI-PET can be applied for staging of metastasized thyroid carcinomas. To date, the data on cervical cancer of unknown primary are sparse but highly interesting as ^{68}Ga-FAPI-PET may detect a significant portion of ^{18}fluoro-deoxyglucose-PET-negative primary tumors.

Fibroblast activation protein inhibitor (FAPI)-PET imaging holds great promise for improving the clinical management of colorectal cancer. High fibroblast activation protein expression is particularly observed in lymph node metastases, in the aggressive Consensus Molecular Subtype 4, in peritoneal metastases, and in tumors that respond poorly to immunotherapy. We have defined six clinical dilemmas in the diagnosis and treatment of colorectal cancer, which FAPI-PET may help solve. Future clinical trials should include patients undergoing tumor resection, allowing correlation of FAPI-PET signals with in-depth histopathological, cellular, and molecular tissue analyses.

Like other major cancers, gastric cancer expresses fibroblast activation protein (FAP) in cancer-associated fibroblasts. Many recent studies have reported the utility and superiority of FAP inhibitor (FAPI)-PET over [^{18}F]fluorodeoxyglucose (FDG)-PET in gastric cancers, from initial staging to recurrence detection. FAPI-PET shows higher accumulation in primary sites and metastatic lesions than does FDG-PET, especially for the detection of peritoneal carcinomatosis. In the case of gastric signet ring cell carcinoma, FAPI-PET showed excellent performance, as uptake is usually weak on FDG-PET in this cohort.

68Ga-FAPI-PET/computed tomography (CT) is a novel PET/CT radiotracer particularly developed for oncologic imaging. Gynecologic malignancies comprise a broad spectrum of entities and, along with breast cancer, constitute cancers occurring exclusively or primarily, respectively, in women. Thus, a tracer designed not only for one but multiple malignancies has theoretic attractions. Even in comparison with 18F-FDG, the current standard oncologic tracer of nuclear medicine, 68Ga-FAPI, has demonstrated advantages in several tumors. As breast cancer, ovarian cancer, and cervical cancer are among the most common tumor types in women and are often accompanied by high morbidity as well as mortality rates, a reliable staging tool is paramount for optimal therapeutic management.

Advances in histopathologic and molecular genetic subtyping of sarcoma will potentially allow identification of novel diagnostic and therapeutic targets for specific subtypes, but a "pan-sarcoma" target is needed. This article provides an overview on expression of one potential candidate, fibroblast activation protein alpha in soft tissue and bone sarcoma, and the resulting application of 68Ga-FAPI as novel imaging probes in these rare tumor entities. Current preclinical and clinical data on 68Ga-FAPI-PET/CT in sarcomas are summarized. 68Ga-FAPI-PET-CT potentially offers important complementary information to be used in diagnostic work-up, assessment of therapy response, and prognostication of soft tissue and bone sarcomas.

The theranostic use of fibroblast activation protein inhibitors (FAPIs) is a novel approach in oncology. Sarcomas are a heterogenous group of rare malignant tumors. Prognosis remains poor in advanced/metastatic disease due to limited therapeutic options. Sarcoma frequently demonstrate high expression of fibroblast activation protein alpha on the tumor cells themselves, in contrast to other solid tumors, where it is mainly expressed on cancer-associated fibroblasts. Consequently, high in vivo uptake of FAPI in PET is observed in sarcoma. Moreover, retrospective case reports and series demonstrated feasibility of FAPI radioligand therapy with signs of tumor response.

Computed tomography (CT), MR imaging, and PET with fluorodeoxyglucose F18/CT are commonly used for radiation therapy planning; however, issues including precise nodal staging on CT or false positive results on PET/CT limit their usability. Clinical trials using fibroblast activation protein ligands for additional imaging have provided promising results regarding staging and target volume delineation—particularly suitable for sarcoma, some gastrointestinal tumors, head and neck tumors, and lung and pancreatic cancer. Although further prospective trials are necessary to identify clinical settings for its application in radiation oncology, fibroblast activation protein inhibitor PET/CT indisputably represents an excellent opportunity for assisting radiotherapy planning.

Tissue injury in nonmalignant human disease can develop from either disproportionate inflammation or exaggerated fibrotic responses. The molecular and cellular fundamental of these 2 processes, their impact on disease prognosis and the treatment concept deviates fundamentally. Consequently, the synchronous assessment and quantification of these 2 processes in vivo is extremely desirable. Although noninvasive molecular techniques such as ^{18}F-fluorodeoxyglucose PET offer insights into the degree of inflammatory activity, the assessment of the molecular dynamics of fibrosis remains challenging. The ^{68}Ga-fibroblast activation protein inhibitor-46 may improve noninvasive clinical diagnostic performance in patients with both fibroinflammatory pathology and long-term CT-abnormalities after severe COVID-19.

Johanna Diekmann and Frank M. Bengel

Several promising applications of cardiac molecular fibroblast activation protein (FAP) imaging are emerging. Myocardial fibrosis plays a key role in the complex process of cardiac remodeling and can lead to adverse clinical outcomes such as left ventricular dysfunction, propensity to arrhythmias, and reduction of perfusion. If fibrosis becomes irreversible, patients can develop heart failure. Therefore identification and early fibrosis treatment is highly warranted. FAP-targeted imaging enables new insights into pathogenesis and treatment response in various cardiac diseases such as myocardial infarction, heart failure or systemic diseases being a new selective biomarker.

Kazuko Kaneda-Nakashima, Yoshifumi Shirakami, Yuichiro Kadonaga, and Tadashi Watabe

Fibroblast activation protein (FAP) was first reported in 1986. However, FAP is not expressed in normal fibroblasts, normal or malignant epithelial cells, or the stroma of benign epithelial tumors. FAP is a cell membrane-bound serine peptidase overexpressed on the surface of cancer-associated fibroblasts and, as such, is a novel target for molecular imaging of several tumors. FAP inhibitors (FAPI) are potential theranostic molecular probes for various cancers. A tumor model expressing FAP was used to verify or confirm the usefulness of FAPI experimentally.

Katharina Lückerath, Marija Trajkovic-Arsic, and Christine E. Mona

Fibroblast activation protein (FAP)-radioligand therapy might be effective in some patients without being curative. FAP-radioligands deliver ionizing radiation directly to FAP$^+$ cancer-associated fibroblasts and, in some cancers, to FAP$^+$ tumor cells; in addition, they indirectly irradiate FAP$^-$ cells in tumor tissue via cross-fire and bystander effects. Here, we discuss the potential to improve FAP-radioligand therapy through interfering with DNA damage repair, immunotherapy, and co-targeting cancer-associated fibroblasts. As the molecular and cellular effects of FAP-radioligands on the tumor and its microenvironment have not been investigated yet, we call for future research to close this gap in knowledge, which prevents the development of more effective FAP-radioligand therapies.

Yuriko Mori, Clemens Kratochwil, Uwe Haberkorn, and Frederik L. Giesel

Fibroblast activation protein (FAP)-targeted radioligand therapy offers a possibility of a novel cancer therapeutic strategy, aiming at tumor stroma1. Early clinical translations of FAP-tracers occurred as early as in the 1990s using antibodies, without substantial achievement further than the clinical phase II trial. The essential step toward the theranostic approach, with a conceptual combination of diagnostic and therapeutic emitters in a specific tracer, began with the implementation of small-molecule FAP-enzyme inhibitors (FAPI) in 2018. Currently, FAPI-04 and FAPI-46, containing

DOTA-chelators with the possibility of radionuclide combination (Ga-68, Y-90, and Lu-177), are the compounds most widely used in the theranostic regimen.

Current State of Clinical Trials and Regulatory Approvals with Fibroblast Activation Protein Targeting Interventions

Sherly Mosessian, Jessica D. Jensen, and Aaron S. Enke

In this article, the authors review the current state of fibroblast activation protein (FAP)-targeted interventions utilizing available data from clinicaltrials.gov. Thirty-seven records were reviewed and demonstrated interventions with imaging studies comprising the largest portion of the active studies in progress, followed by thera-peutic studies using non-radioligand and radioligand therapy. The efforts are in early stages of clinical development; however the field is gaining significant momentum. Completion of existing clincial studies and entrance of new products into the clincial trial phase will shed important light on the clinical utility of these interventions and shape future clinical development efforts.

PET CLINICS

SERIES OF RELATED INTEREST

Advances in Clinical Radiology
Available at: Advancesinclinicalradiology.com
MRI Clinics of North America
Available at: MRI.theclinics.com
Neuroimaging Clinics of North America
Available at: Neuroimaging.theclinics.com
Radiologic Clinics of North America
Available at: Radiologic.theclinics.com

THE CLINICS ARE AVAILABLE ONLINE!
Access your subscription at:
www.theclinics.com

PROGRAM OBJECTIVE

The goal of the *PET Clinics* is to keep practicing radiologists and radiology residents up to date with current clinical practice in positron emission tomography by providing timely articles reviewing the state of the art in patient care.

TARGET AUDIENCE

Practicing radiologists, radiology residents, and other health care professionals who provide patient care utilizing radiologic findings.

LEARNING OBJECTIVES

Upon completion of this activity, participants will be able to:
1. Review the benefits of fibroblast activation protein-α (FAP) as a universal target antigen.
2. Discuss several promising and emerging applications FAP-imaging.
3. Recognize fibroblast activation protein (FAP)-targeted and positron emission tomography (PET) imaging are emerging beyond tumor imaging and represent an excellent opportunity for assisting radiotherapy planning.

ACCREDITATION

The Elsevier Office of Continuing Medical Education (EOCME) is accredited by the Accreditation Council for Continuing Medical Education (ACCME) to provide continuing medical education for physicians.

The EOCME designates this journal-based CME activity for a maximum of 16 *AMA PRA Category 1 Credit*(s)™.Physicians should claim only the credit commensurate with the extent of their participation in the activity.

All other health care professionals requesting continuing education credit for this enduring material will be issued a certificate of participation.

DISCLOSURE OF CONFLICTS OF INTEREST

The EOCME assesses conflict of interest with its instructors, faculty, planners, and other individuals who are in a position to control the content of CME activities. All relevant conflicts of interest that are identified are thoroughly vetted by EOCME for fair balance, scientific objectivity, and patient care recommendations. EOCME is committed to providing its learners with CME activities that promote improvements or quality in healthcare and not a specific proprietary business or a commercial interest.

The planning committee, staff, authors, and editors listed below have identified no financial relationships or relationships to products or devices they or their spouse/life partner have with commercial interest related to the content of this CME activity:

Sebastian Bauer, MD; Frank M. Bengel, MD, FAHA; Haojun Chen, MD, PhD; Phyllis F. Cheung, PhD; Katharina Dendl; Gianpaolo di Santo, MD; Johanna Diekmann, MD; Sjoerd Elias, MD, PhD; Wolfgang P. Fendler, MD; Uwe Haberkorn, MD; Rainer Hamacher, MD; Rodney John Hicks, MB, BS, MD, FRACP; Yuichiro Kadonaga, PhD; Kazuko Kaneda-Nakashima, PhD; Stefan A. Koerber, MD; Onno Kranenburga, PhD; Clemens Kratochwil, MD; Kothainayaki Kulanthaivelu, BCA, MBA; Marnix Lam, MD, PhD; Helena Lanzafame, MD; Qin Lin, MD, PhD; Michelle Littlejohn; Ilektra A. Mavroeidi, MD; Christine E. Mona, PhD; Yuriko Mori, MD; Faud Novruzov, MD; Emil Novruzov, MD; Kim M. Pabst, MD; Yizhen Pang, MD; Manuel Röhrich, MD; Hans-Ulrich Schildhaus, MD; Yoshifumi Shirakami, PhD; Jens T. Siveke, MD; Esther Strating, MD; Long Sun, MD, PhD; Anna Sviridenko, MD; Marija Trajkovic-Arsic, PhD; Anne van de Loo, BSc; Irene Virgolini, MD; Tadashi Watabe, MD, PhD; Hua Wu, MD, PhD; Liang Zhao, MD

The planning committee, staff, authors, and editors listed below have identified financial relationships or relationships to products or devices they or their spouse/life partner have with commercial interest related to the content of this CME activity:

John W. Babich, PhD: Ownership: Ratio Therapeutics, Inc.

Stephen G. DiMagno, PhD: Ownership: Ratio Therapeutics, Inc.

Aaron Enke, BSc: Employee: Clovis Oncology

Frederik L. Giesel, MD, MBA: Advisor: ABX, Telix Pharmaceuticals, SOFIE

Ken Herrmann, MD: Personal fees: Advanced Accelerator Applications, Aktis Oncology, Amgen, Bayer AG, Curium, Endocyte, GE Healthcare, Ipsen, Novartis, Pharma15 Corporattion, Siemens Healthineers, Sirtex, SOFIE, Y-mAbs; Research: BTG Specialty Pharmaceuticals

Jessica D. Jensen, MPH: Employee: POINT Biopharma

Lukas Kessler, MD: Consultant: AAA Pharma, Inc., BTG Specialty Pharmaceuticals

Katharina Lückerath, PhD: Consultant: SOFIE

Sherly Mosessian, PhD: Employee: SOFIE

UNAPPROVED/OFF-LABEL USE DISCLOSURE

The EOCME requires CME faculty to disclose to the participants:

1. When products or procedures being discussed are off-label, unlabelled, experimental, and/or investigational (not US Food and Drug Administration [FDA] approved); and

2. Any limitations on the information presented, such as data that are preliminary or that represent ongoing research, interim analyses, and/or unsupported opinions. Faculty may discuss information about pharmaceutical agents that is outside of FDA-approved labelling. This information is intended solely for CME and is not intended to promote off-label use of these medications. If you have any questions, contact the medical affairs department of the manufacturer for the most recent prescribing information.

TO ENROLL

To enroll in the *PET Clinics* Continuing Medical Education program, call customer service at 1-800-654-2452 or sign up online at http://www.theclinics.com/home/cme. The CME program is available to subscribers for an additional annual fee of USD 239.00

METHOD OF PARTICIPATION

In order to claim credit, participants must complete the following:

1. Complete enrolment as indicated above.
2. Read the activity.
3. Complete the CME Test and Evaluation. Participants must achieve a score of 70% on the test. All CME Tests and Evaluations must be completed online.

CME INQUIRIES/SPECIAL NEEDS

For all CME inquiries or special needs, please contact elsevierCME@elsevier.com.

Preface
Fibroblast Activation Protein as a Diagnostic and Therapeutic Target: Where Do We Go from Here?

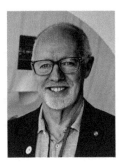
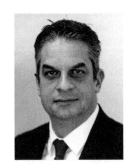
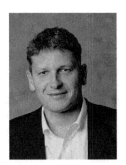

Rodney J. Hicks, MB, BS, MD, FRACP   Frederik L. Giesel, MD, MBA   Ken Herrmann, MD, MBA

Editors

In the twentieth century, cancer was largely considered to result from the outgrowth of malignant epithelial, mesenchymal, hematologic, or neural cells generating carcinomas, sarcomas, lymphoma/leukemias, and gliomas, respectively. However, advances in understanding the interaction between malignant cells and their tumor microenvironment (TME) have revolutionized our understanding of cancers and led to increasingly targeted treatment approaches in the twenty-first century.[1] In particular, the roles of stromal and immune elements are center stage in modern oncology. Elements within the TME clearly interact with epithelial, lymphomatous, glial, or sarcomatous elements to impact tumor progression, invasiveness, and metastasis as well as responsiveness to conventional cancer therapeutics, including chemotherapy and radiotherapy. In solid tumors, cancer-associated fibroblasts (CAFs) play an important role in orchestrating these processes. The origin and function of different subtypes of fibroblast are the focus of intense research.[2] Importantly, the role of fibroblast activation protein (FAP) has come into focus due to both its almost ubiquitous and relatively high expression across most malignancies, and its association with poor prognosis through a combination of increased invasiveness and resistance to therapeutic interventions.[3] Although expressed primarily in the stromal compartment,

FAP is also expressed in some transformed cells, especially sarcoma, as detailed in later discussion.

The development of radiolabeled small-molecule inhibitors of this protein, which are lumped together as fibroblast activation protein inhibitor (FAPI) radiopharmaceuticals, has created huge enthusiasm among the nuclear medicine community with suggestions that these may even compete with the current gold-standard tracer for evaluation, ^{18}F-fluorodeoxyglucose (FDG).[4] In this issue of *PET Clinics*, we have invited experts who have been actively involved in developing or researching the utility of these agents across a broad spectrum of diseases to summarize the current evidence regarding clinical applications of FAP-based imaging probes for diagnosis and, potentially, also for therapy. Although heavily focused on oncologic applications, the emerging role of this target in benign but nevertheless extremely morbid conditions is also highlighted.

To gain an idea of the rapid radiochemistry developments in the field of FAP-targeting radiopharmaceuticals, John Babich, a pioneer in the development of agents in this class, and his colleague Stephen DiMagno have provided a summary of the multitude of agents that have been developed. From the initial series of FAPI agents that were developed in Heidelberg by Tom Lindner and colleagues through to modifications designed to increase target affinity or tissue residence, their

PET Clin 18 (2023) xv–xx
https://doi.org/10.1016/j.cpet.2023.03.006
1556-8598/23/© 2023 Published by Elsevier Inc.

synopsis demonstrates both the ingenuity of modern radiochemists and the reluctance of the nuclear medicine community to stop innovating and just focus on getting an agent into routine clinical practice. With the cost and regulatory hurdles facing the introduction of novel tracers and achieving reimbursement, at some point there needs to be a "winner" (or two, to ensure competitive pricing) in the diagnostic stakes and, perhaps, another couple winners for theranostic application that have sufficient tissue retention to allow prospective dosimetry and delivery of meaningful radiation doses to sites of disease. The potential financial rewards for becoming the agent of choice will, however, likely ensure ongoing competition and, no doubt, further innovation.

The obvious place to start in establishing a diagnostic role for FAPI agents is in cancer settings in which FDG-PET/computed tomography (CT) has recognized limitations either due to low glycolytic activity of the malignancy or high background activity that potentially masks disease detection. One such disease is pancreatic adenocarcinoma, which was one of the first cancers to be recognized as being poorly staged by FDG-PET. Zhao and colleagues describe the advantages of FAPI as an imaging agent in pancreatic cancer, a disease long recognized to be associated with dense desmoplasia, which likely accounts for its high metastatic potential and poor responsiveness to most cancer therapies. Not surprisingly, this was found to be one of the disease groups with the highest expression of FAP[5] and was an obvious cancer in which FAPI agents would be first evaluated. While they review the several studies that have demonstrated a significantly higher uptake of FAPI than FDG in both primary and metastatic lesions, most series have found that significant FDG-avidity with low or absent FAPI uptake can also occur. Given adverse prognostic implications of desmoplasia and the likelihood that the most desmoplastic lesions would also be those most likely to yield higher sensitivity on FAPI than FDG-PET, prior studies have demonstrated that high FDG uptake is an adverse prognostic indicator in pancreatic cancer,[6] just as it is in many other malignancies. This supports the pluralistic nature of prognostic factors in cancer. Consequently, further studies are required to ascertain the prognostic and therapeutic implications of lesions that have discordant FDG-avidity but lack significant FAPI uptake and vice versa.

The role of FAPI in characterizing tumor biology rather than simply having the ability to detect disease sites is a theme that we will return to in our comments on other articles appearing in this issue of PET Clinics. As an additional recurring theme, the lack of specificity of FAP expression is also highlighted with several benign conditions potentially yielding false positive results unless the scans are subjected to appropriate clinical, radiologic, and pathologic correlation. The potential for differential retention of FAPI agents in inflammatory versus malignant tissues, which enables dynamic or delayed imaging protocols to differentiate between pancreatitis and pancreatic adenocarcinoma, may not apply to all available radiopharmaceuticals. For example, the kinetics of small-molecule FAPI agents may differ from those of cyclic peptides. Thus, given the differing pharmacokinetics of the various FAPI radiopharmaceuticals available, design of optimal imaging protocols for each needs to be established.

As another exemplar of a cancer wherein the role of FDG-PET remains uncertain, hepatocellular carcinoma (HCC) is also a cancer for which FAPI imaging has shown promise. While high FDG-avidity has long been known to be associated with adverse prognosis,[7] low uptake related to reduced expression of the rate-limiting glycolytic enzyme hexokinase-II can also occur. The review by Mori and colleagues details recent experience with FAPI-PET/CT in HCC and discusses the other important hepatobiliary cancer, cholangiocarcinoma. The potential for fibrotic changes associated with related benign processes, including cirrhosis and sclerosing cholangitis, to complicate interpretation needs to be considered, but preliminary results look encouraging for both cancer types. However, since most of the series evaluating HCC that have been published thus far have been in Asian populations in which viral causes are dominant, which can occur without severe cirrhotic changes, the role in assessing the development of HCC in alcoholic cirrhosis is unclear. An emerging problem in both the developed and the developing world is obesity, with nonalcoholic steatohepatitis (NASH) thought likely to fuel future increases in the incidence of HCC even as vaccination reduces viral-associated disease.[8] The role of FAPI-PET in the evaluation of HCC arising as a result of NASH will be of interest.

In contradistinction to pancreatic cancer and HCC, head and neck cancers are generally highly FDG-avid. Nevertheless, interpretation can sometimes be compromised by physiologic activity. Despite the recognized benefits of FDG-PET in evaluation of this disparate group of malignancies, few experienced PET readers would disagree that these are among the most difficult studies to interpret due to a combination of high physiologic tracer uptake in lymphoid aggregates within Waldeyer's ring, the frequent occurrence of reactive lymphadenopathy, particularly involving the jugulo-digastric node at the angle of the mandible, and the complex anatomy of the neck and skull base. The frequent occurrence of necrosis in nodal metastases, particularly in carcinomas related to human papillomavirus infection, can lead to interpretative errors if based solely on the intensity of uptake. Contrast-enhanced CT and MR imaging are helpful in identifying such nodes, which often have only a thin rim of viable tumor leading to partial volume effects that reduce apparent FDG-avidity. Nevertheless, imperfect sensitivity remains problematic. Postradiation changes can also be difficult to interpret. In his review, Manuel Röhrich addresses the utility of FAPI-PET in the evaluation of head and neck cancers and its potential to address these limitations of FDG-PET/CT.

Of several disease entities discussed, squamous cell carcinoma appears to have the highest FAP expression with higher uptake often seen in metastatic lesions than observed on FDG-PET, whereas in nasopharyngeal carcinoma, the converse was common. As a result of high tumor-to-background activity ratios, FAPI-PET has been reported to impact radiotherapy planning in a range of head and neck cancers.[9] This has generally been by increasing the planned treatment volume, but whether inclusion of lesions with high FAPI leads to improved local control or has other prognostic implications, including potentially being a predictor of radioresistance, is unknown. Adenoid-cystic carcinoma is an interesting disease entity for FAPI evaluation given its relatively low FDG-avidity and tendency for perineural infiltration extending into the base of the skull, where adjacent physiologic neuronal uptake of FDG can render definition to disease extent difficult. Interestingly, unlike pancreatic cancer where FAPI uptake appears to increase at late time points, washout of FAPI appeared to occur over time in adenoid-cystic carcinomas.[10] Thyroid carcinoma is another example of a malignancy with variable tumor biology and for which FAPI may provide additional information with either prognostic or therapeutic implications beyond merely detecting disease. More studies comparing FAPI with the more common characterization paradigm of combined radioiodine and FDG-PET imaging are awaited.

As a further example of physiologic background activity comprising diagnostic performance of FDG-PET/CT, variable FDG uptake in bowel is a confounding influence in interpretation of FDG-PET/CT and is particularly relevant to gastrointestinal and peritoneal malignancy. Addressing the potential role of FAPI-PET in evaluating colorectal cancer (CRC), Strating and colleagues highlight the advantages of FAPI-PET in primary staging, which relate to the high contrast achieved by virtue of low physiologic uptake in intraabdominal organs. Uptake of FDG in the normal bowel can mask peritoneal seeding, and its detection appears to be a significant advantage of FAPI over FDG, both in the primary diagnostic setting and for surveillance of high-risk patients who would otherwise be subjected to diagnostic laparoscopy. The authors suggest that further studies are required to confirm the utility of FAPI-PET in assessing peritoneal carcinomatosis. Furthermore, they importantly link the uptake of FAPI to tumor biology, recognizing the impact of high FAP expression on prognosis and response to therapy, particularly immunotherapy. Their observation that one of the genomic subtypes of CRC that has a mesenchymal phenotype and poor prognosis has high FAPI-avidity[11] may have implications for therapeutic selection and surveillance strategies. The role of FAPI-PET/CT in potentially selecting patients for FAP-directed therapies also needs to be considered.

Beyond these applications for which there is a developing evidence base, the role of FAPI is promising for several other carcinomas. Watabe and colleagues describe evidence supporting the utility of FAPI agents in the staging of gastric cancer, which, like pancreatic cancer, is known to sometimes have relatively low FDG-avidity, although being less commonly desmoplastic. A particular benefit of this scanning approach is its ability to detect peritoneal carcinomatosis, which is otherwise difficult to detect due to physiologic bowel activity, and poor sensitivity may lead to futile operations. As detailed in the review by Dendl and colleagues, assessment of peritoneal disease may also be a significant advantage in ovarian cancer. Given the utility of MR imaging in the evaluation of peritoneal disease, FAPI-PET/MR imaging may provide incremental diagnostic information relevant to staging and therapeutic planning. The authors of this review also discuss emerging evidence on the utility of FAPI in breast cancer, another disease with variable FDG-avidity. The prognostic significance of high FAPI expression in the various subtypes of breast cancer needs further study. Its role in lobular carcinoma and for detection of disease in radiologically dense breasts, which can have mild but diffusely increased FDG-uptake, will be of interest.

Because of the prevalence of CAF infiltration within the TME, FAPI imaging provides a relatively nonspecific "pan-cancer" target in that the malignant cells remain uncharacterized with lesion detection purely related to the induction of a reactive stroma. An exception to this is the specific expression of FAP in various sarcomas, which arise from mesenchymal cells that include fibroblasts. Lukas Kessler reviews the potential utility of FAPI imaging as a "pan-sarcoma" target. Musing on the extreme heterogeneity in tissues of origin, genomic drivers, and clinical behaviour of this class of malignancy, he details the preliminary experience in this group of diseases and the need for larger and cell-type–specific studies. Of significance, relatively indolent sarcomas can have quite high uptake while significant intralesional variability in FAP expression can occur. For example, studies at his institution have revealed extremely high FAP expression, as reflected by substantially higher maximum standardized uptake value levels in solitary fibrous tumor (SFT) than seen in most sarcomas and almost any carcinomas. Although potentially metastatic, SFTs tend to have a relatively indolent natural history compared with most sarcoma. Accordingly, it behooves the research community to go beyond simply disease detection and to understand the biological significance of high and low FAP expression in sarcoma and how, potentially, this may be complementary to conventional imaging approaches with MR imaging and FDG-PET/CT, which are well-established in the evaluation of these cancers. In addition, being expressed in malignant cells, this might be a particularly important therapeutic target and therefore warrants further evaluation as a theranostic paradigm. Hamacher and colleagues make the case for the targeting of FAP in sarcoma due to its direct expression in the malignant cells themselves. As these cells often exist within a background of relatively acellular matrix, and given low expression in almost all normal tissues, the case for use of alpha emitters, which can deliver high-radiation doses to individual cells, is enhanced, although not specifically addressed by the authors.

In addition to improving detection, the high tumor-to-background activity ratios described in several reviews provide the potential for clearer tumor delineation than achievable with conventional imaging techniques, including that achieved by FDG-PET/CT, particularly when planning locoregional therapies. As detailed by Stefan Koeber, this has implications for radiotherapy planning. This is especially important in areas of complex anatomy wherein avoidance of toxicity in surrounding tissues is compounded by a need to adequately cover disease with sufficient radiation doses to adequately control disease. As radiation therapy becomes more and more conformal, accurate disease definition is vital, first, to demonstrate suitability for aggressive locoregional treatment, and, second, to ensure that all tumors

receive the prescribed radiation dose. Although data supporting the role of FAPI-PET/CT are preliminary, there is a potential for this technology to significantly impact radiotherapy planning in adenoid cystic carcinoma and pancreatic cancer given the known limitations of FDG-PET/CT in both these malignancies. For cancers, like lung cancer, which already has an important and well-validated role in radiation planning,[12] comparison of treatment volumes using each tracer in the same patient will be important to establish whether FAPI-PET/CT or PET/MR imaging will have incremental value in defining radiation treatment volumes or provide incremental predictive or prognostic information that may impact treatment selection or delivery technique.

In the process of evaluating FAPI in patients with cancer, incidental findings of uptake in healing wounds, sites of arthritic involvement, or other nonmalignant process provided recognition that FAPI, like FDG, may be subject to false positive results if considered only to be a cancer probe. However, like FDG, it might have utility in evaluating a range of benign processes that significantly impact human health. These conditions include various autoimmune diseases as detailed by Sviridenko and colleagues. FAP-based PET imaging may have a significant clinical role in monitoring the activity of fibrotic processes as they evolve through an inflammatory phase through active laying down of extracellular material to established fibrosis, analogous to the wound-healing response that eventually leads to scarring. The authors point out that the immediate phase can be negative on FDG but positive on FAPI-PET. This may have therapeutic relevance with the development of various antifibrotic agents. An important multisystem disease that can mimic cancer in which preliminary data are encouraging is IgG4 disease.[13]

Cardiac fibrosis as part of either postischemic remodeling or cardiomyopathy also offers novel potential applications of FAP imaging. Encouraging preclinical data[14] support the clinical use of FAPI radiopharmaceuticals in evaluation of cardiac remodeling in the postmyocardial infarction setting. There is also evidence from incidental cardiac findings in patients undergoing cancer evaluation[15] among numerous other case reports and small series. These include myocarditis related to immune checkpoint inhibitor therapy.[16]

Bengel and Diekmann review the current literature that suggests FAPI-PET/CT may provide incremental information beyond that currently supplied by cardiac MR imaging and echocardiography, particularly with respect to the status of myocardial fibrosis extending beyond the infarct itself into both the ischemic border zone and beyond into the adjacent myocardium, potentially leading to adverse outcomes, including left ventricular impairment and arrhythmia. They speculate that this information may impact postinfarct management, including the use of antifibrotic approaches.

Given the broad potential diagnostic uses of agents targeting FAP and the attraction for also leveraging it therapeutically, nimble preclinical methods are required to evaluate novel agents and assist in the design of clinical protocols. Researchers from Osaka University in Japan, led by Dr Watabe, have provided an excellent summary of the available animal models and various preclinical approaches that are yet to be fully translated into clinical practice. It should be noted that there are significant conceptual limitations of the existing xenograft models in that malignant cells have been transduced to overexpress FAP and, as such, they don't recapitulate human tumors wherein the stroma and not the epithelial cell expresses this target. If desmoplastic stroma exists, it involves host CAFs. Since most immortalized cell lines are relatively rapidly growing, stroma may not have sufficient time to develop before ethical termination of experiments are required. Sarcoma and glioma models are potentially more representative but may lack orthotopic authenticity.

The use of preclinical models to advance the challenges of clinical translation of therapeutic FAP-targeting is addressed by Katharina Lückerath and colleagues. Alluding to the potential for radiation alone being insufficient to control a disease process that leads to intrinsic radioresistance, the authors detail preliminary approaches to enhancing radiobiological effects using various DNA-damage response-modifying agents. Given that desmoplasia can also suppress the immune response to cancers and the effectiveness of chemotherapy, they also discuss combining FAP radioligand therapy with immune modulatory treatments and FAP cotargeting of the TME.

The preliminary data of clinical translation of FAP agents for therapeutic purposes are nicely summarized by Clemens Kratochwil and colleagues. The authors highlight the challenges of relatively low tumor retention of existing agents, which currently favor use of radionuclides with a relatively short half-life. While this is an exciting opportunity, the article details the challenges as well as the future directions of research into FAP-based radioligand therapy.

As several of the articles in this issue of *PET Clinics* can attest, further, preferably prospective, research into the diagnostic and therapeutic roles of FAP-targeting radiopharmaceuticals is needed. Toward this end, authors representing three companies involved in sponsoring such research discuss the status of clinical trials in this domain.

As with all new techniques and technologies, being able to observe for the first time the dynamic process of fibrosis that evolves from initiating events through to an established scar or that accompanies evolution of a tumor deposit from a cluster of cancer cells to a lesion comprising a complex array of stromal and malignant elements, using FAPI imaging, alone or combination with other tracers, to characterize different aspects of tumor biology, and as a potential therapeutic target will need ongoing evidence and will no doubt generate many hypotheses. Some of these will be correct, and others will cause us to ponder anew.

There are two possible outcomes: if the result confirms the hypothesis, you've made a measurement. If the result is contrary to the hypothesis, then you have made a discovery.
—Enrico Fermi

Rodney J. Hicks, MB, BS, MD, FRACP
The Department of Medicine
St Vincent's Medical School
University of Melbourne
Melbourne, Australia

The Department of Medicine
Central Clinical School
the Alfred Hospital
Monash University
Melbourne, Australia

The Melbourne Theranostic Innovation Centre
Level 8, 14-20 Blackwood Street
North Melbourne, Victoria 3051, Australia

Frederik L. Giesel, MD, MBA
Nuclear Medicine
University Hospital Duesseldorf
Duessldorf, Germany

Ken Herrmann, MD, MBA
Nuclear Medicine
Universitätsmedizin Essen
Essen, Germany

E-mail addresses:
rod.hicks@premit.net.au (R.J. Hicks)
Frederik.Giesel@med.uni-duesseldorf.de
(F.L. Giesel)
Ken.Herrmann@uk-essen.de (K. Herrmann)

REFERENCES

1. Hanahan D, Weinberg RA. Hallmarks of cancer: the next generation. Cell 2011;144(5):646–74.
2. Kalluri R. The biology and function of fibroblasts in cancer. Nat Rev Cancer 2016;16(9):582–98.
3. Puré E, Blomberg R. Pro-tumorigenic roles of fibroblast activation protein in cancer: back to the basics. Oncogene 2018;37(32):4343–57.
4. Hicks RJ, Roselt PJ, Kallur KG, et al. FAPI PET/CT: will it end the hegemony of 18F-FDG in Oncology? J Nucl Med 2021;62(3):296–302.
5. Kratochwil C, Flechsig P, Lindner T, et al. Ga-FAPI PET/CT: tracer uptake in 28 different kinds of cancer. J Nucl Med 2019;60(6):801–5.
6. Wang L, Dong P, Shen G, et al. 18F-Fluorodeoxyglucose positron emission tomography predicts treatment efficacy and clinical outcome for patients with pancreatic carcinoma: a meta-analysis. Pancreas 2019;48(8):996–1002.
7. Torizuka T, Tamaki N, Inokuma T, et al. In vivo assessment of glucose metabolism in hepatocellular carcinoma with FDG-PET. J Nucl Med 1995;36(10):1811–7.
8. Ito T, Nguyen MH. Perspectives on the underlying etiology of HCC and its effects on treatment outcomes. J Hepatocell Carcinoma 2023;10:413–28.
9. Syed M, Flechsig P, Liermann J, et al. Fibroblast activation protein inhibitor (FAPI) PET for diagnostics and advanced targeted radiotherapy in head and neck cancers. Eur J Nucl Med Mol Imaging 2020; 47:2836–45.
10. Röhrich M, Syed M, Liew DP, et al. Ga-FAPI-PET/CT improves diagnostic staging and radiotherapy planning of adenoid cystic carcinomas—imaging analysis and histological validation. Radiother Oncol 2021;160:192–201.
11. Strating E, Wassenaar E, Verhagen M, et al. Fibroblast activation protein identifies Consensus Molecular Subtype 4 in colorectal cancer and allows its detection by ^{68}Ga-FAPI-PET imaging. Br J Cancer 2022;127(1):145–55.
12. MacManus M, Everitt S, Hicks RJ. The evolving role of molecular imaging in non-small cell lung cancer radiotherapy. Semin Radiat Oncol 2015;25(2):133–42.
13. Luo Y., Pan Q., Yang H., et al. Fibroblast activation protein targeted PET/CT with 68Ga-FAPI for imaging IgG4-related disease: comparison to 18F-FDG PET/CT, *J Nucl Med*, 62 (2), 2021, 266-271.
14. Langer L.B.N., Hess A., Korkmaz Z., et al. Molecular imaging of fibroblast activation protein after myocardial infarction using the novel radiotracer [^{68}Ga] MHLL1, *Theranostics*, 11 (16), 2021, 7755–7766.
15. Heckmann M.B., Reinhardt F., Finke D., et al. Relationship between cardiac fibroblast activation protein activity by positron emission tomography and cardiovascular disease, *Circ Cardiovasc Imaging*, 13 (9), 2020, e010628.
16. Finke D, Heckmann MB, Herpel E, et al. Early detection of checkpoint inhibitor-associated myocarditis using (68)Ga-FAPI PET/CT. Front Cardiovasc Med 2021;8:614997.

Advanced Fibroblast Activation Protein-Ligand Developments
FAP Imaging Agents: A Review of the Structural Requirements

Stephen G. DiMagno, PhD, John W. Babich, PhD*

KEYWORDS

- Seprase • FAP • Boroproline • Cyanoproline • Cancer-associated fibroblasts

KEY POINTS

- Small molecule inhibitors of fibroblast activation protein-α (FAP) are being developed for radioimaging of FAP expression in humans.
- Small molecule inhibitors of FAP are being developed for targeted radiotherapy of tumors in humans.
- Cyanoproline and boroproline containing FAP inhibitors can be exploited as imaging agents and targeted radiotherapeutics.

INTRODUCTION

Fibroblasts are one of the most abundant cell types in connective tissues. These cells are responsible for tissue homeostasis under normal physiological conditions. When tissues are injured, fibroblasts become activated and differentiate into myofibroblasts, which generate large contractions and actively produce extracellular matrix (ECM) proteins to facilitate wound closure. Both fibroblasts and myofibroblasts play a critical role in wound healing by generating traction and contractile forces, respectively, to enhance wound contraction.

The tumor microenvironment comprises tumor cells and a heterogeneous mix of accessory cells (the tumor stroma), which are critical to tumor development.[1,2] The tumor stroma includes fibroblasts, epithelial cells, endothelial and smooth muscle cells of the vasculature, fat, and immune cells.[3] Although these cells are not malignant, they acquire an altered phenotype allowing them to support and enhance tumor growth. Activated cancer-associated fibroblasts (CAFs) are the primary cellular component of the tumor stroma and have been shown to assist in cancer progression by upregulating the expression of several proteins, including growth and chemotactic factors, angiogenic factors, and matrix metalloproteases.[1–3]

Fibroblast activation protein-α (FAP), also known as seprase (surface expressed protease), is a membrane dipeptidyl peptidase (DPP) of the family of serine proteases. FAP expression is normally restricted to fetal mesenchymal tissue; however, it is selectively expressed in reactive stromal fibroblasts of epithelial cancers and in dermal scars of healing wounds,[4] as well as in liver cirrhosis.[5] The majority of FAP is expressed by activated fibroblasts responding to pathologic situations. FAP is a 170 kDa, type II, integral membrane peptidase in the dipeptidyl peptidase-4 (DPPIV) family of prolyl peptidases, originally defined as the target of a mouse monoclonal antibody, F19.[6] As a type II transmembrane protein, FAP is typically found physically attached to cells

Ratio Therapeutics, Inc., One Design Center Place, Suite# 19-601, Boston, MA 02210, USA
* Corresponding author.
E-mail address: jbabich@ratiotx.com

PET Clin 18 (2023) 287–294
https://doi.org/10.1016/j.cpet.2023.03.002

and with the bulk of the protein, including the catalytic domain, exposed to the extracellular space and accessible to small molecules. Small amounts of soluble FAP are also found in circulation in humans and other mammals.[7,8]

FAP is a nonclassical serine protease, which belongs to the S9B prolyl oligopeptidase subfamily. FAP is most closely related to DPPIV (approximately 50% of their amino acids are identical). The active site of FAP is localized in the extracellular part of the protein and contains a catalytic triad composed of Ser[624], Asp[702], and His[734] in humans and mice.[9] FAP is catalytically active as a 170-kD homodimer and has a dipeptidase and an endopeptidase activity. During the last 2 decades, FAP has attracted increasing attention as a selective marker of CAFs and, more broadly, of activated fibroblasts in tissues undergoing remodeling of their ECM due to chronic inflammation, fibrosis, or wound healing.

FAP is a key component of the tumor microenvironment.[10] A highly consistent feature of tumor stromal fibroblasts or CAFs is the induction of FAP. FAP is a candidate as a universal target antigen because it is reported to be selectively expressed in nearly all solid tumors by a subset of tumor stromal fibroblasts.[11–13] In addition, FAP is expressed on invadopodia of some human breast cancers[14] and melanomas,[15,16] including the human malignant melanoma, LOX, from which it was first identified.[15] Cancer cells that overexpress FAP exhibit an invasive phenotype,[14] serum-free growth,[17] enhanced growth and metastasis in vivo,[18] and exhibit greater microvessel density in the tumor microenvironment.[14] Abrogation of CAF FAP enzyme activity, either through mutagenesis[19] or with a neutralizing antibody,[20] attenuates tumor growth. In summary, CAFs are a dynamic component of the tumor microenvironment that provides mechanical support and controls proliferation and survival, angiogenesis, metastasis, immunogenicity, and resistance to therapies.[21–23]

FAP inhibitors as radioligands for imaging and therapy: The selective expression of FAP on CAFs makes it an attractive target to exploit for noninvasive tumor imaging as well as targeted radiotherapy of via tumor stroma. Clinical trials conducted with [I-131]F19[6] and an [I-131]-radiolabeled humanized version of F19, sibrotuzumab,[24] have demonstrated selective tumor uptake and minimal normal tissue retention in patients with colorectal cancer,[24] thus validating FAP as a molecular target for radioscintigraphy. Although intact antibodies such as sibrotuzumab offer potential for tumor radiotargeting, long circulating half-life and poor tissue penetration limit their

effectiveness as radiodiagnostic and radiotherapeutic agents.

FAP is an atypical serine protease that has both dipeptidyl peptidase and endopeptidase activities, cleaving substrates at a postproline bond. FAP possess both prolyl dipeptidyl peptidase[25,26] as well as gelatinase activity,[16] and a variety of inhibitors of the former catalytic activity has been described.[25–28] Most of these compounds are based on PT-100, a Val-boro-Pro analog, which exhibits antitumor activity in tumor-bearing mice.[28] Although inhibitors of this class are potent, they also block the exopeptidase activity of several other DPPIV family members.[25] To overcome this lack of selectivity, Wolf and colleagues designed compounds, which incorporated a chemical cap on the amino terminus of a Gly-boro-Pro dipeptide.[26] One of their lead compounds, Ac-Gly-boro-Pro, (**Fig. 1**), continues to be recognized by FAP, which displays both exopeptidase and endopeptidase activities but not by several other DPPIV family members that have no endopeptidase activity.[25] In addition, this group demonstrated that potent anti-FAP activity, and selectivity is maintained when significant bulk is added to the amino terminus of Gly-boro-Pro.[26] These observations suggest that it is possible to substitute the amino terminus of Gly-boro-Pro with a chelator capable of coordinating a radioactive metal while retaining affinity for

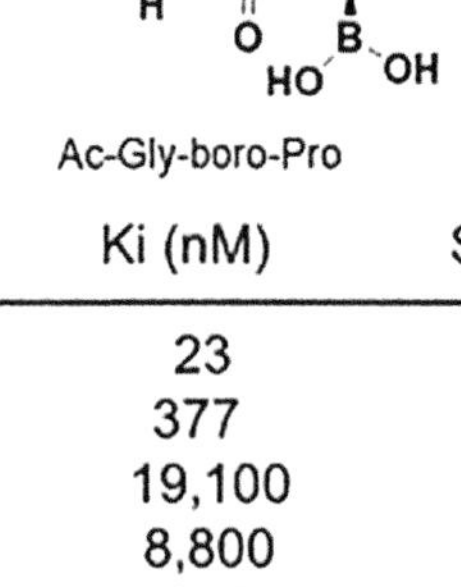

Protease	Ki (nM)	Selectivity
FAP	23	1
DPP-4	377	16.4
DPP-8	19,100	830
DPP-9	8,800	383
APH	575	25
POP	211	9.2
DPP-7	125,000	5434

Fig. 1. Design of R-AA-Pro inhibitors of FAP. TOP: core structure. Middle: Ac-Gly BoroPro. Bottom: Affinity and selectivity of Ac-Gly-BoroPro to FAP and related proteins.

FAP, resulting in a radiopharmaceutical that targets FAP in cancer-associated stromal cells for the potential diagnosis and treatment of cancer.

The activities and specificities of FAP have been investigated using artificial substrates and synthetic peptide libraries,[25,29–32] which revealed a strong preference for FAP cleavage of endopeptidase substrates after glycine-proline (Gly-Pro) motifs. A major hurdle in the study of FAP enzyme activity has been the lack of selective inhibitors against this protease. FAP shares DPP specificity with the enzyme members of the DPP4 family, DPP4, DPP8, and DPP9, as well as endopeptidase specificity with prolyl endopeptidase (PREP). Thus, designing small molecule inhibitors that are selective for FAP over other DPPs and prolyl endopeptidase (PREP) presents a challenge.

Radiolabeled FAP Inhibitors. In 2009, a series of radioiodinated FAP inhibitors for targeting the tumor microenvironment was described based on a series of iodine substituted benzamido-glycine-boronoproline analogs (**Fig. 2**).[33] Iodine was substituted at the 3 positions of the benzene ring, and compounds were assessed for their ability to inhibit the enzymatic activity of recombinant human FAP in a fluorescence-based assay. Among the most active compounds, an ortho-iodine analog (MIP-1231) displayed an IC50 of 6 nM, whereas even more potent para-substituted (MIP-1232)

and meta-substituted (MIP-1233) analogs both had IC50 values of 0.6 nM. To examine the selectivity for FAP over other prolyl peptidases, compounds were tested for their ability to inhibit the enzymatic activity of PREP. The IC50 values of MIP-1231, MIP-1232, and MIP-1233 for PREP were 58, 19, and 7 nM, respectively, with PREP/FAP ratios of 10, 32, and 12, respectively. These data demonstrate that although the para-substituted and meta-substituted compounds have a similar ability to inhibit FAP activity, the para-substituted analog displayed better selectivity. To examine binding to FAP in vivo, human embryonic kidney (HEK-293) cells were stably transfected with the human FAP gene. The equilibrium dissociation constant (Kd) of MIP-1232 for FAP was determined to be 30 nM, whereas there was no specific binding to a nonexpressing clone. The Bmax of the FAP-expressing cells was determined to be approximately 8 pmol/10^6 cells. In addition, MIP-1232 was shown to inhibit the FAP enzymatic activity of the stable FAP-expressing cells. The authors conclude then that radiolabeled FAP inhibitors could be exploited for the diagnosis, staging, prognosis, and potential treatment of solid tumors. Subsequently, Meletta and colleagues described the use of radioiodinated MIP-1232, for its potential to image atherosclerotic plaques.[34] Ex vivo autoradiography showed strong specific accumulation of radiolabeled FAP inhibitor in FAP-positive SK-Mel-187 melanoma xenograft tissue slices while accumulation was negligible in NCI-H69 xenograft tissue slices with low-FAP levels. Binding of the tracer was similar in plaques and normal arteries, hampering its use for atherosclerosis imaging.

In 2013, 2 independent groups reported on the development of potent FAP-selective inhibitors. Poplawski and colleagues reported on potent FAP-selective and PREP-selective inhibitors using boroproline-based compounds (**Fig. 3**).[35] One compound, N-(pyridine-4-carbonyl)-D-Ala-boro-Pro, has a more than 350-fold selectively for FAP over PREP, and with negligible potency against DPP4, DPP8, and DPP9. The University of Antwerp reported on a new class of FAP inhibitors based on an N-(4-quinolinoyl)-Gly-(2-cyanopyrolidine) scaffold.[36] Of the 34 compounds reported on in that study (**Fig. 4**), compound 7 has particular selectivity toward FAP over the related proteases DPP4, DPP8, and DPP9, and is also selective over PREP. Modifications to the quinolinoyl ring improved the selectivity for FAP over PREP,[36] indicating that further developments of this scaffold can yield compounds with more selectivity for FAP.

The pursuit of small molecule inhibitors of FAP as radioligands was bolstered in 2018, by the

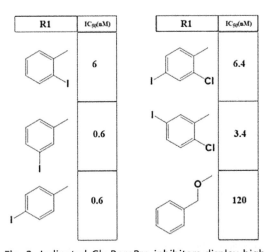

R1	IC$_{50}$(nM)		R1	IC$_{50}$(nM)
	6			6.4
	0.6			3.4
	0.6			120

Fig. 2. Iodinated Gly-BoroPro inhibitors display high affinity for FAP. (*Adapted from* Marquis J, Wang J, Maresca K, Hillier G, Zimmerman C, Joyal J, Babich J; Abstract #4467: Targeting tumor microenvironment with radiolabeled inhibitors of seprase (FAP\ #945;). Cancer Res 1 May 2009; 69 (9_Supplement): 4467.)

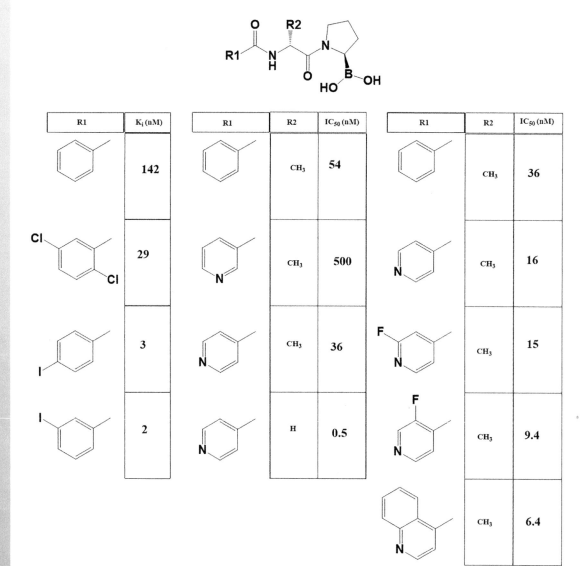

Fig. 3. Structural requirements for FAP affinity and selectivity in Ar-(CO)-D-Ala-BoroPro. (*Data from* Refs.[26,33,35])

Heidelberg group who reported[37] on 2 radioligands based on the N-(4-quinolinoyl)-Gly-(2-cyanopyroli-dine) scaffold previously reported by Jansen and colleagues[36] including an iodinated derivative and a derivative containing the chelate DOTA (2, 2′,2″,2‴-[1,4,7,10-Tetraazacyclododecane-1,4,7, 10-tetrayl] tetraacetic acid) that could potentially be labeled with various radiometals. When the DOTA derivative was labeled with gallium-68 ($t_{1/2}$ = 68 min), this radiolabeled FAP inhibitor (FAPI-02) clearly delineated tumors in animals and in humans with 28 unique cancers being visualized in patient studies. [Ga-68]-FAPI-02 achieved excellent contrast to background as the activity localized only to tumor tissue and was quickly excreted via the renal excretion pathway.[38,39] Since this initial publication, there has been dramatic growth in exploring FAP radiopharmaceuticals for imaging and therapy applications.[40] The remainder of this article will attempt to provide some insights into the structure activity relationship (SAR) of these small molecule inhibitors.

RATIONALE FOR FIBROBLAST ACTIVATION PROTEIN-α INHIBITOR DESIGN

FAP is a serine protease with Gly2-Pro1-cleaving specificity.[41] Wolf and coworkers demonstrated that dipeptides in which Gly was replaced by D-Ala or D-Ser remained substrates for FAP but that the enzyme was highly specific for proline.[30] Early structure-based designs of FAP inhibitors retained these key structural elements and added a third group to extend the peptide chain and provide

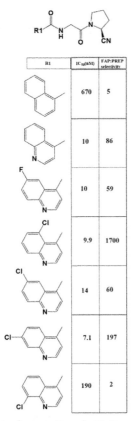

R1	IC₅₀(nM)	FAP:PREP selectivity
	670	5
	10	86
	10	59
	9.9	1700
	14	60
	7.1	197
	190	2

Fig. 4. Impact of aromatic substitution on FAP:PREP selectivity. (*Data from* Jansen K, Heirbaut L, Cheng JD, Joossens J, Ryabtsova O, Cos P, Maes L, Lambeir AM, De Meester I, Augustyns K, Van der Veken P. Selective Inhibitors of Fibroblast Activation Protein (FAP) with a (4- Quinolinoyl)-glycyl-2-cyanopyrrolidine Scaffold. ACS Med Chem Lett. 2013 Mar 18;4(5):491-6.)

specificity. The first potent (23 nM) FAP inhibitor of this class (see **Fig. 1**), Ac-Gly-BoroPro, had good-to-modest selectivity versus other proline-selective peptidases (DPP-4, DPP-7, DPP-8, DPP-9, acyl-peptide hydrolase (APH), and PREP).[25]

Although FAP inhibitors featuring alternative pharmacophores have been prepared, compounds exhibiting the substitution pattern highlighted in **Fig. 1** (R_1 = aromatic, R_2 = H or CH_3, and R_3 = $B(OH)_2$ or CN) are most relevant to potential radiotracer development. The parameter space for each of the key design elements (R_{1-3}) in **Fig. 1** has been probed by medicinal chemistry; potency and selectivity data will be discussed below. These previously published data have been sifted and sorted to emphasize specific trends in the SAR.

Results in **Fig. 3** (left column) from Genentech[26] and Molecular Insight[33] suggest that the R_1 position can accommodate large arenes, and that FAP affinity is correlated with arene size and/or

polarizability. Data in **Fig. 3** (middle column)[35] demonstrate quite convincingly that site-specific (4-position) incorporation of a nitrogen atom in the aryl R_1-substituent results in an increase in potency, which is modest for alanine and quite dramatic in the glycine case. In contrast, a ~ 14-fold loss in affinity is seen on changing the 4-pyridyl substituent to 3-pyridyl, perhaps indicating that a specific interaction of the 4-pyridyl nitrogen, hypothesized to involve a hydrogen bond to Glu^{204} in the FAP active site,[35] overcomes the loss of arene polarizability caused by endocyclic nitrogen. The FAP-inhibition data provided in **Fig. 3** (right column) suggest that the trends seen in the first 2 columns of **Fig. 3** are additive; increasing the size and/or polarizability of the heterocycle increases FAP inhibition. Data collated in **Fig. 4** show that the R_1-substituent properties that increase inhibition in the boronic acid series (R_3 = $B(OH)_2$, see **Fig. 3**) lead to similar effects in the cyanoproline series (CNPro, R_3 = CN, see **Fig. 4**).[36] Once again, introduction of a fluorine atom into the heterocyclic core (see **Fig. 4**, entry 3, 4-(6-fluoroquinolyl) substituent) is well tolerated and occurs without loss of inhibition (although with some decline in selectivity). The similar inhibition observed for the 5-choroquinoloyl, 6-choroquinoloyl, and 7-choroquinoloyl substituents suggests that fluorine substitution at these locations should lead to potent and selective FAP inhibitors.

Finally, it should be noted that a change in R_2 results in diverging trends in the boronic acids and cyano derivatives. Replacement of D-Ala for glycine in the pyridyl and quinolyl series of boronic acids (see **Fig. 3** middle column) leads to a loss of affinity but an increase in selectivity versus similar proteases.[35] In contrast, Gly → D-Ala substitution is associated with an increase in potency and a decrease in selectivity in the 2-cyanopyrrolidine series (data not shown).[36]

IMPROVING RETENTION

For radiotherapeutic applications, tumor retention is a key parameter that is yet to be optimized. Most small molecule inhibitors of the cyanoproline class show relatively rapid renal clearance and modest tumor retention. Moon and coworkers[42] conducted a head-to-head comparison of a dimeric FAP inhibitor [^{68}Ga]Ga-DOTAGA.(SA.FAPi)$_2$ with monomeric [^{68}Ga]Ga-DOTA.SA.FAPi. Inhibition measurements revealed excellent affinity and selectivity with low nanomolar IC50 values for FAP. In PET/computed tomography human studies, significantly higher tumor uptake as well as longer tumor retention could be observed for the dimer. In first in human studies, Ballal and coworkers reported that [^{177}Lu]Lu-DOTAGA.(SA.FAPi)$_2$ exhibited significant tumor retention out to 168 hours in a patient with a follicular variant of papillary carcinoma; accumulation in the normal organs peaked during 24 to 48 hours and decreased significantly by 96 hours after injection.[43] In similar studies, Zhao and coworkers[44] synthesized a Ga-68-labeled FAPI dimer ^{68}Ga-DOTA-2P(FAPI)$_2$ and demonstrated improved potency and tumor retention in preclinical models and in patients with cancer compared with FAPI-46. Zhao and coworkers[45] synthesized the Lu-177 derivative [^{177}Lu]Lu-DOTA-2P(FAPI)$_2$ and demonstrated that improved tumor retention was seen out to 48 hours in a hepatocellular cancer patient-derived xenograft (HCC-PDX) and HT-1080-FAP mouse models. Although the dimer approach seems to result in improved retention, it is not yet clear that uptake and tumor retention are sufficient for effective Lu-177 radiotherapy with these constructs.

Cyclic peptide library screens have identified several FAP-binding radiotherapy candidates that exhibit potential improvements in tumor retention. In first in human studies, Baum and coworkers examined biodistribution and preliminary dosimetry in radiotherapy of adenocarcinomas using [^{177}Lu]Lu-FAP-2286.[46] In several patients, retention of [^{177}Lu]Lu-FAP-2286 in metastases was seen out to 10 days after injection. Treatment with 2.4 GBq of [^{177}Lu]Lu-FAP-2286 resulted in a mixed response after 8 weeks—regression of bone and bone marrow lesions—but overall progressive disease with new evidence of liver metastases. [^{177}Lu]Lu-FAP-2286 is now the subject of a relatively large-scale Phase 1/2 clinical trial (LuMI-ERE, NCT04939610) that will evaluate the safety and efficacy of targeted FAP radiotherapy using this agent. The development of small molecule peptides that show improved engagement and tumor retention indicate that FAP is a potentially addressable target for radioligand therapy.

IMPROVING DELIVERY

Two fundamental elements are required in addition to selective uptake in tumor tissue to consider a new class of targeting ligands as potential radiotherapeutics. These characteristics are significant absolute uptake and prolonged retention in tumor. The former ensuring a significant quantity of the total radioactive drug administered is taken up by tumor cells and the latter ensures sufficient time for the deposition of energy to destroy tumor tissue. Several studies suggest that albumin-binding moieties such as long-chain fatty acids,[47] 4-(p-iodophenyl) alkanoic acid derivatives,[48] as well as ibuprofen derivatives[49] conjugated to various compounds can be used to successfully modulate plasma clearance rates in a predictable manner.

This approach to pharmacokinetic modulation has been applied recently to radiopharmaceuticals and has been shown in some cases to lead to improvements in peak tumor uptake as well as retention, resulting in an improved therapeutic efficacy.[50–52]

This approach has recently been applied to the development of FAP ligands.[53] RPS-309 is a high-affinity FAPα inhibitor with prolonged plasma residence. It is a trifunctional theranostic ligand that targets FAP-α and also reversibly binds albumin and theranostic radiometals.[54] Indeed, [^{177}Lu]Lu-RPS-309 demonstrated a prolonged circulation time through the albumin-binding group as well as high affinity and retention in liposarcoma SW872 tumor-xenografted mice up to 24 hours postinjection. The multifunctional RPS-309 could be a useful tool for the study of the relationship between FAPI structure and substrate activity in the future. Others have followed suit by creating Evans Blue conjugates and other 4-(p-iodophenyl) alkanoic acid derivatives.[55] This approach requires further study as to how it may lead to improved AFP ligands with therapeutic potential.

SUMMARY

The serine protease seprase (surface expressed protease) or FAP has emerged as an attractive therapeutic target in cancer because of its upregulation in several tumor types and relative rarity in healthy tissue. Because FAP is critical to the initiation of metastatic growth, its expression will serve as a molecular marker to detect tumors at an earlier stage of development compared with currently available methods. The design of high-affinity small-molecule FAP inhibitor will allow for noninvasive imaging of activated fibroblasts in patients with cancer. Such compounds are also likely to find broad utility for imaging of various fibrogenic disorders.

The unique expression of FAP in CAFs provides the possibility of targeting a variety of FAP-positive tumors using targeted radiotherapy. Although this area of development is not as advanced as the imaging applications of FAP, the potential to target tumor stroma may have broad application.

CLINICS CARE POINTS

- FAP imaging may have potential for assessing diseases where activated fibroblasts are known to be involved. Such diseases include myocardial remodeling, fibrotic diseases such as liver fibrosis, pulmonary fibrosis, and kidney fibrosis and cancer detection and treatment monitoring.

DISCLOSURE

Dr S.G. DiMagno and Dr J.W. Babich both are inventors on FAP-related technologies and hold equity in Ratio Therapeutics, Inc.

REFERENCES

1. Li H, Fan X, Houghton J. Tumor microenvironment: the role of the tumor stroma in cancer. J Cell Biochem 2007;101(4):805–15.

2. Chen WT, Kelly T. Seprase complexes in cellular invasiveness. Cancer Metastasis Rev 2003;22(2–3):259–69.

3. Tarin D. Role of the host stroma in cancer and its therapeutic significance. Cancer Metastasis Rev 2013;32(3–4):553–66.

4. Jacob M, Chang L, Pure E. Fibroblast activation protein in remodeling tissues, Curr Mol Med, 12 (10), 2012, 1220–1243.

5. Levy MT, McCaughan GW, Marinos G, Gorrell MD. Intrahepatic expression of the hepatic stellate cell marker fibroblast activation protein correlates with the degree of fibrosis in hepatitis C virus infection. Liver 2002;22:93–101.

6. Welt S, Divgi CR, Scott AM, et al. Antibody targeting in metastatic colon cancer: a phase I study of monoclonal antibody F19 against a cell-surface protein of reactive tumor stromal fibroblasts. J Clin Oncol 1994;12(6):1193–203.

7. Lee KN, Jackson KW, Christiansen VJ, et al. Antiplasmin cleaving enzyme is a soluble form of fibroblast activation protein. Blood 2006;107:1397–404.

8. Keane FM, Yao TW, Seelk S, et al. Quantitation of fibroblast activation protein (FAP)-specific protease activity in mouse, baboon and human fluids and organs. FEBS Open Bio 2013;4:43–54.

9. Goldstein LA, Ghersi G, Piñeiro-Sánchez ML, et al. Molecular cloning of seprase: a serine integral membrane protease from human melanoma. Biochim Biophys Acta 1997;1361(1):11–9.

10. O'Brien P, O'Connor BF. Seprase: an overview of an important matrix serine protease. Biochim Biophys Acta 2008;84(9):1130–45.

11. Henry LR, Lee HO, Lee JS, et al. Clinical implications of fibroblast activation protein in patients with colon cancer. Clin Cancer Res 2007;13(6):1736–41.

12. Mori Y, Kono K, Matsumoto Y, et al. The expression of a type II transmembrane serine protease (seprase) in human gastric carcinoma. Oncology 2004;67(5–6):411–9.

13. Iwasa S, Okada K, Chen WT, et al. Increased expression of seprase, a membrane-type serine protease, is associated with lymph node metastasis in human colorectal cancer. Cancer Lett 2005;227(2):229–36.

14. Huang Y, Wang S, Kelly T. Seprase promotes rapid tumor growth and increased microvessel density in a mouse model of human breast cancer. Cancer Res 2004;64(8):2712–6.

15. Monsky WL, Lin CY, Aoyama A, et al. A potential marker protease of invasiveness, seprase, is localized on invadopodia of human malignant melanoma cells. Cancer Res 1994;54(21):5702–10.

16. Piñeiro-Sánchez ML, Goldstein LA, Dodt J, et al. Identification of the 170-kDa melanoma membrane-bound gelatinase (seprase) as a serine integral membrane protease. J Biol Chem 1997;272(12):7595–601.

17. Goodman JD, Rozypal TL, Kelly T. Seprase, a membrane-bound protease, alleviates the serum growth requirement of human breast cancer cells. Clin Exp Metastasis 2003;20(5):459–70.

18. Cheng JD, Dunbrack RL Jr, Valianou M, et al. Promotion of tumor growth by murine fibroblast activation protein, a serine protease, in an animal model. Cancer Res 2002;62(16):4767–72.

19. Cheng JD, Valianou M, Canutescu AA, et al. Abrogation of fibroblast activation protein enzymatic activity attenuates tumor growth. Mol Cancer Ther 2005;4(3):351–60.

20. Ostermann E, Garin-Chesa P, Heider KH, et al. Effective immunoconjugate therapy in cancer models targeting a serine protease of tumor fibroblasts. Clin Cancer Res 2008;14(14):4584–92.

21. Ziani L, Chouaib S, Thiery J. Alteration of the antitumor immune response by cancer-associated fibroblasts. Front Immunol 2018;9:414.

22. Liao Z, Tan ZW, Zhu P, et al. Cancer-associated fibroblasts in tumor microenvironment - accomplices in tumor malignancy. Cell Immunol 2018. https://doi.org/10.1016/j.cellimm.2017.12.003 [pii:S0008-8749(17)30222-30228].

23. Ishii G, Ochiai A, Neri S. Phenotypic and functional heterogeneity of cancer-associated fibroblast within the tumor microenvironment. Adv Drug Deliv Rev 2016;99(Pt B):186–96.

24. Scott AM, Wiseman G, Welt S, et al. A Phase I dose-escalation study of sibrotuzumab in patients with advanced or metastatic fibroblast activation protein-positive cancer. Clin Cancer Res 2003;9(5):1639–47.

25. Edosada CY, Quan C, Wiesmann C, et al. Selective inhibition of fibroblast activation protein protease based on dipeptide substrate specificity. J Biol Chem 2006;281(11):7437–44.

26. Tran T, Quan C, Edosada CY, et al. Synthesis and structure-activity relationship of N-acyl-Gly-, N-acyl-Sar- and N-blocked-boroPro inhibitors of FAP, DPP4, and POP. Bioorg Med Chem Lett 2007;17(5):1438–42.

27. Gilmore BF, Lynas JF, Scott CJ, et al. Dipeptide proline diphenyl phosphonates are potent, irreversible inhibitors of seprase (FAPalpha). Biochem Biophys Res Commun 2006;346(2):436–46.

28. Adams S, Miller GT, Jesson MI, et al. PT-100, a small molecule dipeptidyl peptidase inhibitor, has potent antitumor effects and augments antibody-mediated cytotoxicity via a novel immune mechanism. Cancer Res 2004;64(15):5471–80.

29. Aertgeerts K, Levin I, Shi L, et al. Structural and kinetic analysis of the substrate specificity of human fibroblast activation protein Alpha. J Biol Chem 2005;280:19441–4.

30. Edosada CY, Quan C, Tran T, et al. Peptide substrate profiling defines fibroblast activation protein as an endopeptidase of strict Gly(2)-Pro(1)-cleaving specificity. FEBS Lett 2006;580:1581–6.

31. Jambunathan K, Watson DS, Endsley AN, et al. Comparative analysis of the substrate preferences of two post-proline cleaving endopeptidases, prolyl oligopeptidase and fibroblast activation protein alpha. FEBS Lett 2012;586:2507–12.

32. Huang S, Fang R, Xu J, et al. Evaluation of the tumor targeting of a FAPalpha-based doxorubicin prodrug. J Drug Target 2011;19:487–96.

33. Marquis J, Wang J, Maresca K, et al. Abstract #4467: targeting tumor microenvironment with radiolabeled inhibitors of seprase (FAP\ #945;). Cancer Res 2009;69(9_Supplement):4467.

34. Meletta R, Müller Herde A, Chiotellis A, et al. Evaluation of the radiolabeled boronic acid-based FAP inhibitor MIP-1232 for atherosclerotic plaque imaging. Molecules 2015;20(2):2081–99.

35. Poplawski SE, Lai JH, Li Y, et al. Identification of selective and potent inhibitors of fibroblast activation protein and prolyl oligopeptidase. J Med Chem 2013;56:3467–77.

36. Jansen K, Heirbaut L, Cheng JD, et al. Selective inhibitors of fibroblast activation protein (FAP) with a (4-quinolinoyl)-glycyl-2-cyanopyrrolidine scaffold. ACS Med Chem Lett 2013;4(5):491–6.

37. Loktev A, Lindner T, Mier W, et al. A tumor-imaging method targeting cancer-associated fibroblasts. J Nucl Med 2018;59(9):1423–9.

38. Kratochwil C, Flechsig P, Lindner T, et al. 68 Ga-FAPI PET/CT: tracer uptake in 28 different kinds of cancer. J Nucl Med 2019;60(6):801–5.

39. Giesel FL, Kratochwil C, Lindner T, et al. 68Ga-FAPI PET/CT: biodistribution and preliminary dosimetry estimate of 2 DOTA-containing FAP-targeting agents in patients with various cancers. J Nucl Med 2019; 60(3):386–92.

40. Lindner T, Giesel FL, Kratochwil C, et al. Radioligands targeting fibroblast activation protein (FAP). Cancers 2021;13(22):5744.

41. Aertgeerts K, Levin I, Shi L, et al. Structural and kinetic analysis of the substrate specificity of human fibroblast activation protein α. J Biol Chem 2005; 280:19441–4.

42. Moon ES, Ballal S, Yadav MP, et al. Fibroblast Activation Protein (FAP) targeting homodimeric FAP inhibitor radiotheranostics: a step to improve tumor uptake and retention time. Am J Nucl Med Mol Imaging 2021;11(6):476–91.

43. Ballal S, Yadav MP, Moon ES, et al. First-in-human results on the biodistribution, pharmacokinetics, and dosimetry of [177Lu]Lu-DOTA.SA.FAPi and [177Lu]Lu-DOTAGA.(SA.FAPi)2. Pharmaceuticals (Basel) 2021;14(12):1212.

44. Zhao L, Niu B, Fang J, et al. Synthesis, preclinical evaluation, and a pilot clinical PET imaging study of 68Ga-labeled FAPI dimer. J Nucl Med 2022; 63(6):862–8.

45. Zhao L, Chen J, Pang Y, et al. Development of fibroblast activation protein inhibitor-based dimeric radiotracers with improved tumor retention and antitumor efficacy. Mol Pharm 2022;19(10):3640–51.

46. Baum RP, Schuchardt C, Singh A, et al. Feasibility, biodistribution, and preliminary dosimetry in peptide-targeted radionuclide therapy of diverse adenocarcinomas using 177Lu-FAP-2286: first-in-humans results. J Nucl Med 2022;63(3):415–23.

47. Bhat M, Jatyan R, Mittal A, et al. Opportunities and challenges of fatty acid conjugated therapeutics. Chem Phys Lipids 2021;236:105053.

48. Dumelin CE, Trüssel S, Buller F, et al. A portable albumin binder from a DNA-encoded chemical library. Angew Chem Int Ed Engl 2008;47(17):3196–201.

49. Manoharan M, Inamati GB, Lesnik EA, et al. Improving antisense oligonucleotide binding to human serum albumin: dramatic effect of ibuprofen conjugation. Chembiochem 2002;3:1257–60.

50. Kelly JM, Amor-Coarasa A, Ponnala S, et al. Albumin-binding PSMA ligands: implications for expanding the therapeutic window. J Nucl Med 2019;60(5): 656–63.

51. Kelly J, Amor-Coarasa A, Ponnala S, et al. Trifunctional PSMA-targeting constructs for prostate cancer with unprecedented localization to LNCaP tumors. Eur J Nucl Med Mol Imaging 2018;45(11):1841–51.

52. Kelly JM, Amor-Coarasa A, Ponnala S, et al. A single dose of 225Ac-RPS-074 induces a complete tumor response in a LNCaP xenograft model. J Nucl Med 2018. https://doi.org/10.2967/jnumed.118.219592 [pii:jnumed.118.219592].

53. Zhang X, Chen D, Babich JW, et al. In Vivo imaging of fibroblast activity using a 68Ga-labeled fibroblast activation protein alpha (FAP-α) inhibitor: study in a mouse rotator cuff repair model. J Bone Joint Surg Am 2021;103(10):e40.

54. Kelly JM, Jeitner TM, Ponnala S, et al. A trifunctional theranostic ligand targeting fibroblast activation protein-α (FAPα). Mol Imaging Biol 2021. https://doi.org/10.1007/s11307-021-01593-1.

55. Xu M, Zhang P, Ding J, et al. Albumin binder-conjugated fibroblast activation protein inhibitor radiopharmaceuticals for cancer therapy. J Nucl Med 2022;63(6):952–8.

Fibroblast Activation Protein Inhibitor PET in Pancreatic Cancer

Liang Zhao, MD[a,b,1], Yizhen Pang, MD[a,b,1], Long Sun, MD, PhD[a],
Qin Lin, MD, PhD[b], Hua Wu, MD, PhD[a], Haojun Chen, MD, PhD[a,*]

KEYWORDS

- FAPI • FDG • PET • Pancreatic cancer • Oncologic management

KEY POINTS

- Pancreatic cancer is typically characterized by intense desmoplastic reactions, resulting in intense fibroblast activation protein (FAP) expression in the tumor stroma.
- ^{68}Ga-FAP inhibitor (FAPI) PET often yields a higher radiotracer uptake and tumor-to-background ratio than ^{18}F-fluorodeoxyglucose PET in primary tumors, involved lymph nodes, and bone and visceral metastases enhancing sensitivity.
- FAPI PET/computed tomography (CT) may offer additional information for the oncologic management of patients with pancreatic cancer, including more accurate TNM staging and improved radiotherapy planning.
- FAPI PET/CT results should be carefully evaluated because increased FAPI uptake may also be observed in benign conditions, including pancreatitis, pancreatic tuberculosis, IgG4-related disease, and serous cystadenoma.

INTRODUCTION

The estimated worldwide incidence and cancer-associated mortality of pancreatic cancer were about 496,000 and 466,000, respectively, according to the 2020 Global Cancer Statistics.[1] The most common (90%) histological subtype of pancreatic cancer is pancreatic ductal adenocarcinoma (PDAC); other subtypes include neuroendocrine tumor, acinar cell carcinoma, and pancreatoblastoma. The symptoms in most early-stage pancreatic cancer are atypical, complicating the diagnosis. Because this disease is usually diagnosed at an advanced stage and as systemic treatment options are rarely curative, the 5-year overall survival rate is less than 10%.[2]

Pancreatic cancer is typically characterized by intense desmoplastic reactions surrounding the cancer cells. The characteristic stromal desmoplastic response plays a key role in tumor invasion, metastasis, and drug resistance.[3–5] The stromal component comprises up to 80% of the pancreatic tumor mass.[6] Generated from the pancreatic stellate cells, cancer-associated fibroblasts (CAFs) are the predominant component of the tumor stroma.[7] Once activated, CAFs perform secretory and contractile functions in tumor development. Fibroblast activation protein (FAP) is an

[a] Department of Nuclear Medicine and Minnan PET Center, Xiamen Cancer Center, The First Affiliated Hospital of Xiamen University, School of Medicine, Xiamen University, 55 Zhenhai Road, Siming District, Xiamen 361003, China; [b] Department of Radiation Oncology, Xiamen Cancer Center, Xiamen Key Laboratory of Radiation Oncology, The First Affiliated Hospital of Xiamen University, School of Medicine, Xiamen University, 55 Zhenhai Road, Siming District, Xiamen 361003, China
[1] First authors contributed equally to this article.
* Corresponding author.
E-mail address: leochen0821@foxmail.com

PET Clin 18 (2023) 295–308
https://doi.org/10.1016/j.cpet.2023.02.001
1556-8598/23/© 2023 Elsevier Inc. All rights reserved.

important biomarker that is highly expressed on the surfaces of CAFs. Moreover, it is a key factor in extracellular matrix formation, angiogenesis, cancer cell invasion, and immunosuppression.[8,9] Therefore, FAP is an attractive target for tumor imaging and therapy in pancreatic cancer.

FIBROBLAST ACTIVATION PROTEIN INHIBITOR PET/COMPUTED TOMOGRAPHY AND PET/MR IMAGING IN THE DIAGNOSIS OF PANCREATIC CANCER

Although it is the most widely used PET tracer in nuclear oncology, ^{18}F-fluorodeoxyglucose(^{18}F-FDG) has several limitations in the diagnosis and staging of pancreatic cancer.[10] First, ^{18}F-FDG PET/computed tomography (CT) sometimes yields false-negative results in the detection of small, isodense pancreatic cancers.[11] Second, ^{18}F-FDG PET/CT has a low-to-moderate sensitivity in the evaluation of metastatic lymph nodes (LNs). It underestimates the N (node) stage, limiting its utility in the surgical planning for patients with pancreatic cancer.[10] Furthermore, ^{18}F-FDG PET/CT exhibits poor performance in the detection of liver metastases and peritoneal carcinomatosis, which are common forms of metastasis in pancreatic cancer.[12,13]

In recent years, whole-body integrated ^{18}F-FDG PET/MR imaging modality has become available for clinical use. This system shows many potential advantages over PET/CT, including inherently higher soft-tissue contrast, multiparametric imaging capabilities, and lower radiation exposure.[14] For its use in pancreatic cancer, a previous study has demonstrated that ^{18}F-FDG PET/MR could potentially serve as an alternative to ^{18}F-FDG PET/CT plus multidetector CT in the preoperative assessment of resectability and staging of pancreatic cancer, thereby shortening the workup period for the determination of therapeutic strategy.[15] Another research demonstrated that ^{18}F-FDG PET/MR imaging was useful in differentiating pancreatic cancer from benign lesions.[16] In addition, it was helpful in evaluating relationship between lesions and surrounding tissues as well as in detecting extra benign cysts.[17]

Fibroblast Activation Protein as a Target for Imaging of Pancreatic Cancer

Given the limitations of ^{18}F-FDG, alternative radiotracers and imaging targets have been explored for the diagnosis of pancreatic cancer. As FAP is overexpressed on the CAFs of 90% of the types of malignant epithelial cancer and exhibits negative/low expression in healthy tissues, it has attracted much attention as a pan-cancer marker.[18,19] Recently, a series of quinoline-based FAP inhibitors (FAPIs) have been developed and these have yielded encouraging results in preclinical and clinical molecular imaging studies.[20–22] In a preclinical study, a patient-derived orthotopic xenograft model of pancreatic adenocarcinoma displayed a significantly higher tumor-to-muscle ratio with ^{68}Ga-FAPI-04 than with ^{18}F-FDG.[23] The favorable image contrast obtained with ^{68}Ga-FAPI PET/CT may allow its clinical use for the detection of early-stage pancreatic cancer. The first report of a clinical FAPI PET study on pancreatic cancer was published in 2018. In that translational study, ^{68}Ga-FAPI (FAPI-02) PET/CT exhibited intense radiotracer uptake in pancreatic tumor lesions but low uptake in normal organs.[20] In a subsequent clinical investigation of a larger patient cohort, ^{68}Ga-FAPI (FAPI-04) PET/CT exhibited intense radiotracer uptake and favorable tumor-to-background contrast ratios in various cancers, including pancreatic cancer (maximum standardized uptake value [SUVmax] > 10 in pancreatic cancer, n = 51).[24] In a study reported by Rohrich and colleagues,[25] 19 patients with PDAC (7 primary, 12 progressive/recurrent) demonstrated intense ^{68}Ga-FAPI (FAPI-04) uptake in the primary tumors (SUVmax: 13.37 ± 5.45), LN metastases (SUVmax: 14.13 ± 8.50), and distant metastases (SUVmax: 7.34 ± 2.48). These first experiences of ^{68}Ga-FAPI PET/CT in pancreatic cancer highlight its potential use in tumor staging, recurrence detection, and individual oncologic management. Moreover, the clear tumor boundary definition derived via ^{68}Ga-FAPI PET/CT may improve the delineation of gross tumor volume (GTV) for precise radiotherapy planning. However, it should be noted that inflammatory uptake distal to the primary that may sometimes obscure tumor boundaries, and dynamic imaging of FAPI PET/CT could differentiate these changes from tumor.[25,26]

Comparison of ^{68}Ga-FAPI and ^{18}F-FDG Uptake in Pancreatic Cancer

As a promising PET tracer for imaging of pancreatic cancers, the comparison between FAPI and FDG is of interest. In the first systematic, clinical comparison of ^{68}Ga-FAPI PET/CT and ^{18}F-FDG in various types of cancer, the ^{68}Ga-FAPI (FAPI-04) uptake in pancreatic cancer was significantly higher than that of ^{18}F-FDG (SUVmax: 17.5 vs 4.8, $P = .043$, n = 4).[27] Moreover, the higher lesion detection rate of ^{68}Ga-FAPI PET/CT resulted in an upstaging of the TNM stage in 2 of the 4 patients (compared with ^{18}F-FDG PET/CT). Similar observations were made in several contemporaneous case studies that ^{68}Ga-FAPI PET/CT was superior

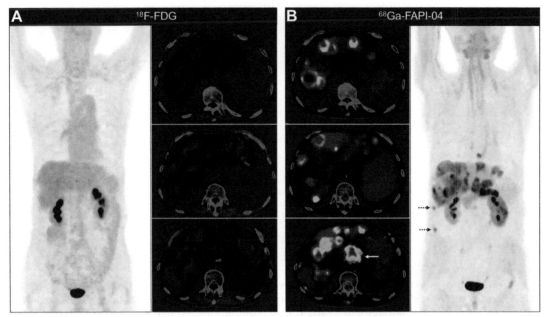

Fig. 1. A 75-year-old man with pancreatic adenocarcinoma underwent ^{18}F-FDG and ^{68}Ga-FAPI-04 PET/CT for initial staging. (*A*) Besides moderate metabolic activity in the head of the pancreas, ^{18}F-FDG PET/CT revealed multiple hypoattenuating lesions in the liver with low-to-moderate metabolic activity. (*B*) ^{68}Ga-FAPI-04 PET/CT exhibited much higher tracer uptake in both the primary (*solid arrow*) and metastatic lesions. Moreover, abnormal foci were observed on the mesentery, which were negative on ^{18}F-FDG PET/CT. (*From* Chen H., et al., Usefulness of [(68)Ga]Ga-DOTA-FAPI-04 PET/CT in patients presenting with inconclusive [(18)F]FDG PET/CT findings. Eur J Nucl Med Mol Imaging. 2021;48(1):73-86.)

to ^{18}F-FDG PET/CT for the detection of visceral metastases from pancreatic cancer, including liver and peritoneal metastases[28–31] **(Fig. 1)**.

In the first head-to-head comparative study in pancreatic cancer (^{68}Ga-FAPI-04 vs ^{18}F-FDG), ^{68}Ga-FAPI PET/CT exhibited significantly higher radiotracer uptake than ^{18}F-FDG in primary tumors (SUVmax, 21.4 vs 4.8; $P < .001$), involved LNs (SUVmax, 8.6 vs 2.7; $P < .001$), liver metastases (SUVmax, 7.4 vs 3.7; $P < .001$), peritoneal metastases (SUVmax, 8.4 vs 2.8; $P < .001$), and bone metastases (SUVmax, 10.6 vs 2.3; $P = .001$).[26] In contrast to ^{18}F-FDG, ^{68}Ga-FAPI was not taken up by the brain tissue, and exhibited lower background activity in the liver, heart, and gastrointestinal tract. ^{68}Ga-FAPI PET/CT yielded a favorable image contrast with low background activity throughout the body **(Fig. 2)**.[26] Regarding the diagnostic accuracy, ^{68}Ga-FAPI PET/CT exhibited significantly higher sensitivity than ^{18}F-FDG PET/CT in the detection of primary tumors (100% vs 73%), involved LNs (82% vs 59%), and bone and visceral metastases (92% vs 44%).[26] The encouraging results from that study further highlight the clinical value of FAPI PET/CT for the diagnosis of pancreatic cancer, especially for the detection of involved LNs and bone and visceral metastases.

Multisequence MR imaging provides more information and yields superior soft-tissue contrast than CT scans do, and integrated PET/MR imaging may overcome the limitation of PET/CT in the evaluation of LN and visceral metastases.[32,33] Zhang and colleagues recently introduced ^{68}Ga-FAPI (FAPI-04) PET/MR imaging for the diagnosis of pancreatic cancer and compared the results with those of ^{18}F-FDG PET/CT. Unsurprisingly, the results suggested that ^{68}Ga-FAPI PET/MR imaging was superior to ^{18}F-FDG PET/CT for the diagnosis of pancreatic cancer, especially for the detection of suspicious LN metastases (42 vs 30, $P < .001$; **Fig. 3**).[34] Consistent with previous results, the primary tumors exhibited significantly higher uptake of ^{68}Ga-FAPI than ^{18}F-FDG (SUVmax, 12.58 vs 8.78). Interestingly, density differences were not observed in 75% (12/16) of primary pancreatic lesions on the CT scans, whereas abnormal signals were observed in all (16/16) primary lesions on multiparameter MR imaging, which helped to enhance the confidence in the interpretation of primary tumors. Moreover, multisequence MR imaging led to the detection of more liver metastases than ^{18}F-FDG (256 vs 181, $P < .001$). However, unlike results in a previous study, ^{18}F-FDG PET detected a greater number of liver metastases

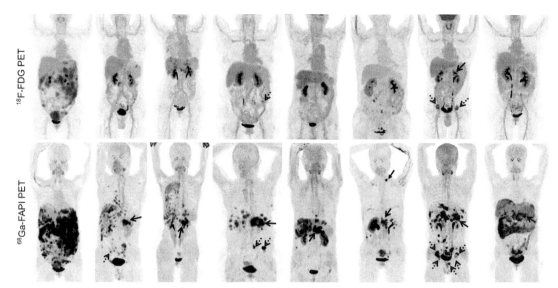

Fig. 2. Representative maximum intensity projection images of paired ^{18}F-FDG and ^{68}Ga-FAPI PET/CT in patients with pancreatic cancer. *Solid arrows* indicate the primary tumor, *Dotted arrows* indicate bone metastases, *Arrowhead* indicate lymph node metastases. (*From* Pang Y., et al., Positron emission tomography and computed tomography with [(68)Ga]Ga-fibroblast activation protein inhibitors improves tumor detection and staging in patients with pancreatic cancer. Eur J Nucl Med Mol Imaging. 2022;49(4):1322-1337.)

than ^{68}Ga-FAPI PET in the study by Chen and colleagues[30] (181 vs 104, $P < .001$). Therefore, ^{68}Ga-FAPI PET combined with hybrid MR imaging is a promising imaging modality for the evaluation of both primary and metastatic lesions but ^{18}F-FDG PET/CT can detect some lesions with low FAP expression.

Impact of FAPI PET/CT in TNM Staging and Oncological Management

Only 20% of patients with pancreatic cancer are suited for surgery; as a result, chemotherapy and targeted therapy are crucial in the treatment of this disease.[35] However, chemotherapy usually

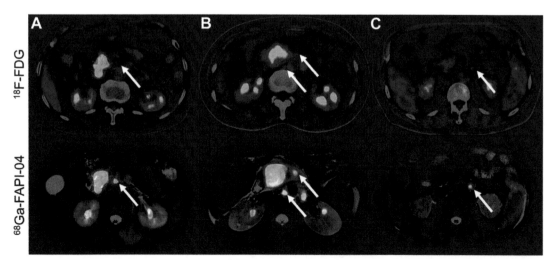

Fig. 3. Three patients (*A*, *B*, and *C*) with ^{68}Ga-FAPI-positive but ^{18}F-FDG-negative uptake in lymph nodes (*arrows*). (*From* Zhang Z., et al., Comparison of the diagnostic efficacy of (68)Ga-FAPI-04 PET/MR and (18)F-FDG PET/CT in patients with pancreatic cancer. Eur J Nucl Med Mol Imaging. 2022;49(8):2877-2888.)

yields a low clinical response, short overall survival, and moderate toxicity in pancreatic cancer.[36] Comprehensive assessment of a patient's disease status followed by individualized treatment may improve the survival. As FAPI PET/CT is superior to ^{18}F-FDG PET/CT in the detection of primary and metastatic lesions, it may offer additional information in the oncologic management of patients with pancreatic cancer.

In the first study of the clinical impact of ^{68}Ga-FAPI PET/CT in patients with PDAC (n = 19), ^{68}Ga-FAPI PET/CT led to changes in TNM staging in 10 of 19 (53%) patients compared with contrast-enhanced (CE) CT.[25] Of the 12 patients with recurrent/progressive disease, 8 patients were upstaged and 1 was downstaged. Among the other 7 treatment-naïve patients, TNM staging was upstaged in one. Changes in oncologic

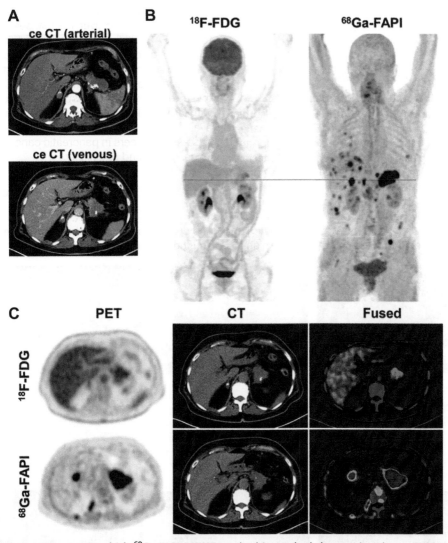

Fig. 4. Representative case in which ^{68}Ga-FAPI PET/CT resulted in marked changes in primary TNM staging (up-staging) compared with CE-CT and ^{18}F-FDG PET/CT. (*A*) Axial images of PDAC and the liver in the arterial (upper image) and venous (lower image) phase of a CE-CT scan. (*B*) Maximum intensity projection ^{18}F-FDG and FAPI PET/CT images. (*C*) Axial ^{18}F-FDG and FAPI PET/CT images of the same patient at the level (*blue line* in *B*) of the pancreatic tumor mass and another suspicious FAPI accumulation in a projection of the perihepatic lymph node. Metastases, which had been revealed by FAPI PET/CT, were confirmed via biopsy of a pulmonary lesion; it was diagnosed as metastasis of the PDAC. This research was originally published in JNM. Rohrich M., et al., Impact of (68)Ga-FAPI PET/CT Imaging on the Therapeutic Management of Primary and Recurrent Pancreatic Ductal Adenocarcinomas. J Nucl Med. June 2021, 62(6) 779-786; DOI: https://doi.org/10.2967/jnumed.120.253062. © SNMMI.

management occurred in 7 out of 19 (37%) patients (**Fig. 4**). In another study, with 23 patients who underwent paired ^{18}F-FDG and ^{68}Ga-FAPI PET/CT for initial staging, ^{68}Ga-FAPI PET/CT resulted in TNM upstaging in 6 out of 23 (26%) patients (N stage in 7 patients and M stage in 5).[26] It also resulted in a modified therapeutic regimen in 2 out of 23 patients (9%) compared with ^{18}F-FDG, and in only 1 patient compared with CE-CT (1 out of 23, 4%). However, owing to the limited numbers of patients from those studies, we are unable to definitively comment on the role of FAPI PET/CT in clinical management of pancreatic cancer at this point, and we eagerly await further investigations.

FAPI PET/CT in the Discrimination of Suspicious Pancreatic Lesions

Apart from cancer staging, FAPI PET may also be used for the discrimination of suspicious mass lesions of the pancreas. An intraductal papillary mucinous neoplasm (IPMN) is a benign cystic lesion in the ducts of the pancreas, and PDAC may originate from an IPMN. However, it is very challenging to differentiate between malignant and benign IPMNs via conventional imaging modalities. In a recent study of 25 patients with cystic pancreatic lesions, malignant IPMNs and PDACs had higher

^{68}Ga-FAPI uptakes than low-grade IPMNs and other benign cystic lesions (**Fig. 5**).[37] Therefore, the lower radiotracer uptake of ^{68}Ga-FAPI by pancreatic lesions may be indicative of benign disease and help clinicians to avoid unnecessary surgical treatment of nonmalignant pancreatic IPMNs.[37]

Other radiolabeled FAPI agents have been used for the imaging of pancreatic cancer. For example, in a translational study of a patient with pancreatic cancer, the tumor lesions could be clearly visualized via ^{99m}Tc-FAPI-34 SPECT.[38] Considered together, except for one study in which ^{18}F-FDG PET detected more liver metastases than ^{68}Ga-FAPI,[34] FAPI PET was superior to FDG PET for the detection of primary tumors and distant metastases, which may improve the clinical staging and lead to an optimal treatment strategy. However, these results warrant prospective clinical studies with large patient samples for the comprehensive evaluation of the diagnostic accuracy of FAPI-based radiotracers in pancreatic cancer, including its sensitivity and specificity.

PROGNOSTIC VALUE OF FAPI PET IN PANCREATIC CANCER

The prognosis of pancreatic cancer remains poor, and the number of deaths was approximately with

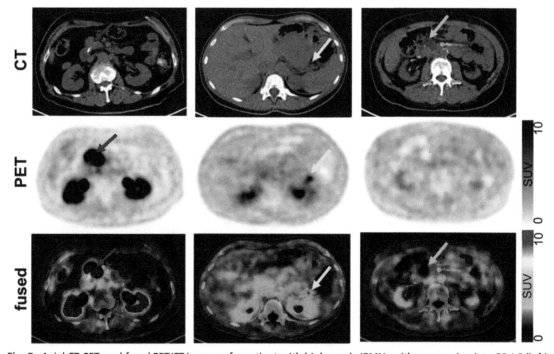

Fig. 5. Axial CT, PET, and fused PET/CT images of a patient with high-grade IPMNs with progression into PDAC (left), a patient with a high-grade IPMN without PDAC (middle), and a patient with low-grade IPMN (right). Arrows indicate the pathologies. This research was originally published in JNM. Lang M., et al. Static and dynamic (68)Ga-FAPI PET/CT for the detection of malignant transformation of intraductal papillary mucinous neoplasia of the pancreas. J Nucl Med. February 2023, 64(2) 244-251; DOI: https://doi.org/10.2967/jnumed.122.264361. © SNMMI.

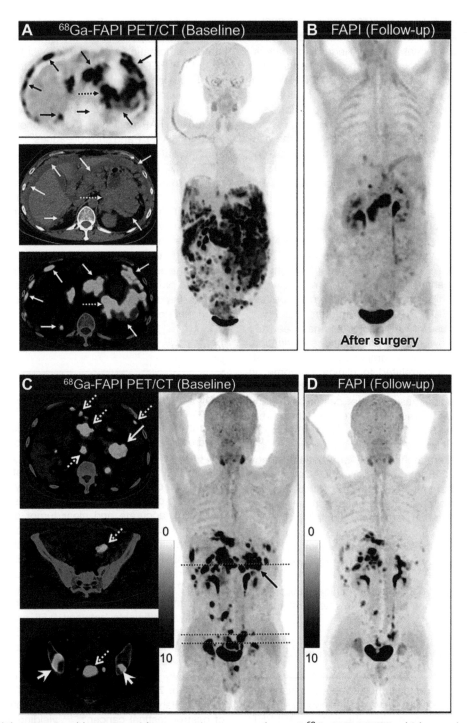

Fig. 6. (*A*) A 55-year-old woman with pancreatic cancer underwent ^{68}Ga-FAPI PET/CT, which revealed a mass lesion with increased ^{68}Ga-FAPI uptake in the tail of pancreas (*dotted arrow*), and several abnormal foci in the mesentery and omentum (*solid arrows*). The patient subsequently underwent a distal pancreatectomy plus cytoreductive surgery of the peritoneal carcinomatosis and adjuvant nab-paclitaxel plus gemcitabine chemotherapy. (*B*) Follow-up ^{68}Ga-FAPI PET/CT (3 months after surgery) revealed an excellent response with decreased ^{68}Ga-FAPI activity in the abdomen and pelvis. (*C*) A 53-year-old man with known pancreatic ductal adenocarcinoma (with signet-ring cell features) underwent ^{68}Ga-FAPI PET/CT, revealing intensive radiotracer uptake in the primary lesion (*solid arrow*), bone metastases (*arrowheads*), and peritoneal carcinomatosis (*dotted arrows*). (*D*) Follow-up ^{68}Ga-FAPI PET/CT after 2 cycles of chemotherapy revealed a partial response (measurable target lesions,

the number of diagnoses (466,000 vs 496,000) in 2020.[1] The incidence and death rate has not declined in recent years. Regarding cancer-related deaths, pancreatic cancer ranked seventh and breast cancer ranked third in 2020.[1] However, pancreatic cancer was projected to be the third leading cancer-associated death, possibly surpassing breast cancer, by 2025.[39]

As a functional molecule that allows for the visualization of the tumor metabolic activity, the parameters derived from ^{18}F-FDG PET/CT are prognostically useful in the clinical setting. For example, in a meta-analysis of 23 studies (1762 patients), a higher SUVmax in the primary tumor was significantly associated with a poorer survival.[40] Similarly, metabolic tumor volume and total lesion glycolysis, parameters derived from ^{18}F-FDG PET/CT, were independent prognostic factors in pancreatic cancer in a retrospective study.[41] Similar prognostic value may be expected of FAPI PET/CT parameters. However, the clinical use of FAPI molecules has been too short to allow robust prognostic stratification. Nevertheless, there is ample evidence that FAP expression is correlated to clinical outcome. In preclinical studies, FAP played an important role in tumor angiogenesis, cancer cell invasion, and immune suppression.[8,9] Moreover, the tumor stroma may be a barrier for chemotherapy in pancreatic cancer.[42] In a retrospective study, multiplex immunohistochemistry-based image analysis of 215 treatment-naïve PDACs revealed that patients with FAP-dominant, fibroblast-rich stroma exhibited poorer prognosis than patients with collagen-rich stroma.[43] Similarly, Shi and colleagues[44] reported that high expression of FAP was correlated to an unfavorable prognosis in 134 patients with PDAC. Therefore, we speculate that parameters derived from FAPI PET/CT may be associated with the clinical outcome in pancreatic cancer. However, this warrants further investigation.

Use of Fibroblast Activation Protein Inhibitor for Response Assessment

Early evaluation of the tumor response to therapy is important. Recently, several preliminary studies were conducted to explore the role of FAPI PET/CT in the evaluation of the response of pancreatic cancer to therapy. For example, Zhao and colleagues[31] reported that one patient with metastatic pancreatic cancer underwent follow-up ^{68}Ga-FAPI PET/CT (3 months after treatment) for tumor response evaluation to cytoreductive surgery and adjuvant chemotherapy. Their study revealed a large therapeutic response, visualized as decreasing FAPI activity, in the peritoneal metastases (**Fig. 6** A-B). Pang and colleagues[26] reported on another patient who underwent follow-up ^{68}Ga-FAPI PET/CT (2 cycles after treatment) for evaluation of tumor response to chemotherapy. They revealed a partial response (decreased FAPI uptake) in most metastatic lesions (**Fig. 6**C, D). Therefore, we speculate that FAPI PET/CT may be useful for the evaluation of the tumor response, particularly to chemotherapy. The next step is to assess the usefulness of PET/CT in early prognostication in patients with pancreatic cancer. A study addressing this specific question would be an important contribution.

Impact of FAPI PET/CT in Radiotherapy Planning

In inoperable cases, radiotherapy, such as stereotactic body radiotherapy, is an alternative strategy for locally recurrent pancreatic cancer.[45] CE-CT is the current reference standard for the diagnosis of pancreatic cancer and target volume delineation for radiotherapy planning. However, with poor sensitivity (0.7) and specificity (0.8), postoperative anatomical changes or fibrosis in locally recurrent pancreatic cancer can be difficult to assess.[46,47] Therefore, accurate and clear tumor delineation with a molecular imaging modality may be of assistance in radiotherapy planning. The first study of the use of FAPI PET/CT for the automatic delineation of tumors in GTV contouring yielded encouraging results in 7 patients with locally recurring tumors.[48] Significant differences were observed (mean dice similarity coefficients between 0.55 and 0.65) in the GTVs manually determined via CE-CT by 6 radiation oncologists, whereas no significant differences were observed in automatically assigned FAPI-GTVs and 4 of the 6 manually contoured GTVs (**Fig. 7**). The value of FAPI PET/CT in radiotherapy planning was also explored in other types of gastrointestinal cancer,[49–51] yielding improved target volume delineation in esophageal, rectal,

38% decrease in the sum of the longest diameters). (*From* Zhao L., et al., Use of 68Ga-FAPI PET/CT for Evaluation of Peritoneal Carcinomatosis Before and After Cytoreductive Surgery. Clin Nucl Med. 2021;46(6):491-493. From Pang Y., et al., Positron emission tomography and computed tomography with [(68)Ga]Ga-fibroblast activation protein inhibitors improves tumor detection and staging in patients with pancreatic cancer. Eur J Nucl Med Mol Imaging. 2022;49(4):1322-1337.)

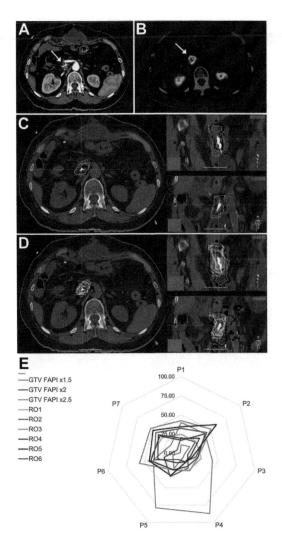

Fig. 7. (*A, B*) Contrast-enhanced CT and ^{68}Ga-FAPI PET/CT images in a 66-year-old patient with locally recurrent pancreatic cancer. The local tumor recurrence is adjacent to a surgical clip, as marked by the white arrow. (*C*) GTVs determined by 6 different radiation oncologists (different colors), delineated on a conventional CT image. An axial slice is shown on the left, and sagittal and coronal slices are shown on the upper and lower right, respectively. (*D*) Automated contoured GTVs with three different FAPI thresholds (red: 1.5, green: 2.0, black: 2.5). For comparative purposes, the GTVs manually defined by the radiation oncologists in panel (*C*) are superimposed in light blue. (*E*) Spider plot comparing mean GTVs (cubic centimeter) of individual patients (P1–7) as contoured manually using conventional CT by 6 different radiation oncologists (RO1–6). In addition, 3 different automatically contoured GTVs using FAPI-PET/CT are displayed. (*From* Liermann J., et al., Impact of FAPI-PET/CT on Target Volume Definition in Radiation Therapy of Locally Recurrent Pancreatic Cancer. Cancers (Basel). 2021;13(4).)

and anal cancer. Thus, FAPI PET/CT is a promising imaging modality for the improvement of GTV delineation and for decreasing interobserver variability in pancreatic cancer, especially in cases presenting with inconclusive CE-CT findings.

INCREASED FIBROBLAST ACTIVATION PROTEIN INHIBITOR UPTAKE IN NONMALIGNANT PANCREATIC LESIONS

When considering the clinical use of FAPI PET/CT in the differential diagnosis and management of malignant pancreatic lesions, oncologists must be aware of the danger of false-positive results.[52] Chronic pancreatitis and/or tumor-induced pancreatitis/cholangitis may result in intense FAPI uptake (on the standard scan, 60 minutes after injection) in the whole pancreas in patients with pancreatic cancer.[28,53] For example, among 11 patients who had undergone no or only partial pancreatectomy before ^{68}Ga-FAPI PET/CT, 8 exhibited homogeneously elevated ^{68}Ga-FAPI uptake in the rest of pancreas.[25] Pang and colleagues[26] reported a similar phenomenon in nearly half of patients (12 out of 26) with newly diagnosed pancreatic cancer. Similarly, in a recent study by Zhang and colleagues,[34] 16 patients with pancreatic cancer exhibited elevated tracer uptake in the adjacent pancreatic tissue. The intense FAPI uptake in patients with chronic pancreatitis may mask tumor activity related to pancreatic cancer. Therefore, careful attention is required when evaluating FAPI PET/CT images in patients with pancreatitis who may have pancreatic cancer.

As a solution, an additional, delayed scan may improve discrimination of noncancerous and cancerous lesions, as malignant tumors usually exhibit further increases in radiotracer uptake on the delayed scans, whereas benign lesions usually exhibit decreases.[54] The use of dual-time scanning for discrimination of PDAC from pancreatitis was first reported by Röhrich and colleagues,[25] revealing a slightly increased FAPI uptake in PDAC and a decreased uptake in pancreatitis in 2 patients (**Fig. 8**A). The hypothesis of a differential uptake over time in PDAC and pancreatitis was further evaluated by Pang and colleagues, performing an additional, 3-hour-delayed ^{68}Ga-FAPI PET scan in 6 patients with pancreatic cancer. All 6 dual-time FAPI PET scans revealed a stable ^{68}Ga-FAPI uptake in pancreatic tumors (SUVmax, 20.4 vs 20.1; $P = .249$) but decreased uptake in noncancerous lesions (SUVmax, 18.6 vs 13.7; $P = .028$; **Fig. 8**B), which was consistent with earlier findings.[26] Therefore, the differences in uptake kinetics of ^{68}Ga-FAPI may help differentiate pancreatic cancer from pancreatitis, a hypothesis

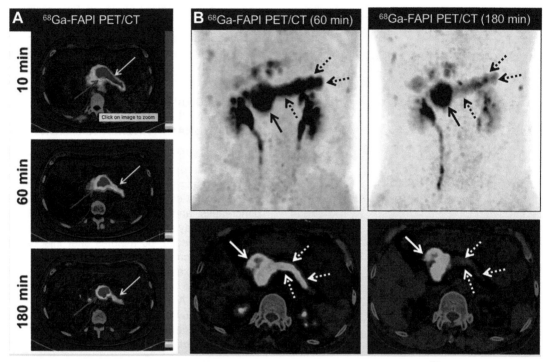

Fig. 8. (*A*) Examples of tumor-related (*red arrow*) and pancreatitis-related (*yellow arrow*) ^{68}Ga-FAPI uptake 10, 60, and 180 min after administration. (*B*) Representative ^{68}Ga-FAPI PET/CT images of pancreatic cancer (*solid arrow*) and pancreatitis (*dotted arrow*) at 60 and 180 min. (This research was originally published in JNM. Rohrich M., et al., Impact of (68)Ga-FAPI PET/CT Imaging on the Therapeutic Management of Primary and Recurrent Pancreatic Ductal Adenocarcinomas. J Nucl Med. June 2021, 62(6) 779-786; DOI: https://doi.org/10.2967/jnumed.120. 253062. © SNMMI. *From* Rohrich M., et al., Impact of (68)Ga-FAPI PET/CT Imaging on the Therapeutic Management of Primary and Recurrent Pancreatic Ductal Adenocarcinomas. J Nucl Med. 2021;62(6):779-786.)

that should be systematically evaluated in a larger patient cohort.

Besides ~~chronic~~ pancreatitis, other benign pancreatic diseases may also cause increased FAPI uptake and be mistaken for pancreatic malignancy. Sun and colleagues[55] reported one case of intense ^{68}Ga-FAPI uptake in the head of pancreas, initially suspected of pancreatic malignancy but finally diagnosed as pancreatic tuberculosis via postoperative histopathology (**Fig. 9**A). Intense ^{68}Ga-FAPI uptake may also be observed in pancreatic pseudocysts, sites of earlier pancreatitis,[52] and serous cystadenoma (**Fig. 9**B).[56] Besides these, immunoglobulin G4-related disease (IgG4-RD) affects multiple organs, and is histopathologically characterized by "storiform" fibrosis. Therefore, intense FAPI uptake was observed in the pancreas of a patient with IgG4-RD (**Fig. 9**C).[57] Such false-positive results indicate that focally elevated uptake in the pancreas should not be deemed a result of pancreatic malignancy without proper differential diagnosis of benign lesions, which includes clinical radiological, and

preferably pathological correlation to confirm or exclude malignancy.[55–57]

SUMMARY

FAPI PET has yielded promising results in the diagnosis of pancreatic cancer, generally exhibiting higher radiotracer uptake than, and superior sensitivity to FDG PET in the detection of primary tumors, involved LNs, and liver/bone/peritoneal metastases. As a result, FAPI may yield better performance than ^{18}F-FDG in terms of TNM staging. The role of FAPI PET in guiding clinical management of patients with pancreatic cancer requires further investigation. In addition, the use of FAPI PET in tumor therapeutic response evaluation and early prognostication in such patients is of interest. As such, well-designed prospective trials, including head-to-head comparisons, more extensive studies, randomized controlled trials, and histopathological examinations are needed to clarify the usefulness of FAPI PET imaging in pancreatic cancer.

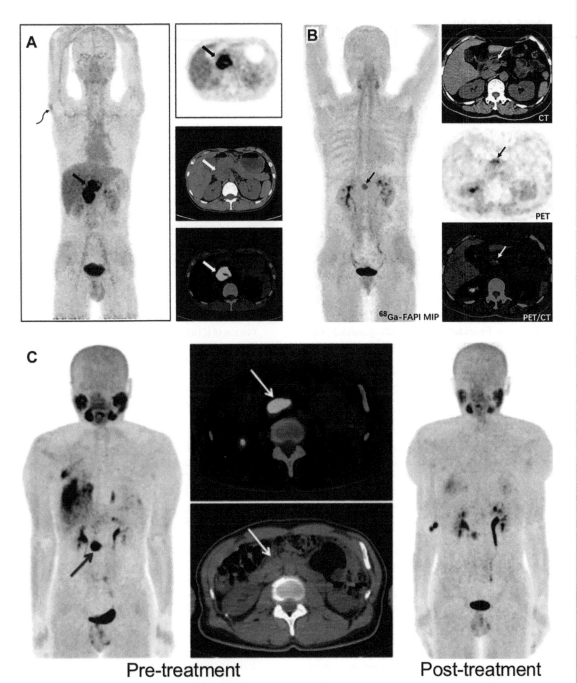

Pre-treatment   **Post-treatment**

Fig. 9. (*A*) Maximum intensity projection (MIP) and axial images of ^{68}Ga-FAPI PET/CT revealed abnormal ^{68}Ga-FAPI uptake in the right shoulder joint (*curved arrow*) and in the region of the pancreatic head (*straight arrow*). However, postoperative pathological results demonstrated the presence of tuberculosis. (*B*) MIP and axial images of ^{68}Ga-FAPI PET/CT revealed abnormal ^{68}Ga-FAPI uptake in the pancreatic head (*arrow*). The histopathological results of the surgical specimen resulted in a diagnosis of serous cystadenoma of the pancreas. (*C*) Pretreatment and posttreatment ^{68}Ga-FAPI PET/CT images of a 58-year-old man with IgG4-related disease. (*From* Sun R., et al., 68Ga-FAPI and 18F-FDG PET/CT Findings in a Patient With Pancreatic Tuberculosis Mimicking Malignant Tumor. Clin Nucl Med. 2022;47(7):653-654. From Xu W., et al., Serous Cystadenoma of the Pancreas Showing Increased Uptake on 68Ga-FAPI PET/CT. Clin Nucl Med. 2022. From Luo Y., et al., IgG4-related disease revealed by (68)Ga-FAPI and (18)F-FDG PET/CT. Eur J Nucl Med Mol Imaging. 2019;46(12):2625-2626.)

CLINICS CARE POINTS

- Compared to contrast-enhanced CT and 18F-FDG PET/CT, FAPI PET/CT led to significant changes in staging and clinical management in patients with pancreatic cancer, especially in detecting local recurrence, liver and peritoneal metastases.

DECLARATION OF INTERESTS AND SOURCE OF FUNDING

This study is supported by the National Natural Science Foundation of China, China (82071961), Key Scientific Research Program for Yong Scholars in Fujian (2021ZQNZD 016), Fujian Natural Science Foundation for Distinguished Yong Scholars (2022J01310623), Fujian Research and Training Grants for Young and Middle-aged Leaders in Healthcare, and Key Medical and Health Projects in Xiamen (3502Z20209002).

REFERENCES

1. Sung H, Ferlay J, Siegel RL, et al. Global cancer statistics 2020: GLOBOCAN estimates of incidence and mortality worldwide for 36 cancers in 185 countries. CA Cancer J Clin 2021;71(3):209–49.
2. Siegel RL, Miller KD, Jemal A. Cancer statistics, 2020. CA Cancer J Clin 2020;70(1):7–30.
3. Gao Z, Wang X, Wu K, et al. Pancreatic stellate cells increase the invasion of human pancreatic cancer cells through the stromal cell-derived factor-1/CXCR4 axis. Pancreatology 2010;10(2–3):186–93.
4. Nielsen SR, Quaranta V, Linford A, et al. Macrophage-secreted granulin supports pancreatic cancer metastasis by inducing liver fibrosis. Nat Cell Biol 2016;18(5):549–60.
5. Provenzano PP, Cuevas C, Chang AE, et al. Enzymatic targeting of the stroma ablates physical barriers to treatment of pancreatic ductal adenocarcinoma. Cancer Cell 2012;21(3):418–29.
6. Erkan M, Michalski CW, Rieder S, et al. The activated stroma index is a novel and independent prognostic marker in pancreatic ductal adenocarcinoma. Clin Gastroenterol Hepatol 2008;6(10):1155–61.
7. Apte MV, Haber PS, Applegate TL, et al. Periacinar stellate shaped cells in rat pancreas: identification, isolation, and culture. Gut 1998;43(1):128–33.
8. Lee HO, Mullins SR, Franco-Barraza J, et al. FAP-overexpressing fibroblasts produce an extracellular matrix that enhances invasive velocity and directionality of pancreatic cancer cells. BMC Cancer 2011;11:245.
9. Kawase T, Yasui Y, Nishina S, et al. Fibroblast activation protein-alpha-expressing fibroblasts promote the progression of pancreatic ductal adenocarcinoma. BMC Gastroenterol 2015;15:109.
10. Strobel O, Buchler MW. Pancreatic cancer: FDG-PET is not useful in early pancreatic cancer diagnosis. Nat Rev Gastroenterol Hepatol 2013;10(4):203–5.
11. Buchs NC, Buhler L, Bucher P, et al. Value of contrast-enhanced 18F-fluorodeoxyglucose positron emission tomography/computed tomography in detection and presurgical assessment of pancreatic cancer: a prospective study. J Gastroenterol Hepatol 2011;26(4):657–62.
12. Zhao L, Pang Y, Luo Z, et al. Role of [(68)Ga]Ga-DOTA-FAPI-04 PET/CT in the evaluation of peritoneal carcinomatosis and comparison with [(18)F]-FDG PET/CT. Eur J Nucl Med Mol Imaging 2021;48(6):1944–55.
13. Hong SB, Choi SH, Kim KW, et al. Diagnostic performance of [(18)F]FDG-PET/MRI for liver metastasis in patients with primary malignancy: a systematic review and meta-analysis. Eur Radiol 2019;29(7):3553–63.
14. Paspulati RM, Gupta A. PET/MR imaging in cancers of the gastrointestinal tract. Pet Clin 2016;11(4):403–23.
15. Joo I, Lee JM, Lee DH, et al. Preoperative assessment of pancreatic cancer with FDG PET/MR imaging versus FDG PET/CT plus contrast-enhanced multidetector CT: a prospective preliminary study. Radiology 2017;282(1):149–59.
16. Xing H, Ding H, Hou B, et al. The performance comparison of (18)F-FDG PET/MRI and (18)F-FDG PET/CT for the identification of pancreatic neoplasms. Mol Imaging Biol 2022;24(3):489–97.
17. Nagamachi S, Nishii R, Wakamatsu H, et al. The usefulness of (18)F-FDG PET/MRI fusion image in diagnosing pancreatic tumor: comparison with (18)F-FDG PET/CT. Ann Nucl Med 2013;27(6):554–63.
18. Chen X, Song E. Turning foes to friends: targeting cancer-associated fibroblasts. Nat Rev Drug Discov 2019;18(2):99–115.
19. Hofheinz RD, al-Batran SE, Hartmann F, et al. Stromal antigen targeting by a humanised monoclonal antibody: an early phase II trial of sibrotuzumab in patients with metastatic colorectal cancer. Onkologie 2003;26(1):44–8.
20. Loktev A, Lindner T, Mier W, et al. A tumor-imaging method targeting cancer-associated fibroblasts. J Nucl Med 2018;59(9):1423–9.
21. Lindner T, Loktev A, Altmann A, et al. Development of quinoline-based theranostic ligands for the targeting of fibroblast activation protein. J Nucl Med 2018;59(9):1415–22.

22. Loktev A, Lindner T, Burger EM, et al. Development of fibroblast activation protein-targeted radiotracers with improved tumor retention. J Nucl Med 2019; 60(10):1421–9.

23. Zhang H, An J, Wu P, et al. The application of [(68) Ga]-labeled FAPI-04 PET/CT for targeting and early detection of pancreatic carcinoma in patient-derived orthotopic xenograft models. Contrast Media Mol Imaging 2022;2022:6596702.

24. Kratochwil C, Flechsig P, Lindner T, et al. 68)Ga-FAPI PET/CT: tracer uptake in 28 different kinds of cancer. J Nucl Med 2019;60(6):801–5.

25. Rohrich M, Naumann P, Giesel FL, et al. Impact of (68)Ga-FAPI PET/CT imaging on the therapeutic management of primary and recurrent pancreatic ductal adenocarcinomas. J Nucl Med 2021;62(6): 779–86.

26. Pang Y, Zhao L, Shang Q, et al. Positron emission tomography and computed tomography with [(68)Ga] Ga-fibroblast activation protein inhibitors improves tumor detection and staging in patients with pancreatic cancer. Eur J Nucl Med Mol Imaging 2022;49(4): 1322–37.

27. Chen H, Pang Y, Wu J, et al. Comparison of [(68)Ga] Ga-DOTA-FAPI-04 and [(18)F] FDG PET/CT for the diagnosis of primary and metastatic lesions in patients with various types of cancer. Eur J Nucl Med Mol Imaging 2020;47(8):1820–32.

28. Deng M, Chen Y, Cai L. Comparison of 68Ga-FAPI and 18F-FDG PET/CT in the imaging of pancreatic cancer with liver metastases. Clin Nucl Med 2021; 46(7):589–91.

29. Kaghazchi F, Divband G, Amini H, et al. 68 Ga-FAPI-46 and 18 F-FDG in advanced metastatic pancreatic cancer. Clin Nucl Med 2022;47(10):e666–9.

30. Chen H, Zhao L, Ruan D, et al. Usefulness of [(68) Ga]Ga-DOTA-FAPI-04 PET/CT in patients presenting with inconclusive [(18)F]FDG PET/CT findings. Eur J Nucl Med Mol Imaging 2021;48(1):73–86.

31. Zhao L, Pang Y, Wei J, et al. Use of 68Ga-FAPI PET/ CT for evaluation of peritoneal carcinomatosis before and after cytoreductive surgery. Clin Nucl Med 2021;46(6):491–3.

32. Sagiyama K, Watanabe Y, Kamei R, et al. Multiparametric voxel-based analyses of standardized uptake values and apparent diffusion coefficients of soft-tissue tumours with a positron emission tomography/magnetic resonance system: preliminary results. Eur Radiol 2017;27(12):5024–33.

33. Yeh R, Dercle L, Garg I, et al. The role of 18F-FDG PET/CT and PET/MRI in pancreatic ductal adeno-carcinoma. Abdom Radiol (NY) 2018;43(2): 415–34.

34. Zhang Z, Jia G, Pan G, et al. Comparison of the diagnostic efficacy of (68) Ga-FAPI-04 PET/MR and (18)F-FDG PET/CT in patients with pancreatic cancer. Eur J Nucl Med Mol Imaging 2022;49(8):2877–88.

35. von Ahrens D, Bhagat TD, Nagrath D, et al. The role of stromal cancer-associated fibroblasts in pancreatic cancer. J Hematol Oncol 2017;10(1):76.

36. Goldstein D, El-Maraghi RH, Hammel P, et al. nab-Paclitaxel plus gemcitabine for metastatic pancreatic cancer: long-term survival from a phase III trial, J Natl Cancer. Inst 2015;107(2).

37. Lang M., Spektor A.M., Hielscher T., et al., Static and dynamic (68)Ga-FAPI PET/CT for the detection of malignant transformation of intraductal papillary mucinous neoplasia of the pancreas, J Nucl Med, 64(2), 2022, 244–251.

38. Lindner T, Altmann A, Kramer S, et al. Design and development of (99m)Tc-labeled FAPI tracers for SPECT imaging and (188)Re therapy. J Nucl Med 2020;61(10):1507–13.

39. Ferlay J, Partensky C, Bray F. More deaths from pancreatic cancer than breast cancer in the EU by 2017. Acta Oncol 2016;55(9–10):1158–60.

40. Wang L, Dong P, Shen G, et al. 18F-Fluorodeoxyglu-cose positron emission tomography predicts treatment efficacy and clinical outcome for patients with pancreatic carcinoma: a meta-analysis. Pancreas 2019;48(8):996–1002.

41. Lee JW, Kang CM, Choi HJ, et al. Prognostic value of metabolic tumor volume and total lesion glycolysis on preoperative (1)(8)F-FDG PET/CT in patients with pancreatic cancer. J Nucl Med 2014;55(6):898–904.

42. Hosein AN, Brekken RA, Maitra A. Pancreatic cancer stroma: an update on therapeutic targeting strategies. Nat Rev Gastroenterol Hepatol 2020;17(8): 487–505.

43. Ogawa Y, Masugi Y, Abe T, et al. Three distinct stroma types in human pancreatic cancer identified by image analysis of fibroblast subpopulations and collagen. Clin Cancer Res 2021;27(1):107–19.

44. Shi M, Yu DH, Chen Y, et al. Expression of fibroblast activation protein in human pancreatic adenocarcinoma and its clinicopathological significance. World J Gastroenterol 2012;18(8):840–6.

45. Koong AC, Christofferson E, Le QT, et al. Phase II study to assess the efficacy of conventionally fractionated radiotherapy followed by a stereotactic radiosurgery boost in patients with locally advanced pancreatic cancer. Int J Radiat Oncol Biol Phys 2005;63(2):320–3.

46. Balaj C, Ayav A, Oliver A, et al. CT imaging of early local recurrence of pancreatic adenocarcinoma following pancreaticoduodenectomy. Abdom Radiol (NY) 2016;41(2):273–82.

47. Daamen LA, Groot VP, Goense L, et al. The diagnostic performance of CT versus FDG PET-CT for the detection of recurrent pancreatic cancer: a systematic review and meta-analysis. Eur J Radiol 2018;106:128–36.

48. Liermann J, Syed M, Ben-Josef E, et al. Impact of FAPI-PET/CT on target volume definition in radiation

therapy of locally recurrent pancreatic cancer. Cancers 2021;13(4):796.

49. Zhao L, Chen S, Chen S, et al. 68)Ga-fibroblast activation protein inhibitor PET/CT on gross tumour volume delineation for radiotherapy planning of oesophageal cancer. Radiother Oncol 2021;158: 55–61.

50. Koerber SA, Staudinger F, Kratochwil C, et al. The role of (68)Ga-FAPI PET/CT for patients with malignancies of the lower gastrointestinal tract: first clinical experience. J Nucl Med 2020;61(9):1331–6.

51. Ristau J, Giesel FL, Haefner MF, et al. Impact of primary staging with fibroblast activation protein specific enzyme inhibitor (FAPI)-PET/CT on radio-oncologic treatment planning of patients with esophageal cancer. Mol Imaging Biol 2020;22(6): 1495–500.

52. Zhang X, Song W, Qin C, et al. Non-malignant findings of focal (68)Ga-FAPI-04 uptake in pancreas. Eur J Nucl Med Mol Imaging 2021;48(8):2635–41.

53. Gong W, Yang X, Wu J, et al. 68Ga-FAPI PET/CT imaging of multiple muscle metastases of pancreatic cancer. Clin Nucl Med 2022;47(1):73–5.

54. Wada R, Kamiya T, Fujino K, et al. [Creation and evaluation of educational programs for additional delayed scan of FDG-PET/CT]. Nihon Hoshasen Gijutsu Gakkai Zasshi 2017;73(11):1119–24.

55. Sun R, Huang Z, Wei J, et al. 68Ga-FAPI and 18F-FDG PET/CT findings in a patient with pancreatic tuberculosis mimicking malignant tumor. Clin Nucl Med 2022;47(7):653–4.

56. Xu W., Zhao L., Meng T., et al., Serous cystadenoma of the pancreas showing increased uptake on 68Ga-FAPI PET/CT, Clin Nucl Med, 47(12), 2022, 1095-1098.

57. Luo Y, Pan Q, Zhang W. IgG4-related disease revealed by (68)Ga-FAPI and (18)F-FDG PET/CT. Eur J Nucl Med Mol Imaging 2019;46(12):2625–6.

The Diagnostic Value of Fibroblast Activation Protein Imaging in Hepatocellular Carcinoma and Cholangiocellular Carcinoma

Emil Novruzov, MD[a],*, Yuriko Mori, MD[a], Fuad Novruzov, MD[b]

KEYWORDS

- Hepatocellular carcinoma • Cholangiocellular carcinoma • FAPI PET • FAP imaging
- Fibroblast activation protein

KEY POINTS

- Fibroblast activation protein (FAP) imaging seems to be a very promising molecular imaging agent for diagnostic workup of primary liver malignancies.
- Current studies indicate the added diagnostic value of FAP inhibitor (FAPI) tracer in the detection of both intrahepatic and extrahepatic lesions of primary liver malignancies compared with conventional radiologic imaging modalities as well as the current state-of-the-art pan-cancer agent [18F] FDG.
- The early clinical studies report the potential of discrimination of primary and secondary liver malignancies with respect to dynamic FAPI uptake pattern of lesions.

BACKGROUND

Hepatocellular carcinoma (HCC) is the most common primary liver malignancy with worldwide high incidence and mortality. In more than 90% of cases, HCC arise from a cirrhotic liver that is mostly induced by viral diseases (HBV, HCV) and especially in developed countries alcoholic steatohepatitis (ASH) and non-alcoholic steatohepatitis (NASH) and to a lesser extent, inherited metabolic disorders such as hemochromatosis, porphyria, and type-1 glycogen storage diseases. The surgical resection of local disease by partial hepatectomy or orthotopic liver transplantation (OLT) is the only curative options. The pretransplant radiological criteria, known as Milan criteria, indicate an OLT in HCC patients with a single tumor up to 5 cm in diameter or two to three tumors 3 cm in diameter and no evidence of macroscopic vascular invasion, as such cases demonstrated benefit with 5-year and recurrence-free survival rates after OLT of 75% and 83%, respectively.[1,2]

In contrast, cholangiocellular carcinoma (CCC) is a very rare cancer entity with a high mortality due to insidious onset. The only curative option is a surgical resection in early-stage diagnosis which accounts only for 20% of patients.[3,4]

In addition, the liver is the first target organ for metastases (secondary liver malignancy) of colorectal cancer and several other malignancies, which is, however, beyond the scope of this review.

THE DIAGNOSTIC VALUE AND LIMITATIONS OF THE STANDARD-OF-CARE IMAGING WITH [18F]FDG PET/CT SCAN

In patients with HCC, [18F]FDG PET/CT scan shows no better diagnostic accuracy than conventional

a Department of Nuclear Medicine, Medical Faculty, Heinrich-Heine-University, University Hospital Dusseldorf, Moorenstrasse 5, Dusseldorf 40225, Germany; b Department of Nuclear Medicine, Azerbaijan National Centre of Oncology, M. Xiyabani Street No. 137, Baku, Azerbaijan
* Corresponding author.
E-mail address: Emil.novruzov@med.uni-duesseldorf.de

PET Clin 18 (2023) 309–314
https://doi.org/10.1016/j.cpet.2023.02.011
1556-8598/23/© 2023 Elsevier Inc. All rights reserved.

imaging modalities in primary staging and seems to be particularly limited in the case of well-differentiated tumors. [18F]FDG PET/CT scan shows only a slightly better diagnostic performance in restaging regarding local relapse (pooled sensitivity and specificity of 65% and 95%, respectively) and a similar diagnostic accuracy in detecting extrahepatic lesions (pooled sensitivity and specificity of 46% and 95%, respectively) in comparison with conventional imaging modalities. [18F]FDG diagnostic is generally hampered by well-known limitations such as relatively high false-negative rate due to high physiological uptake in liver tissue, lack of specificity, that is, cirrhotic liver and lower Warburg effect of HCC lesions than other tumors. Nonetheless, [18F]FDG imaging allows a reliable outcome prediction with respect to local ablative therapies and OLT, as well-differentiated tumors, as aforementioned, with relatively lower [18F]FDG uptake have better prognosis.[1-4]

Especially in detecting extrahepatic lesions of CCC such as regional nodal and distant metastases, [18F]FDG PET/CT scan has been proven to be superior to conventional imaging modalities in restaging with a sensitivity and specificity of 90.1% and 83.5%, respectively, whereas the diagnostic accuracy in detecting primary lesions in the initial workup is not convincing with a sensitivity and specificity of 91.7% and 51.3%, respectively.[5] The studies indicate a sensitivity and specificity rate of 88.4% and 69.1%, respectively, for diagnostic workup of nodal staging. One of the potential limitations of the use of [18F]FDG imaging in patients with CCC may be the false-positive results related to biliary stenting, biliary sepsis and local infection, and also small local infiltrative pattern, making the interpretation of [18F]FDG PET/CT results challenging. An accurate diagnostic tool would spare patients from unnecessary surgical operations and guide the correct treatment choice (surgery vs chemotherapy).[4]

CANCER-ASSOCIATED FIBROBLAST AND ITS ROLE IN CARCINOGENESIS OF HEPATOCELLULAR CARCINOMA AND CHOLANGIOCELLULAR CARCINOMA

The liver carcinogenesis has been proved to be promoted by the so-called desmoplastic response which involves abnormal activity of an epithelial neoplasia to modulate the tumor stroma via over-stimulation and overproduction of stromal fibroblasts. The cancer-associated fibroblasts (CAFs) of liver originate from quiescent hepatic stellate cells because of a sustained wound-healing response to chronic liver injury. CAFs have been demonstrated to play a pivotal role in the tumorigenesis of hepatic cells by mediating cross-talk between tumor cells and tumor stroma as has been shown with other epithelial malignancies.[1,6]

CCC is also characterized by a rich desmoplastic tumor stroma with abundant number of CAFs, which leads to aggressive tumor behavior by modulating tumor growth, progression, and therapy resistance through interactive autocrine and paracrine signaling pathways.[7]

FIBROBLAST ACTIVATION PROTEIN OVEREXPRESSION AND FIBROBLAST ACTIVATION PROTEIN LIGANDS IN PET IMAGING

Fibroblast activation protein (FAP), a member of dipeptidyl peptidase-family, is a type II transmembrane serine protease with collagenase activity on cell membranes of CAFs, which regulates extracellular matrix hemostasis. This has been shown to be overexpressed in the stroma of more than 90% of epithelial-derived tumors and their metastases as well as in fetal mesenchymal tissues, healing wounds after endometrial detachment in adults, chronic inflammatory or fibrosing processes, and organ reconstruction sites. FAP overexpression correlates directly with rapid progression and metastasis and poor prognosis, which makes it a promising target for both diagnostic and therapeutic purposes.[8,9]

FAP PET imaging has been performed by quinoline-based small-molecule FAP inhibitors (FAPIs), which show high affinity for FAP with favorable pharmacokinetics and labeled by ^{68}Ga or ^{18}F. To date, several derivatives, such as FAPI-04, FAPI-46, and FAPI-74, have been developed and tested successfully with very promising results especially for tumor entities with lower diagnostic accuracy on [18F]FDG imaging, for example, HCC and especially in local staging of CCC, which makes FAPI imaging to a valid alternative to the current pan-cancer tracer [18F]FDG. Moreover, FAPI imaging offers new avenues due to high diagnostic potential in the assessment of chronic inflammatory and fibrotic processes.[9] For instance, in HCC, the prolonged CAF activation caused by chronic inflammatory changes in liver tissue, usually due to concurrent viral infection such as hepatitis B or C, even in cases with sustained viral response, highlights the potential role of FAP imaging for the evaluation of liver fibrosis or even for screening hepatic carcinogenesis in addition to diagnostic workup regarding tumor management.[1,6]

CURRENT STATE OF THE RESEARCH IN FIBROBLAST ACTIVATION PROTEIN IMAGING

Kratochwil and colleagues[10] reported initially a moderate to high [^{68}Ga]Ga-FAPI uptake in HCC and CCC lesions coupled with negligible background uptake in normal tissue with a subsequent sharp imaging contrast (**Fig. 1**). Subsequently, a series of studies with small cohorts were conducted mostly on basis of an intraindividual comparison with [^{18}F]FDG PET imaging with very promising results regarding both intrahepatic and extrahepatic lesions (**Table 1**).

In a retrospective, monocentric study, Wang and colleagues[11] reported a better sensitivity rate in detection of primary liver malignancy compared with [^{18}F]FDG imaging (96% vs 65%) (**Fig. 2**). The prospective monocentric study with 20 patients by Shi and colleagues[12] demonstrated similar results in favor of [^{68}Ga]Ga-FAPI imaging (100% vs 58.8%). The results of Siripongsatian and colleagues presented a similar picture with an excellent accuracy of [^{68}Ga]Ga-FAPI imaging regarding the detection of primary and regional lymph node metastases in comparison to [^{18}F]FDG imaging both in HCC and CCC (sensitivity 100% vs 58%), whereas [^{68}Ga]Ga-FAPI imaging detected more distant metastatic lesions than [^{18}F]FDG imaging. In addition, [^{68}Ga]Ga-FAPI uptake in CCC seemed to be higher than in HCC in terms of SUV$_{max}$ and TBR, quite consistent with the results of

Kratochwil and colleagues[3,10] (**Fig. 3**). Guo and colleagues[13] investigated 32 patients with primary liver malignancies (20 HCC and 12 CCC) as part of a single-center post hoc retrospective analysis of data obtained from a prospective parent study, which demonstrated [^{68}Ga]Ga-FAPI imaging outperforming [^{18}F]FDG imaging both in detecting intrahepatic lesions (96% vs 65%) and overall malignant lesions including extrahepatic lesions (87.4% vs. 65.0%). Zhang and colleagues conducted an interesting prospective study that included only patients with [^{18}F]FDG negative (non-avid) primary liver malignancies (20 HCC and 5 CCC), excluding patients with inflammatory hepatic lesions. They reported a sensitivity and an overall diagnostic accuracy of 96.0% and 83.8%, respectively. Although the study by Kosmala and colleagues[14,15] demonstrated upstaging in 66.7% and treatment changes in 50.0% in patients with HCC compared with conventional imaging modalities in a small patient cohort.

Of note, the intensity of tracer uptake between primary and secondary liver malignancies does not seem to differ substantially, which might be overcome by using dynamic [^{68}Ga]Ga-FAPI PET combined with kinetic modeling exploiting the

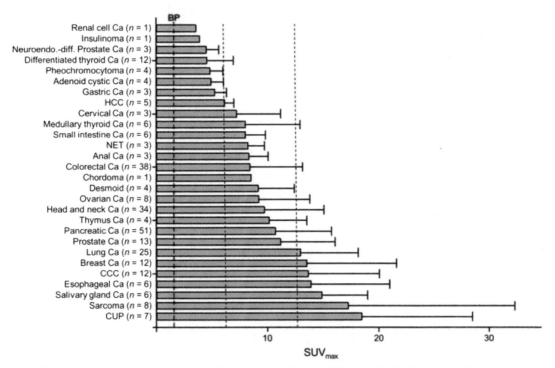

Fig. 1. Illustration of FAPI uptake among various tumor entities emphasizing the high tumor-to-background ratio in terms of blood pool (BP). Ca, cancer; CCC, cholangiocellular carcinoma; CUP, carcinoma of unknown primary; HCC, hepatocellular carcinoma; NET, neuroendocrine tumor. This research was originally published in JNM. Kratochwil C et al., 68Ga-FAPI PET/CT: Tracer Uptake in 28 Different Kinds of Cancer. J Nucl Med. 2019 Jun;60(6):801-805. © SNMMI.

Table 1
An overview of the included studies about the diagnostic performance of fibroblast activation protein inhibitor in patients with hepatocellular carcinoma and cholangiocellular carcinoma

Authors, Year	Country	Type of Study	Radiopharmaceuticals	Number of Included Cases	Comparison of Diagnostic Accuracy
Siripongsatian et al,[3] 2022	Thailand	Retrospective monocentric	[18F]F-FDG vs [68Ga]Ga-FAPI-46	27 (13 HCC and 14 CCC)	FAPI > FDG
Wang et al,[8] 2021	China	Retrospective monocentric	[18F]F-FDG vs [68Ga]Ga-FAPI-04	25	FAPI > FDG
Shi et al,[9] 2021	China	Prospective monocentric	[18F]F-FDG vs [68Ga]Ga-FAPI-04	20	FAPI > FDG
Guo et al,[10] 2021	China	Retrospective monocentric	[18F]F-FDG vs [68Ga]Ga-FAPI-04	32 (20 HCC and 12 CCC)	FAPI > FDG
Zhang et al,[11] 2022	China	Prospective monocentric	[18F]F-FDG vs [68Ga]Ga-FAPI	25 (20 HCC and 5 CCC)	FAPI > FDG
Kosmala et al,[12] 2022	Germany	Retrospective monocentric	CT or MR imaging vs [68Ga]Ga-FAPI-04	6	FAPI > CT/MR imaging

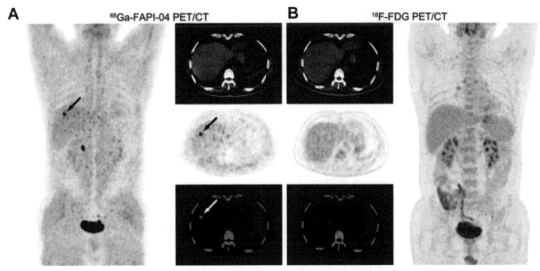

Fig. 2. Intraindividual comparison of [^{68}Ga]Ga-FAPI-04 and [^{18}F]F-FDG PET/CT scan in a 53-year-old male patient with moderately differentiated HCC. (*A*) A small tumor lesion with strong FAPI uptake in the right lobe of the liver (*black* and *white arrows*, SUV$_{max}$: 7.36, TBR: 6.03). (*B*) The tumor lesion with a slight [^{18}F]FDG uptake cannot be detected due to poor TBR (SUV$_{max}$: 2.36, TBR: 1.31). *From* Wang H, Zhu W, Ren S, Kong Y, Huang Q, Zhao J, Guan Y, Jia H, Chen J, Lu L, Xie F, Qin L. 68Ga-FAPI-04 Versus 18F-FDG PET/CT in the Detection of Hepatocellular Carcinoma. Front Oncol. 2021 Jun 25;11:693640.

distinct blood supply of HCC (predominantly over hepatic artery rather than portal vein) from other secondary hepatic lesions, suggesting that dynamic [^{68}Ga]Ga-FAPI PET imaging had potential for the accurate noninvasive diagnosis of liver malignancies.[16,17] Furthermore, this acquisition strategy might theoretically be applied to small suspected tumor lesions in liver tissue to distinguish them from fibrotic nodules in patients with advanced stage cirrhotic liver tissue, where a lower TBR than usual is expected. The potential added diagnostic value of dynamic tracer uptake pattern would be therefore mainly expected in developed countries, where HCC incidence is predominantly associated with cirrhotic livers. In developing countries, particularly in Asia, HCC

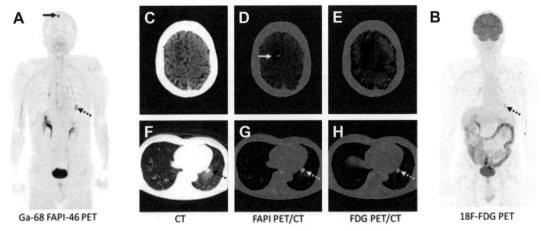

Fig. 3. Metachronous brain and lung metastases after right hepatectomy and adjuvant chemotherapy in a 67-year-old man with CCC at follow-up 6 months after completion of therapy (*A, C, D*). [^{68}Ga]Ga-FAPI-46 PET/CT scan reveals a brain metastasis (*arrow*) in the right high parasagittal frontal area with perilesional brain edema (*B, E*). [^{18}F]F-FDG PET/CT scan shows no detection of brain metastasis. The pulmonal metastasis seems to be both [^{68}Ga]Ga-FAPI-46 and [^{18}F]FDG avid (*arrow dot*) (*A, B, F–H*). *From* Siripongsatian D, Promteangtrong C, Kunawudhi A, Kiatkittikul P, Boonkawin N, Chinnanthachai C, Jantarato A, Chotipanich C. Comparisons of Quantitative Parameters of Ga-68-Labelled Fibroblast Activating Protein Inhibitor (FAPI) PET/CT and [18F]F-FDG PET/CT in Patients with Liver Malignancies. Mol Imaging Biol. 2022 Oct;24(5):818-829.

incidence is relatively high in non-cirrhotic livers due to the higher prevalence of viral disease.

OUTLOOK

In conclusion, due to the clinical and methodological heterogeneity of the included studies, the current state of research does not allow definitive conclusions about the use of [68Ga]Ga-FAPI imaging in primary liver malignancies.[18] Yet, the first clinical studies indicate a substantial added value of [68Ga]Ga-FAPI imaging both for detection of intrahepatic and extrahepatic lesions, making it a very strong candidate as the future modality of choice in tumor staging, image-guided radiotherapy, and perhaps even in molecular imaging-guided distinguishing between various liver tumors by evaluation of tracer uptake pattern. However, large-scale, prospective studies with histological validation are warranted for this purpose.

CLINICS CARE POINTS

- FAPI PET/CT has already been recognized as an alternative pan-cancer imaging probe with theranostic potential.
- Among other epithelial malignancies, also for HCC & CCC, there is growing evidence for the utility of FAPI imaging.

CONFLICT OF INTEREST

The authors declare no conflict of interest.

REFERENCES

1. Kubo N, Araki K, Kuwano H, et al. Cancer-associated fibroblasts in hepatocellular carcinoma. World J Gastroenterol 2016;22(30):6841–50.
2. Asman Y, Evenson AR, Even-Sapir E, et al. [18F]fludeoxyglucose positron emission tomography and computed tomography as a prognostic tool before liver transplantation, resection, and loco-ablative therapies for hepatocellular carcinoma. Liver Transplant 2015;21(5):572–80.
3. Siripongsatian D, Promteangtrong C, Kunawudhi A, et al. Comparisons of quantitative parameters of Ga-68-labelled fibroblast activating protein inhibitor (FAPI) PET/CT and [18F]F-FDG PET/CT in patients with liver malignancies. Mol Imaging Biol 2022;24(5):818–29.
4. Liao X, Wei J, Li Y, et al. 18F-FDG PET with or without CT in the diagnosis of extrahepatic metastases or local residual/recurrent hepatocellular carcinoma. Medicine (Baltim) 2018;97(34):e11970.
5. Lamarca A, Barriuso J, Chander A, et al. 18F-fluorodeoxyglucose positron emission tomography (18FDG-PET) for patients with biliary tract cancer: systematic review and meta-analysis. J Hepatol 2019;71(1):115–29.
6. Dhar D, Baglieri J, Kisseleva T, et al. Mechanisms of liver fibrosis and its role in liver cancer. Exp Biol Med (Maywood) 2020;245(2):96–108.
7. Sirica AE, Gores GJ. Desmoplastic stroma and cholangiocarcinoma: clinical implications and therapeutic targeting. Hepatology 2014;59(6):2397–402.
8. Huang R, Pu Y, Huang S, et al. FAPI-PET/CT in cancer imaging: a potential novel molecule of the century. Front Oncol 2022;12:854658.
9. Dendl K, Schlittenhardt J, Staudinger F, et al. The role of fibroblast activation protein ligands in oncologic PET IMAGING. Pet Clin 2021;16(3):341–51.
10. Kratochwil C, Flechsig P, Lindner T, et al. 68Ga-FAPI PET/CT: tracer uptake in 28 different kinds of cancer. J Nucl Med 2019;60(6):801–5.
11. Wang H, Zhu W, Ren S, et al. 68Ga-FAPI-04 versus 18F-FDG PET/CT in the detection of hepatocellular carcinoma. Front Oncol 2021;11:693640.
12. Shi X, Xing H, Yang X, et al. Comparison of PET imaging of activated fibroblasts and 18F-FDG for diagnosis of primary hepatic tumours: a prospective pilot study. Eur J Nucl Med Mol Imaging 2021;48(5):1593–603.
13. Guo W, Pang Y, Yao L, et al. Imaging fibroblast activation protein in liver cancer: a single-center post hoc retrospective analysis to compare [68Ga]Ga-FAPI-04 PET/CT versus MRI and [18F]-FDG PET/CT. Eur J Nucl Med Mol Imaging 2021;48(5):1604–17.
14. Zhang J, He Q, Jiang S, et al. [18F]FAPI PET/CT in the evaluation of focal liver lesions with [18F]FDG non-avidity. Eur J Nucl Med Mol Imaging 2022. https://doi.org/10.1007/s00259-022-06022-1. Epub ahead of print. PMID: 36346437.
15. Kosmala A, Serfling SE, Schlötelburg W, et al. Impact of 68 Ga-FAPI-04 PET/CT on staging and therapeutic management in patients with digestive system tumors. Clin Nucl Med 2023;48(1):35–42.
16. Koerber SA, Staudinger F, Kratochwil C, et al. The role of 68Ga-FAPI PET/CT for patients with malignancies of the lower gastrointestinal tract: first clinical experience. J Nucl Med 2020;61(9):1331–6.
17. Geist BK, Xing H, Wang J, et al. A methodological investigation of healthy tissue, hepatocellular carcinoma, and other lesions with dynamic 68Ga-FAPI-04 PET/CT imaging. EJNMMI Phys 2021;8(1):8.
18. Treglia G, Muoio B, Roustaei H, et al. Head-to-head comparison of fibroblast activation protein inhibitors (FAPI) radiotracers versus [18F]F-FDG in oncology: a systematic review. Int J Mol Sci 2021;22(20):11192.

Fibroblast Activation Protein Inhibitor PET Imaging in Head and Neck Cancer

Manuel Röhrich, PhD, MD (German PD)

KEYWORDS

- FAPI-PET • Head and neck cancer • Oral squamous cell carcinomas • Hypopharynx carcinomas
- PET • Adenoid cystic carcinoma • ACC • Thyroid cancer

KEY POINTS

- ^{68}Ga-fibroblast activation protein inhibitor (FAPI)-PET is a promising new imaging method for head and neck cancers including oral squamous cell carcinomas, hypopharynx carcinomas, adenoid cystic carcinomas, thyroid cancer, and cervical cancer of unknown primary.
- For oral squamous cell carcinomas, hypopharynx carcinomas, and adenoid cystic carcinomas, ^{68}Ga-FAPI-PET adds substantial diagnostic information to established imaging modalities such as ultrasound, computed tomography, MR imaging, and [18]fluoro-deoxyglucose (^{18}F-FDG)-PET regarding primary tumors, which impact radiotherapy planning. The incremental value of ^{68}Ga-FAPI-PET for N and M staging of these tumors is not well characterized yet.
- ^{68}Ga-FAPI-PET can be applied for staging of metastasized thyroid carcinomas. Further research is needed to further characterize the diagnostic value of ^{68}Ga-FAPI-PET for this entity.
- To date, the data on cervical cancer of unknown primary are sparse but highly interesting because ^{68}Ga-FAPI-PET may detect a significant portion of primary tumors, which are ^{18}F-FDG-PET-negative or obscured by uptake in lymphoid aggregates.

INTRODUCTION: OVERVIEW OF HEAD AND NECK CANCERS

The term "head and neck cancers" summarizes malignancies of the oral cavity (including lip, tongue, buccal cavity, palate, and salivary glands), of the nasopharynx, of the oropharynx, of the hypopharynx, the larynx and of the outer neck, especially thyroid cancer, and cancer of unknown primary that manifests as cervical lymph node metastasis. Histologically, most head and neck cancers are squamous cell carcinomas (SCCs) originating from the mucosal surface of the oral cavity or the pharynx. Adenocarcinomas and sarcomas occur less frequently.[1] Adenoid cystic carcinomas (ACCs) are a rare subclass of epithelial head and neck tumors with a mixed adenoid and cystic histologic appearance and perineural growth pattern.[2] Head and neck cancers typically occur in elderly patients and account for approximately 3% of all cancers and 1.5% of all cancer deaths. Main risk factors for the development of head and neck cancers are long-time use of tobacco and alcohol and infections with human papilloma virus (HPV) type 16, especially for oropharyngeal cancers in younger patients. After history and physical examination and radiological cross-sectional imaging, diagnosis is confirmed by biopsy of primary tumors or cervical lymph node metastases. Staging of head and neck cancers is performed according to the American Joint Committee of Cancer and the Union for International Cancer Control staging systems using the TNM (tumor, node, metastasis) system depending

Department of Nuclear Medicine, University Hospital Heidelberg, INF 400, 69120, Heidelberg, Germany
E-mail address: manuel.roehrich@med.uni-heidelberg.de

PET Clin 18 (2023) 315–323
https://doi.org/10.1016/j.cpet.2023.02.002

on the anatomic site of tumors.[3] For oropharyngeal cancer, assessment of the HPV-16 status is necessary due to improved prognosis for HPV-positive oropharyngeal cancers. Treatment of head and neck cancers comprises surgery, radiotherapy, and systemic oncological treatments and depends on TNM staging, anatomic site, and surgical accessibility of the tumors.

NORMAL ANATOMY AND IMAGING TECHNIQUE
Anatomic Considerations

In general, the assessment of head and neck tumors is challenging because the anatomic regions, in which these tumors occur (skull base, oral cavity, pharyngeal spaces, larynx and outer neck) contain numerous delicate anatomic structures, which are located close to each other. The skull base with its numerous foramina and corresponding cranial nerves is frequently hard to assess in clinical routine because differences in density, MR imaging appearance and contrast enhancement of healthy tissues and invaded structures are frequently relatively subtle. This is relevant especially for adenoid cystic carcinomas, which grow slowly but are characterized by the invasion of surrounding structures and perineural spread. With respect to oral cavity and pharyngeal spaces and larynx, it must be considered that as well physiologic contrast enhancement as physiologic glucose metabolism of lymphoid tissue in the nasopharynx, tonsils, and sublingual and retrolingual locations may hamper the diagnosis of tumors due to reduced contrast. Cervical lymph nodes of all regions represent another daily challenge for diagnostic radiologists and nuclear physicians because they frequently seem enlarged in computed tomography (CT)/MR imaging morphology or [18]fluoro-deoxyglucose (^{18}F-FDG)-avid due to local inflammatory changes, especially in the jugulodigastric node. The significance of these findings—in particular the question of suspected malignancy—must be evaluated for each individual patient under consideration of all available imaging data and clinical information. The assessment of the thyroid gland with respect to thyroid cancer, especially the assessment of thyroid nodules, is a classic field of discussion in diagnostic nuclear medicine and neuroendocrine medicine because a wide spectrum of the differential diagnoses (among them adenomas, inflammation, degenerative changes) must be considered and cannot always be clearly differentiated by the clinically established imaging techniques (ultrasound [US], scintigraphies, CT, and MR imaging).

Imaging Technique

Established imaging modalities for the staging of head and neck cancers comprise CT, MR imaging, US, and ^{18}F-FDG-PET.[4] CT is the first-line modality for imaging of neck masses due to its ability to asses all types of tissues, its widespread availability and its low cost. US is the favorable modality for imaging of thyroid gland nodules and superficial cervical lymph nodes due to its high resolution but is not suitable for imaging of deeper layers of the neck. MR imaging is particularly preferable for imaging of intracranial and intraspinal pathologic conditions because it allows good tissue characterization and definition of tumor margins due to high contrasts, especially in soft tissues. ^{18}F-FDG-PET has shown high sensitivity and specificity for the detection of occult, recurrent, and metastatic head and neck cancers in primary and recurrent settings but lacks detailed anatomic information and thus requires synopsis with high-resolution CT or MR imaging. Other PET tracers than ^{18}F-FDG that visualize hypoxia (eg, ^{18}F-fluoromisonidazole) and proliferation (^{18}F-FLT) have been applied to head and neck tumors in specialized centers but have not become part of the clinical routine.[5]

Since the development of [68]Gallium (^{68}Ga) and [18]Fluorine (^{18}F)-labeled PET-tracers based on fibroblast activation protein inhibitors (FAPIs), these tracers have mainly been applied as tumor-imaging agents in a large variety of cancers—among them different types of head and neck cancers—that show FAP expression. The intense expression of FAP in various head and neck cancers particularly oropharyngeal cancers and adenoid cystic carcinomas has been validated by immunohistochemical studies[6,7] (**Fig. 1**). To date, several studies have focused on ^{68}Ga-FAPI-PET in different head and neck cancers, and here, we summarize their results on the most frequently addressed entities of these studies: oral SCCs, nasopharynx carcinomas, adenoid cystic carcinomas, thyroid cancers, and cancer of unknown primary presenting as lymph node metastasis. We will describe imaging properties, the potential impact of FAPI-PET on staging and radiotherapy planning, and—if available—first results of comparisons with other imaging modalities, particularly ^{18}F-FDG.

PROTOCOLS

With respect to ^{68}Ga-FAPI-PET in general, a definite consensus regarding the optimal injected activity, acquisition time, and FAPI-tracer variant has not been achieved yet. It has been shown

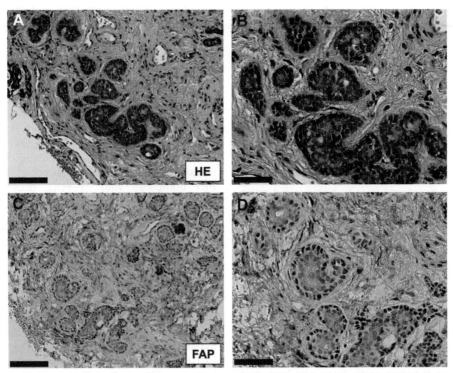

Fig. 1. Target validation in ACC: (*A, B*) Hematoxylin and eosin (HE) staining and (*C, D*) FAP-immunohistochemistry of an ACC. FAP is strongly expressed in the stromal compound and negative in the neoplastic cell clusters. Scale bars: 100 μm for *A*, and *C* and 50 μm for *B*, and *D*. (*From* Rohrich M, Syed M, Liew DP, et al. (68)Ga-FAPI-PET/CT improves diagnostic staging and radiotherapy planning of adenoid cystic carcinomas-Imaging analysis and histologic validation. Radiother Oncol. Jul 2021;160:192-201.)

that the injection of 200 megabecquerel (MBq) FAPI-2 or FAPI-4 lead to equivalent doses of approximately 3 to 4 mSv, which are comparable with examination with widely used PET tracers such as ^{18}F-FDG, ^{68}Ga-DOTATATE, and ^{68}Ga-PSMA-11.[8] In all the studies summarized in this article, PET images were acquired 1 hour after injection but earlier acquisition times seem feasible.[9,10] In most studies investigating head and neck cancers that have been reported thus far, ^{68}Ga-FAPI-04 has been used, However, Röhrich and colleagues demonstrated in their analysis of ACC that other FAPI-variants (FAPI-2, FAPI-46, and FAPI-74) also led to high tumor uptake and low background activity.

IMAGING FINDINGS/PATHOLOGY
Oral Squamous Cell Cancers

In an initial analysis of 14 head and neck cancers (without information on specific tumor sites), of which 12 had histologically confirmed SCC, Syed and colleagues demonstrated that the low signal of ^{68}Ga-FAPI-PET in healthy tissues and the high ^{68}Ga-FAPI-avidity of head and neck tumors lead to high-contrast images of both the primary tumors and lymph node metastases in the head and neck region, as well as of distant metastatic lesions. In another study specifically focusing on oral SCC, Linz and colleagues analyzed ^{18}F-FDG-PET, MR imaging, and ^{68}Ga-FAPI-PET performed in 10 patients with newly diagnosed oral SCC. In this study, high tumor uptake within oral SCC was reported but background tissues were not analyzed.[11] Chen and colleagues analyzed preoperative staging with ^{18}F-FDG and ^{68}Ga-FAPI-PET and included 36 treatment-naïve patients with oral SCC in their analysis. They also found high tumor-to-background ratios for oral SCC lesions on ^{68}Ga-FAPI-PET.[12]

Nasopharyngeal Carcinomas

Zhao and colleagues compared tracer uptake and staging results ^{68}Ga-FAPI-PET and ^{18}F-FDG in 45 patients with nasopharyngeal carcinomas (39 primary, 6 recurrent). They found higher ^{68}Ga-FAPI than ^{18}F-FDG uptake in primary tumors, lymph node metastases, and distant metastases.[13]

Quin and colleagues performed a prospective head-to-head comparison of ^{68}Ga-FAPI-PET/MR imaging and ^{18}F-FDG/MR imaging in 15 patients with nasopharyngeal carcinoma. In contrast to the results of Zhao and colleagues, they found lower ^{68}Ga-FAPI-PET uptake than ^{18}F-FDG uptake in primary tumors but the difference was not statistically significant. Lymph nodes showed significantly lower ^{68}Ga-FAPI-PET uptake than ^{18}F-FDG uptake.[14]

Adenoid Cystic Carcinomas

Röhrich, Syed and colleagues performed a retrospective analysis of ^{68}Ga-FAPI-PET of 12 ACCs (7 primary, 5 recurrent) and reported high tracer uptake and excellent tumor-to-background ratios for primary and recurrent ACCs. Metastatic lesions showed lower uptake than primary tumors but still markedly elevated compared with peritumoral tissue. With respect to FAPI kinetics over time, ACCs showed slightly decreasing uptake but increasing tumor-to-background ratios.[7]

Thyroid Cancer

Chen and colleagues applied ^{68}Ga-FAPI-PET to 24 patients with radioiodine refractory differentiated thyroid cancers. They found moderate ^{68}Ga-FAPI-uptake in lymph node, bone and lung, and metastatic lesions.[15] Fu and colleagues analyzed ^{68}Ga-FAPI-PET and ^{18}F-FDG-PET in 35 patients with metastatic differentiated thyroid cancer. They found high ^{68}Ga-FAPI-uptake in cervical, axillary, and mediastinal lymph node metastases but only slight ^{68}Ga-FAPI-uptake in pulmonary metastases.[16] There are single case studies on the application of ^{68}Ga-FAPI-PET in metastatic medullary thyroid cancers but these reports are too preliminary to draw any conclusions.[17] Comparative studies using FAPI-PET, ^{18}F FDG-PET, or Iodine imaging for thyroid cancer have not been performed to date.

Cervical Cancer of Unknown Primary

Only one study focusing on ^{68}Ga-FAPI-PET for cervical cancer of unknown primary (CUP) exits, in which the authors analyzed ^{68}Ga-FAPI-PET in 18 patients in whom ^{18}F-FDG had failed to identify a head and neck primary. They describe intense ^{68}Ga-FAPI tracer uptake in both the detected primary tumors (frequently located in areas with high physiologic ^{18}F-FDG-uptake, eg, the tonsils) and lymph node and bone metastases.[18]

CLINICAL APPLICATIONS
Staging of Oral Squamous Cell Cancer and Comparison with Other Imaging Modalities

In their multimodal imaging study of oral SCC, Linz and colleagues compared sensitivity and specificity of ^{68}Ga-FAPI-PET and ^{18}F-FDG and found identical detection of primary tumors, a slightly lower sensitivity of ^{68}Ga-FAPI-PET for the detection of metastases but marginally higher specificity for the detection of lymph node metastases. Compared to MR imaging, PET imaging with both tracers had slight diagnostic advantages. Chen and colleagues found that the primary tumor sites of all patients included were equally well detected by ^{68}Ga-FAPI-PET and ^{18}F-FDG-PET. With respect to nodal metastases, they found advantageous diagnostic accuracy of ^{68}Ga-FAPI-PET compared with ^{18}F-FDG, especially with regard to its markedly higher specificity. The patients included had no distant metastases, so that no statement on the diagnostic performance of ^{68}Ga-FAPI-PET with respect to M status was possible.

Staging of Nasopharyneal Carcinomas and Comparison with Other Imaging Modalities

Zhao and colleagues compared, in their above-mentioned study, the diagnostic performance, PET-based volumetric parameters, and staging based on ^{68}Ga-FAPI-PET and ^{18}F-FDG-PET. The sensitivity for the detection of primary tumors did not significantly differ between both tracers but ^{68}Ga-FAPI-PET-based gross tumor volumes (GTVs) and ^{68}Ga-PET-based total lesion FAPI (TL-FAPI) (calculated as mean standardized uptake value [SUVmean] * GTV) were significantly higher compared with ^{18}F-FDG-based GTV and total lesion glycolysis. With respect to lymph node metastases and distant metastases, the detection rate of ^{68}Ga-FAPI-PET was higher than that of ^{18}F-FDG. TNM staging based on ^{68}Ga-FAPI-PET compared with ^{18}F-FDG-PET was altered in 28% (T), 3% (N), and 5% (M) of the patients and additional metastases were detected in 41% of the patients implying that ^{68}Ga-FAPI-PET may be have marked impact on the staging of NPC.

Quin and colleagues also compared staging of NPC based on ^{68}Ga-FAPI-PET and ^{18}F-FDG-PET. Although the absolute tumor uptake of ^{68}Ga-FAPI was lower than that of ^{18}F-FDG, ^{68}Ga-FAPI was superior to ^{18}F-FDG with respect to T staging as significantly lower background activity improved the evaluation of tumor boundaries and skull-based and intracranial invasion. The authors did not draw any definitive conclusions on N and M staging due to missing histopathological confirmation but found more ^{18}F-FDG-positive than ^{68}Ga-FAPI-positive lymph nodes and more metastasis-suspicious ^{68}Ga-FAPI-uptake than ^{18}F-FDG-uptake.

Staging of Adenoid Cystic Carcinomas and Comparison with Other Imaging Modalities

As ACCs are known to be ^{18}F-FDG-negative in many cases, Röhrich, Syed and colleagues compared ^{68}Ga-FAPI-PET-based and contrast-enhanced CT and MR imaging-based staging of ACCs. Herein, they found that additional ^{68}Ga-FAPI-PET led to the detection of new metastases in 5 out of 12 patients compared with CT/MR imaging alone. A head-to-head comparison between ^{68}Ga-FAPI-PET and ^{18}F-FDG-PET for imaging ACCs does not exist to date. However, Liew, Röhrich and colleagues correlated ^{68}Ga-FAPI-PET and MR imaging (contrast enhanced T1-weighted and T2-weighted sequences) signal intensities in ACCs and could show that ^{68}Ga-FAPI signaling is an independent signal and not a surrogate marker of MR imaging sequences.[19]

Staging of Thyroid Carcinomas and Comparison with Other Imaging Modalities

Because the systematic analyses of ^{68}Ga-FAPI-PET of thyroid cancer focus on the metastatic — and thus postthyroidectomy setting, no data on eventual benefit of ^{68}Ga-FAPI-PET for the assessment of primary manifestations of thyroid cancer are available. Fu and colleagues report that lymph node and pulmonary metastases exhibit higher ^{68}Ga-FAPI-avidity than ^{18}F-FDG-avidity but the diagnostic accuracy for the detection of lymph node and distant metastases did not differ between both tracers. Chen and colleagues did not perform a head-to-head comparison of ^{68}Ga-FAPI-PET and ^{18}F-FDG-PET in their study but determined the patient-wise detection rate of ^{68}Ga-FAPI-PET for metastatic disease and correlated ^{68}Ga-FAPI-uptake of metastatic lesions with CT-based growth rates and thyroglobulin levels. They report ^{68}Ga-FAPI-positive metastases in 87.5% of all patients. ^{68}Ga-FAPI-uptake was positively correlated with growth rates but showed no correlation with thyroglobulin levels.

Assessment of Cervical Cancer of Unknown Primary

In their abovementioned study, Gu and colleagues found ^{68}Ga-FAPI-positive primary tumors in 7 out of 18 cases, in which ^{18}F-FDG-PET had not revealed any potential primary sites. All these tumors were head and neck tumors. The detection and signal intensities of lymph node metastases and bone metastases were almost equal for ^{68}Ga-FAPI-PET and ^{18}F-FDG-PET.

Potential Impact of ^{68}Ga-FAPI-PET on Radiotherapy Planning of Head and Neck Tumors

In their abovementioned analysis, Syed and colleagues could show that ^{68}Ga-FAPI-PET had significant impact on the radiotherapy planning of head and neck tumors meaning that the volume and the anatomic coverage of GTVs were changed substantially compared with CT-based radiotherapy planning.[20] Similar findings regarding GTV delineation have been reported by Röhrich, Syed and colleagues for ACCs.[7] Here, the authors point out that subtle findings, such as perineural spread and invasion of small foramina at the skull base, which are relevant for GTV countering, are well depicted in ^{68}Ga-FAPI-PET imaging. In another study on ^{68}Ga-FAPI-PET-based radiotherapy planning of pharyngeal and laryngeal carcinomas, Wegen and colleagues showed that ^{68}Ga-FAPI-PET resulted in greater GTVs than ^{18}F-FDG-PET-based or CT-based planning.[21]

DIAGNOSTIC CRITERIA

Due to the still limited database available for oncologic ^{68}Ga-FAPI-PET and given the possibility of nonmalignant ^{68}Ga-FAPI-uptake,[22] ^{68}Ga-FAPI-PET scans should always be interpreted with caution and in the context of morphologic imaging and clinical information in order to avoid overdiagnosis. Most of the studies summarized here report average SUVmax values in the range of 11 to 21 for head and neck cancers including ACCs. The average uptake of lymph node metastases was considerably lower (average SUVmax in the range 9–11) and distant metastases showed the same tendency toward lower SUVmax values. Especially lymph node and distant metastases of thyroid cancer seem to be less ^{68}Ga-FAPI-avid than metastases of oral SCC, nasopharynx carcinomas, and ACCs. Considered together, for primaries of head and neck cancers, SUVmax values lower than 10 should challenge the assumption of malignancy and consideration of differential diagnoses. However, for lymph node and distant metastases, lower ^{68}Ga-FAPI-uptake should still be considered suspicious for malignancy.

DIFFERENTIAL DIAGNOSIS

Although ^{68}Ga-FAPI-PET has been introduced as a tumor tracer, it has been shown that a large variety of nononcological pathologic conditions including fibrotic, inflammatory, reactive, and degenerative processes are ^{68}Ga-FAPI-avid, and the assessment of ^{68}Ga-FAPI-positive structures and lesions can be challenging. Morphologic

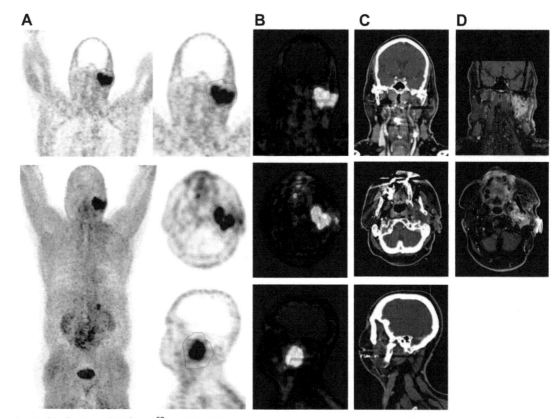

Fig. 2. (*A, B*) MIP and CT-fused ^{68}Ga-FAPI-PET images showing precise tracer uptake of a parotid carcinoma and very-low background activity. (*C, D*) conventional contrast-enhanced CT and contrast-enhanced MR imaging showing diffuse tumor infiltration making differentiation between tumor and healthy tissue difficult and subjective. MIP, maximum intensity projection. (*From* Syed M, Flechsig P, Liermann J, et al. Fibroblast activation protein inhibitor (FAPI) PET for diagnostics and advanced targeted radiotherapy in head and neck cancers. Eur J Nucl Med Mol Imaging. Nov 2020;47(12):2836-2845.)

correlation with cross-sectional imaging and the inclusion of clinical information is crucial for avoiding overdiagnosis based on ^{68}Ga-FAPI-PET. Important differential diagnoses with respect to the head and neck area region are the following.

- Lymph nodes with low or intermediate ^{68}Ga-FAPI-uptake should be interpreted with caution. Although recent studies found that ^{68}Ga-FAPI-uptake of chronic inflammatory lymph nodes is significantly lower than ^{18}F-FDG-uptake,[23] inflammatory or reactive uptake should still be considered as an alternative to lymph node metastases.
- Bone or joint associated uptake requires CT-imaging and/or MR imaging morphologic correlation as degenerative lesions can exhibit high ^{68}Ga-FAPI-uptake and mimic bone metastases.
- As head and neck cancers frequently undergo radiotherapy, irradiation-induced inflammation

of the tumor bed is a possible reason for increased ^{68}Ga-FAPI-uptake. The role of FAPI in the postradiotherapy setting, especially the optimal time span between the end of radiotherapy and ^{68}Ga-FAPI-PET requires further clarification.
- Similarly, patients that have undergone surgery regularly show wound healing associated ^{68}Ga-FAPI-uptake in the resection area, which can last for several months.
- In radioiodine refractory differentiated thyroid cancers, increased uptake of parotid and submaxillary gland was observed in 7 out of 24 patients, which was attributed to atrophy of these glands after radioiodine treatment.
- Luo and colleagues report ^{68}Ga-FAPI-positivity of lacrimal and salivary glands due to the involvement into IgG4-related disease.[23] Even though this is a rare differential

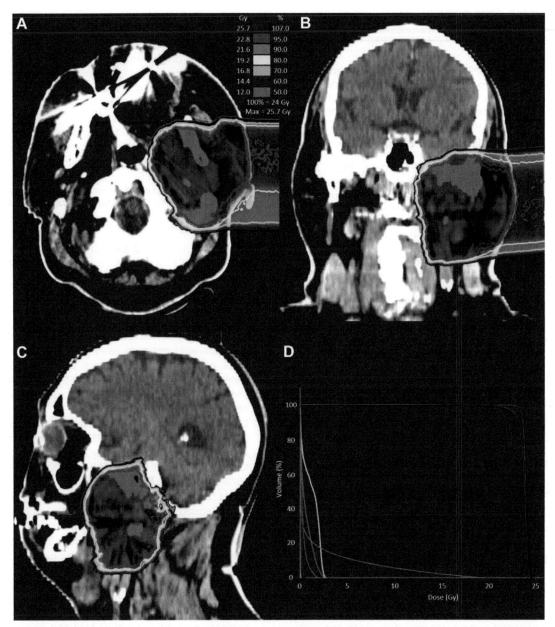

Fig. 3. Radiation treatment plan of the patient presented in **Fig. 2** with (*A*) axial, (*B*) coronal, (*C*) sagittal dose distribution, and (*D*) dose volume histogram. (*From* Syed M, Flechsig P, Liermann J, et al. Fibroblast activation protein inhibitor (FAPI) PET for diagnostics and advanced targeted radiotherapy in head and neck cancers. Eur J Nucl Med Mol Imaging. Nov 2020;47(12):2836-2845.)

diagnosis, it should be considered in cases of symmetric increased uptake in these glands.

CASE STUDY PRESENTATION

A 64 year-old male patient presented with mucoepidermoid carcinoma of the left parotid gland and received ^{68}Ga-FAPI-PET in addition to contrast-enhanced CT and contrast enhanced MR imaging to support radiotherapy planning. Intense and precise tracer accumulation significantly facilitated automated target volume delineation for radiotherapy planning compared with conventional imaging in this case as illustrated by **Figs. 2** and **3**.

CLINICS CARE POINTS

- ^{68}Ga-FAPI-PET is a promising new imaging method for head and neck cancers including oral SCCs, hypopharynx carcinomas, adenoid cystic carcinomas, thyroid cancer, and cervical cancer of unknown primary.

- Most studies on head and neck cancers suggest that ^{68}Ga-FAPI-PET has high potential for imaging of regularly highly ^{68}Ga-FAPI-avid primary tumors including the assessment of the local tumor extent and the involvement of surrounding structures. When ^{68}Ga-FAPI-PET was compared head-to-head with ^{18}F-FDG-PET, authors considered ^{68}Ga-FAPI-PET favorable for primary tumors. With respect to lymph node and distant metastases, the results are sparse, and especially for the comparison between ^{68}Ga-FAPI-PET and ^{18}F-FDG-PET, no definitive conclusions can be drawn from the existing data.

- The findings on ^{68}Ga-FAPI-PET with respect to cervical CUP are exciting as in a substantial portion of patients without suspicious findings in ^{18}F-FDG-PET primary tumors were detected by ^{68}Ga-FAPI-PET. Additional projects focusing on cervical and other CUP with higher numbers of patients are needed to confirm these promising initial findings.

DECLARATION OF INTERESTS

I declare that no commercial or financial conflicts of interest regarding this article exist.

REFERENCES

1. Chow LQM. Head and neck cancer. N Engl J Med 2020;382(1):60–72.
2. Coca-Pelaz A, Rodrigo JP, Bradley PJ, et al. Adenoid cystic carcinoma of the head and neck–An update. Oral Oncol 2015;51(7):652–61.
3. Huang SH, O'Sullivan B. Overview of the 8th Edition TNM Classification for head and neck cancer. Curr Treat Options Oncol 2017;18(7):40.
4. Junn JC, Soderlund KA, Glastonbury CM. Imaging of head and neck cancer with CT, MRI, and US. Semin Nucl Med 2021;51(1):3–12.
5. Marcus C, Subramaniam RM. Role of non-FDG-PET/CT in head and neck cancer. Semin Nucl Med 2021;51(1):68–78.
6. Mona CE, Benz MR, Hikmat F, et al. Correlation of (68)Ga-FAPi-46 PET biodistribution with FAP expression by immunohistochemistry in patients with solid cancers: interim analysis of a prospective

7. translational Exploratory study. J Nucl Med 2022;63(7):1021–6.
7. Rohrich M, Syed M, Liew DP, et al. 68)Ga-FAPI-PET/CT improves diagnostic staging and radiotherapy planning of adenoid cystic carcinomas - imaging analysis and histological validation. Radiother Oncol 2021;160:192–201.
8. Giesel FL, Kratochwil C, Lindner T, et al. 68)Ga-FAPI PET/CT: biodistribution and preliminary dosimetry Estimate of 2 DOTA-Containing FAP-targeting agents in patients with various cancers. J Nucl Med 2019;60(3):386–92.
9. Ferdinandus J, Kessler L, Hirmas N, et al. Equivalent tumor detection for early and late FAPI-46 PET acquisition. Eur J Nucl Med Mol Imaging 2021;48(10):3221–7.
10. Glatting FM, Hoppner J, Liew DP, et al. Repetitive early FAPI-PET acquisition comparing FAPI-02, FAPI-46 and FAPI-74: methodological and diagnostic implications for malignant, inflammatory and degenerative lesions. J Nucl Med 2022. https://doi.org/10.2967/jnumed.122.264069.
11. Linz C, Brands RC, Kertels O, et al. Targeting fibroblast activation protein in newly diagnosed squamous cell carcinoma of the oral cavity - initial experience and comparison to [(18)F]FDG PET/CT and MRI. Eur J Nucl Med Mol Imaging 2021;48(12):3951–60.
12. Chen S, Chen Z, Zou G, et al. Accurate preoperative staging with [(68)Ga]Ga-FAPI PET/CT for patients with oral squamous cell carcinoma: a comparison to 2-[(18)F]FDG PET/CT. Eur Radiol 2022;32(9):6070–9.
13. Zhao L, Pang Y, Zheng H, et al. Clinical utility of [(68)Ga]Ga-labeled fibroblast activation protein inhibitor (FAPI) positron emission tomography/computed tomography for primary staging and recurrence detection in nasopharyngeal carcinoma. Eur J Nucl Med Mol Imaging 2021;48(11):3606–17.
14. Qin C, Liu F, Huang J, et al. A head-to-head comparison of (68)Ga-DOTA-FAPI-04 and (18)F-FDG PET/MR in patients with nasopharyngeal carcinoma: a prospective study. Eur J Nucl Med Mol Imaging 2021;48(10):3228–37.
15. Chen Y, Zheng S, Zhang J, et al. 68)Ga-DOTA-FAPI-04 PET/CT imaging in radioiodine-refractory differentiated thyroid cancer (RR-DTC) patients. Ann Nucl Med 2022;36(7):610–22.
16. Fu H, Wu J, Huang J, et al. 68)Ga fibroblast activation protein inhibitor PET/CT in the detection of metastatic thyroid cancer: comparison with (18)F-FDG PET/CT. Radiology 2022;304(2):397–405.
17. Kuyumcu S, Isik EG, Sanli Y. Liver metastases from medullary thyroid carcinoma detected on (68)Ga-FAPI-04 PET/CT. Endocrine 2021;74(3):727–8.
18. Gu B, Xu X, Zhang J, et al. The added value of (68)Ga-FAPI PET/CT in patients with head and neck

cancer of unknown primary with (18)F-FDG-Negative findings. J Nucl Med 2022;63(6):875–81.

19. Liew DP, Rohrich M, Loi L, et al. FAP-specific signalling is an independent diagnostic approach in ACC and not a surrogate marker of MRI sequences. Cancers 2022;14(17). https://doi.org/10.3390/cancers14174253.

20. Syed M, Flechsig P, Liermann J, et al. Fibroblast activation protein inhibitor (FAPI) PET for diagnostics and advanced targeted radiotherapy in head and neck cancers. Eur J Nucl Med Mol Imaging 2020; 47(12):2836–45.

21. Wegen S, van Heek L, Linde P, et al. Head-to-Head comparison of [(68) Ga]Ga-FAPI-46-PET/CT and [(18)F]F-FDG-PET/CT for radiotherapy planning in head and neck cancer. Mol Imaging Biol 2022. https://doi.org/10.1007/s11307-022-01749-7.

22. Kessler L, Ferdinandus J, Hirmas N, et al. Pitfalls and Common findings in (68)Ga-FAPI PET: a pictorial analysis. J Nucl Med 2022;63(6):890–6.

23. Luo Y, Pan Q, Yang H, et al. Fibroblast activation protein-targeted PET/CT with (68)Ga-FAPI for imaging IgG4-related disease: comparison to (18)F-FDG PET/CT. J Nucl Med 2021;62(2):266–71.

Fibroblast Activation Protein Inhibitor-PET Imaging in Colorectal Cancer

Esther Strating, MD[a], Anne van de Loo, BSc[a], Sjoerd Elias, MD, PhD[b], Marnix Lam, MD, PhD[c],*, Onno Kranenburg, PhD[a],*

KEYWORDS

- Colorectal cancer • Fibroblast activation protein • Fibroblast activation protein inhibitor • PET
- Peritoneal metastases

KEY POINTS

- Based on fibroblast activation protein (FAP) expression patterns in colorectal cancer, distinct focus areas for applying fibroblast activation protein inhibitor (FAPI)-PET are defined.
- FAPI-PET may improve lymph node staging at first diagnosis.
- FAPI-PET provides a novel diagnostic tool for identifying the aggressive Consensus Molecular Subtype 4.
- FAPI-PET detects peritoneal metastases that are invisible using conventional imaging and may therefore have value as a tool to select patients for surgery and monitor therapy response.
- High FAP expression is associated with resistance to immunotherapy, suggesting that FAPI-PET may help predict response to immunotherapy.

INTRODUCTION

Colorectal cancer (CRC) is one of the leading causes of cancer-related mortality.[1] In the last decades our understanding of the pathophysiology of CRC has advanced, resulting in more therapeutic options for localized and metastatic disease.[2] However, 5-year survival for CRC with distant metastasis is still only ~15%.[3] The focus of cancer research has shifted from a cancer cell-centric view to a more holistic view in which the interaction of cancer cells with the tumor microenvironment (TME) sustains and promotes tumor growth.[4] Aside from cancer cells, the TME consists of extracellular matrix (ECM), endothelial cells, immune cells, and cancer-associated fibroblasts (CAFs). CAFs play an important role in CRC

initiation, progression, metastasis, and therapy resistance.[5] CAFs influence tumor behavior by secreting growth factors, by shaping the ECM and through their influence on immune cells. An important CAF marker is fibroblast activation protein (FAP). FAP is a cell surface serine protease that can cleave various peptides and ECM molecules.[6] Physiologically, FAP is expressed during embryogenesis[7] and wound healing.[8] In healthy adult tissues FAP expression is minimal. However, FAP is overexpressed by CAFs in the stroma of many different solid tumors.[9] As such, FAP is an attractive target for molecular imaging, especially for tumor types with a high amount of reactive stroma. Various FAP inhibitors (FAPIs) were developed that are now primarily used as molecular imaging tools.[10] The high affinity of FAPIs for

[a] Division of Imaging and Cancer, Laboratory Translational Oncology, University Medical Center Utrecht, Utrecht University, Heidelberglaan 100, 3584 CX, G.04.2.28, Utrecht, the Netherlands; [b] Department of Epidemiology, Julius Center for Health Sciences and Primary Care, University Medical Center Utrecht, Utrecht University, Heidelberglaan 100, 3584 CX, STR.6.131, Utrecht, the Netherlands; [c] Department of Radiology and Nuclear Medicine, University Medical Center Utrecht, Utrecht University, Heidelberglaan 100, 3584 CX, E.01. 1.32, Utrecht, the Netherlands
* Corresponding authors.
E-mail addresses: m.lam@umcutrecht.nl (M.L.); o.kranenburg@umcutrecht.nl (O.K.)

PET Clin 18 (2023) 325–335
https://doi.org/10.1016/j.cpet.2023.02.003
1556-8598/23/© 2023 Elsevier Inc. All rights reserved.

FAP, the selective expression of FAP in tumor tissue, and the rapid clearance of FAPIs from the circulation yields a high contrast in FAPI-PET imaging.[10]

But FAP is more than just an attractive target for molecular imaging. For instance, FAP has been implicated in tumor cell migration through ECM remodeling and has pro-angiogenic and immuno-suppressive effects in the TME.[6] Furthermore, high FAP expression is associated with worse overall survival in many epithelial cancers, including CRC.[11]

Based on FAP expression patterns in CRC, distinct focus areas for applying FAPI-PET can be defined, which could contribute to improving the clinical management of CRC. In this review, we define six specific clinical dilemmas (**Fig. 1**) in the diagnosis and treatment of CRC in which FAPI-PET may have value, and highlight important aspects regarding future clinical study design.

FAPI-PET IMAGING IN COLORECTAL CANCER

Several retrospective cohort studies on FAPI-PET imaging in patients with CRC have been performed (**Table 1**). Most of these studies focused on staging and restaging, often comparing FAPI-PET to conventional imaging and ^{18}F-fluorodeoxyglucose-PET (FDG-PET). FAPI-PET showed higher maximum standardized uptake value (SUVmax) values[12] and better sensitivity and specificity for detecting primary tumors, lymph node metastases, and distant metastases,[13–15] often leading to a change in clinical management.[16–18] Overall, FAPI-PET imaging seems a promising tool for improving the clinical management of patients with CRC. However, these studies are limited by heterogeneous patient populations and lack of correlation between the histopathological diagnosis of resected tissues and FAPI-PET signal. More prospective trials in specified groups of patients with CRC, comparing

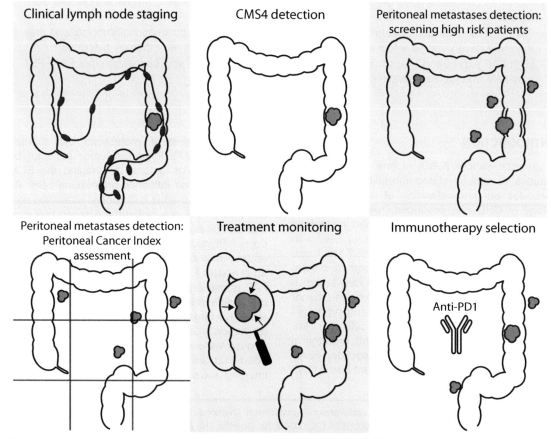

Fig. 1. Six clinical dilemmas in the diagnosis and treatment of CRC in which FAPI-PET may have value. (1) Conventional imaging modalities have a poor sensitivity and specificity for clinical lymph node staging. (2) The Consensus Molecular Subtype 4 shows inter- and intra-tumor heterogeneity complicating the interpretation of biopsy-based diagnostics. (3) Peritoneal metastases are notoriously difficult to detect using conventional imaging. This complicates early diagnosis in high-risk patients, (4) selection for curative treatment through assessment of the peritoneal cancer index (PCI), and (5) treatment monitoring. (6) Currently used biomarkers perform poorly in predicting response to immunotherapy in patients with MSI-H metastatic CRC. The *arrows* indicate tumor shrinkage.

Table 1
An overview of all published fibroblast activation protein inhibitor-PET data in patients with colorectal cancer

First Author	FAPI	No. of pts. Total/CRC	Comparison to	Main Findings
Qin et al,[18] 2022	^{68}Ga-FAPI-04	120/38	FDG-PET Conventional imaging	In a subgroup analysis of patients with CRC the diagnostic accuracy for FAPI-PET was 97.4% ($n = 38$), for FDG-PET 90.9% ($n = 11$) and for conventional imaging 63.9% ($n = 36$). There was a significant difference between FAPI-PET and conventional imaging ($P < .001$), but the difference between FAPI and FDG was not significant.
Kömek et al,[13] 2022	^{68}Ga-FAPI-04	39/39	FDG-PET Histopathological examination	The diagnostic accuracy of FAPI-PET was higher than that of FDG-PET for primary tumors (100% vs 92.1%, $P = .031$) and lymph node metastases (95% vs 80.5%, $P = .022$). There was no significant difference in diagnostic accuracy between FAPI-PET and FDG-PET for peritoneal metastases (100% vs 89.7%, $P = .125$).
Elboga et al,[12] 2022	^{68}Ga-FAPI-04	37/13	FDG-PET	The median SUV_{max} of FAPI-PET was higher than that of FDG-PET for primary tumors (13.2 vs 7.5, $P < .001$), lymph node metastases (8.3 vs 3.9, $P = .006$), liver metastases (8.5 vs 4.7, $P = .002$), peritoneal metastases (8.1 vs 2.6, $P < .001$) and bone metastases (13.4 vs 0, $P = .018$). There was no significant difference for lung metastases (4.5 vs 4.0, $P = .109$). No CRC subgroup analysis was performed.
Pang et al,[17] 2020	^{68}Ga-FAPI-04	35/8	FDG-PET	In treatment naïve patients FAPI-PET led to upstaging in 21% compared with FDG-PET. The sensitivity of FAPI-PET was significantly higher than FDG-PET for the detection of primary tumors (100% vs 53%, $P = .004$), lymph node metastases (79% vs 54%, $P < .001$) and bone and visceral metastases (89% vs 57%, $P < .001$). No CRC subgroup analysis was performed.
Sahin et al,[15] 2021	^{68}Ga-FAPI-04	31/15	FDG-PET	The sensitivity for the detection of liver metastases was higher for FAPI-PET compared with FDG-PET (96.6% vs 70.8%). In a subgroup analysis, the tumor-to-background ratio of CRC liver metastases was significantly higher for FAPI than for FDG (4.5 vs 1.3, $P = .00$).

(continued on next page)

Table 1
(continued)

First Author	FAPI	No. of pts. Total/CRC	Comparison to	Main Findings
Zhao et al,[14] 2021	^{68}Ga-FAPI-04	46/10	FDG-PET	In a subgroup analysis of patients with CRC, FAPI-PET showed a significantly higher median SUV of peritoneal metastases than FDG-PET (10.14 vs 3.86, $P = .028$). The median peritoneal cancer index score derived from FAPI-PET imaging was higher than that derived from FDG-PET but this difference was not significant (6 vs 3, $P = .068$).
Koerber et al,[16] 2020	^{68}Ga-FAPI-04 ^{68}Ga-FAPI-46	22/15	Conventional imaging	FAPI imaging caused a high, medium, and low change in oncologic or radio oncologic management in 19%, 33%, and 29%, respectively.
Kratochwil et al,[20] 2019	^{68}Ga-FAPI-04	38 CRC lesions	–	Colorectal cancer showed an intermediate average SUV_{max} activity (SUV range 6 to 12).
All combined		330/138		Overall, FAPI-PET imaging results in higher SUVmax values, improved tumor to background ratios and a higher sensitivity for the detection of primary CRC and distant metastases, compared with conventional imaging and FDG-PET.

FAPI activity with ex vivo histopathological, cellular, and molecular tissue analyses, are needed. For a more detailed description of the CRC FAPI cohorts, we refer the reader to a recent review by Cheng and colleagues.[19]

Lymph Node Metastases

Disease staging according to the tumor, node, metastasis (TNM) classification is essential for the treatment selection of patients with solid tumors, including CRC. Because of imaging limitations in terms of sensitivity, there is no proven benefit of more precise preoperative clinical lymph node staging in patients with CRC who undergo radical resection. In this patient group, the pathologic N-stage currently determines the indication for adjuvant chemotherapy. However, in specific patient groups, accurate clinical lymph node staging can be of great value, for example, in patients who present with low-risk T1 CRC. These patients can be treated with curative endoscopic resection. Nonetheless, approximately 10% of patients with T1 tumors have lymph node metastases for which a radical resection is necessary.[21] Current risk stratification models based on histologic characteristics classify more than 50% of all T1 tumors as high risk with an indication for radical resection. This results in an unnecessary surgical resection of more than 40% of T1 CRC.[22] Furthermore, the potential benefit of neoadjuvant chemotherapy in stage II/III CRC has renewed interest in clinical lymph node staging.[23,24] In rectal cancer specifically, clinical lymph node staging is far more important as patients receive neoadjuvant chemoradiotherapy based on clinical TNM-staging (T3-4 and/or N+).[25]

Clinical lymph node status is assessed based on the size, shape, irregularity of the border, and heterogeneity of the signal on computed tomography (CT) or MR imaging. With current imaging modalities the sensitivity and specificity range from 41% to 56% and 67% to 87% respectively.[26] The poor accuracy of clinical lymph node detection may therefore lead to undertreatment as well as overtreatment.

To determine if FAPI-PET could play a role in improving clinical N-staging, the stroma content of 126 lymph node metastases from 73 patients with stage III colon cancer was assessed.[27] Only 2% of lymph node metastases were classified as stroma-negative (<5% stroma content), whereas 98% were stroma-positive. Unfortunately, no FAP immunohistochemistry was performed, so the number of FAP-positive lymph node metastases could not be established. Another study looked at FAP expression of lymph node metastases ($n = 227$).[28] Here only ~30% were classified as FAP-positive according to a semiquantitative scale.[29] It is currently impossible to judge how the scores of both methods correlate with signals on an FAPI-PET scan.

A study comparing FAPI-PET activity of lymph node metastases with histopathological diagnosis of resected lymph nodes in CRC, found a sensitivity and specificity of 90% and 100% for the detection of lymph node metastases by FAPI-PET in 17 patients with colon cancer.[13] Only one patient was wrongly classified as lymph node metastases negative, the remaining patients were classified as true positive ($n = 10$) or true negative ($n = 6$). FDG-PET performed worse in detecting lymph node metastases with 80% sensitivity and 81.8% specificity. More prospective clinical studies in colon and rectal cancer, comparing FAPI lymph node metastases detection with pathologic examination of resected lymph nodes for tumor positivity, are needed. In these studies, it is essential that lymph nodes visible on imaging can be directly correlated to specific lesions within the resection specimen and that FAP expression in such lesions is determined by immunohistochemistry or other, more quantitative, methods such as enzyme-linked immunosorbent assay. This will help define the correlation between the level of FAP expression in lymph nodes and FAPI activity on PET.

Consensus Molecular Subtype 4 detection

A relatively new classification system, the Consensus Molecular Subtypes (CMS) distinguishes four subtypes (CMS1–4), based on recurrent gene expression patterns.[30] The CMS framework can be used to gain more insight in tumor biology, guide drug development, and provide better survival estimates and treatment selection. In the localized disease stage, patients with CMS4 tumors have the worst prognosis and benefit least from adjuvant systemic therapy.[31] CMS4 is often referred to as the "mesenchymal subtype" due to atypically high expression of mesenchymal genes. Currently available CMS diagnostic tests require tumor tissue samples. However, the interpretation of biopsy-based CMS diagnosis is complicated by variability of

CMS status between lesions in individual patients,[32] between regions within one lesion[33,34] and over time as a result of chemotherapy.[35] The development of CMS4-targeted therapy strategies requires a robust and clinically applicable diagnostic test for assessment of CMS4 status of all lesions in individual cancer patients. Although gene profiling costs are decreasing, genomic technologies are not widely accessible in clinical practice and do not obviate the need for accurate staging.

A possible solution would be to diagnose CMS4 status by using a radiotracer that enables the quantitative assessment of CMS4 in vivo by whole-body molecular imaging as well as providing more accurate disease staging than conventional imaging approaches. We have previously shown that FAP mRNA expression can identify CMS4 with very high specificity and sensitivity (area under the receiver operation characteristic [AUROC] > 0.91).[33] To use FAPI-PET molecular imaging to diagnose the CMS4 subtype, there has to be a strong correlation between FAP expression and tracer signal. So far, several studies have shown a significant positive correlation between FAPI activity on PET and FAP expression in tumor tissue ($r = 0.43$ to 0.94),[36–38] suggesting that FAPI-PET imaging is a promising diagnostic tool to identify CMS4.

The next step will be to conduct a clinical study that will correlate FAPI activity in primary tumors and metastatic lesions to CMS4 classification based on gene expression data of tumor biopsies. An important aspect of such a clinical study is to address CMS heterogeneity by taking multiregion biopsies of each lesion. Molecular imaging has a unique capability for demonstrating the heterogeneity of tumor targets on a whole-body scale. A possible endpoint to assess the diagnostic accuracy could be the AUROC of tumor-level FAPI uptake for the CMS4 subtype.

Peritoneal metastases detection

CRC metastasizes to the peritoneum in approximately 10% of all patients.[39] In approximately half of the cases peritoneal metastases (PM) are detected at initial diagnosis (synchronous PM), whereas the other half develops in the period after primary tumor resection (metachronous PM). PM development is associated with a very poor prognosis and high morbidity. Cytoreductive surgery (CRS) combined with hyperthermic intra-peritoneal chemotherapy (HIPEC) can be curative, but only in patients with limited peritoneal disease.[40,41] Conventional imaging modalities perform poorly in detecting PM.[42] Diagnostic laparoscopy (DLS) can be applied to screen for metachronous PM development, but this procedure leaves important intra- and extra-abdominal regions unexamined. Moreover, the procedure can lead to the seeding of abdominal wall metastases within the laparoscopy wound.[43] This illustrates the need for developing non-invasive, sensitive methods for the early detection of metachronous PM.

An important tool for selecting patients with synchronous or metachronous PM who might benefit from CRS-HIPEC is the peritoneal cancer index (PCI), a semiquantitative measure of intraperitoneal tumor load.[44,45] The PCI is a composite score of tumor load in 13 anatomically defined intra-abdominal regions. DLS is currently the clinical standard for PCI assessment. However, with the current patient selection strategies, CRS is discontinued in up to 30% to 40% of the procedures due to an unexpectedly high PCI score observed during surgery.[46,47] Therefore, improved patient selection strategies, for instance, based on PCI assessment by pre-operative non-invasive imaging, are urgently needed.

We recently showed that PM in CRC are a near-homogeneous entity of CMS4 and that FAP is highly expressed by myofibroblasts in virtually all PM.[33,48,49] In addition, the first clinical studies on FAPI-PET imaging of PM show promising results: In a cohort of 46 patients with PM from various primary tumor types, FAPI PET/CT showed a higher PCI score and better sensitivity for the detection of PM than FDG-PET/CT.[14] A second study comparing FAPI and FDG activity in 35 patients with gastric, duodenal or CRC, the sensitivity of FAPI PET/CT to detect distant metastasis (including PM) was 89% compared with 57% for FDG.[17] This could in part be due to the lower physiologic uptake of FAPI in the abdominal cavity compared with FDG, resulting in higher tumor-to-background ratios for FAPI.[13] Although most studies used FAPI-PET/CT for imaging of PM, FAPI PET/MR imaging may provide advantages given the superiority of MR imaging over CT for the detection and quantification of CRC PM.[50]

The homogenous nature of FAP expression in PM and the favorable clinical experience thus far, strongly suggest that FAPI-PET may have value in the detection and quantification of PM.

Screening high-risk patients

Early detection of PM is essential to increase eligibility for CRS-HIPEC, and hence cure rate. In patients who are at high risk of developing metachronous PM, for instance, those who present with a pT4 or a perforated primary tumor, DLS is routinely applied as a PM detection strategy.[51] The COLOPEC-2 study (NCT03413254) aims to

assess whether a *second-look* DLS (a DLS within 6 to 9 months after curative resection of a pT4 tumor) in this patient category may improve early PM detection.[52] Based on the above rationale, FAPI-PET may have value in the early detection of metachronous PM in high-risk patients. To assess such value, we propose a study in patients with a pT4 or perforated tumor, who will receive an FAPI-PET scan in addition to DLS to detect PM after surgical removal of the primary tumor. The goal of such a study would be to compare the diagnostic accuracy of early PM detection by either method.

Peritoneal cancer index assessment

The homogeneously high expression of FAP in PM suggests that FAPI-PET could serve as a quantitative noninvasive diagnostic tool for PCI assessment. To determine the potential value of FAPI-PET in PCI assessment, we propose a study in patients who are considered eligible for surgery during routine diagnostic workup, based on PCI assessment by DLS and/or routine imaging. The study should compare PCI values generated by FAPI-PET and by routine assessment in relation to the golden standard 'true' histopathological PCI, which is determined after surgical removal of all PM. To accurately assess the specificity of FAPI-PET imaging for PCI determination, it is important that all FAPI-PET positive lesions are resected for pathologic investigation. The quantitative nature of the PET signal would provide an unbiased selection tool and a solid basis for developing a standardized (center-independent) procedure for selecting patients for surgery. To further increase standardization, threshold-based segmentation tools can be used to quantify the molecular imaging tumor volume of FAPI-PET (MITV-FAPI).

Therapy response monitoring of peritoneal metastases

Currently PM are detected at a stage in which only approximately 20% to 25% of patients can be treated with CRS/HIPEC. The remaining patient group will be offered palliative chemotherapy. Unfortunately, the benefit of systemic therapy in patients with PM is much lower compared with other metastatic sites.[53] Because PM are difficult to image with conventional imaging modalities, chemotherapy regimens are often administered without a good method for response monitoring. Moreover, this has led to the active exclusion of patients with PM from clinical trials.[54] Therefore, new imaging techniques to monitor PM response to systemic therapies are urgently needed. We recently provided proof-of-concept that FAPI-

PET may be used to document the response of PM to systemic chemotherapy (**Fig. 2**). Only a few studies have been published on FAPI-PET response evaluation of systemic therapy.[55,56] In a pilot study of four patients receiving induction chemotherapy for locally advanced pancreatic cancer, a decrease of FAPI-PET SUVmax correlated with histopathological regression and R0 status.[55] Another study used FAPI-PET to measure response to FAP targeting chimeric antigen receptor (CAR)-T cells in a murine model of lung cancer.[56]

A potential pitfall of measuring therapy response with FAPI-PET is the generation of fibrotic tissue as a result of systemic therapy.[57] The activated fibroblasts in such tissues may express FAP and this could confound FAPI-PET-based response measurements. Indeed, post-treatment fibrotic reactions have been detected by FAPI-PET.[18,58] Therefore, the value of FAPI PET in evaluating the response of PM to standard chemotherapy and to novel drug combinations will need to be thoroughly assessed.

In the Dutch CAIRO6 study (NCT02758951), half of the patients with operable PM receive systemic chemotherapy before CRS/HIPEC.[59] Such a study would be an ideal setting to test FAPI-PET imaging for treatment monitoring of PM. In this study, a number of these patients would receive an FAPI-PET scan before the start of neoadjuvant chemotherapy and before surgical resection of the treated tumor. Pre- and posttreatment FAPI activity can then be compared and be related to the histopathologic tumor response and to the presence of (potentially therapy-induced) FAP-positive fibrotic tissue.

Pressurized intraperitoneal aerosol chemotherapy (PIPAC) of inoperable PM provides another clinical setting in which the potential value of FAPI-PET in response evaluation may be determined. In PIPAC, oxaliplatin is locally vaporized, to improve

Before start systemic chemotherapy (FOLFIRI-B)

Two months after start therapy

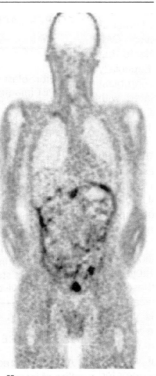
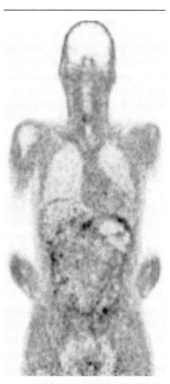

Fig. 2. A 71-year-old man underwent a ^{68}Ga-FAPI-PET/CT for possible PM recurrence. The FAPI-PET showed diffuse tracer activity along the peritoneum (*small arrows*) and intense activity in lower left ventral abdominal wall (*large arrow*) suspect for disease recurrence. The patient subsequently received systemic chemotherapy for 2 months. Disease evaluation with FAPI-PET showed a reduction of tracer activity that correlated with clinical response. From Strating E, Wassenaar E, Verhagen M, et al. Fibroblast activation protein identifies Consensus Molecular Subtype 4 in colorectal cancer and allows its detection by 68Ga-FAPI-PET imaging. Br J Cancer. 2022;(February):1-11.

drug distribution, within the abdomen in multiple cycles usually 6 weeks apart.[60] The repeated access to the peritoneal cavity in patients receiving PIPAC treatment allows longitudinal sampling of tumor tissue, and hence, assessment of histopathological tumor responses over time. The addition of FAPI-PET scans to PIPAC study protocols would allow a direct comparison of response evaluation by FAPI-PET, by routine radiological procedures, and by histopathology.

Selecting Patients for Immunotherapy

Metastatic CRC (mCRC) with a deficient mismatch repair system (dMMR)/microsatellite instability-high (MSI-H) phenotype is characterized by a high tumor mutational burden, yielding potentially antigenic tumor neoantigens. As a result, such tumors are often recognized by the patient's immune system, and they are characterized by a high amount of tumor-infiltrating lymphocytes. Patients with MSI-H mCRC show a good response to treatment with immunotherapy. However, only 5% of patients with mCRC have dMMR/MSI-H tumors. Furthermore, approximately 40% to 50% of patients with MSI-H mCRC who are treated with immunotherapy show an objective response.[61,62] Tools accurately predicting response to immunotherapy are currently lacking. However, CAF gene signatures are upregulated in patients that fail to respond to immunotherapy.[63] Especially gene signatures expressed by the myofibroblast subset of CAFs (myCAFs) are associated with immunotherapy resistance.[64–66] In CRC, FAP is an excellent marker of myCAFs.[33,67] High FAP expression measured by FAPI could therefore possibly predict resistance to immunotherapy in dMMR/MSI-H patients. In metastatic gastric cancer FAP mRNA expression was a good predictor of immunotherapy failure with an AUROC of 0.733.[68] Furthermore patients that did not respond to PD-1 inhibition had a higher pretreatment activity of FAPI ($P = .0149$).[68]

Preclinical studies in which CAF-targeting therapies were combined with immunotherapy have shown promising results.[69–71] Some of these strategies are currently further tested in clinical trials, in which adequate patient selection is vital. In this respect, FAPI-PET could have value as a tool to select patients for the combination therapy. Furthermore, the therapeutic potential of FAPI can be exploited by administering FAP-targeted radioligand therapy with the aim of increasing tumor neoantigens and immune influx and thereby sensitizing the tumor to immunotherapy.[72,73]

Prospective clinical studies are needed to assess whether FAPI activity can help predict response to immunotherapy in dMMR/MSI-H patients. In such studies pretreatment FAPI-PET scans and subsequent FAPI-PET scans during and after treatment may be correlated with the radiologic response to treatment, and with currently used biomarkers predicting immunotherapy response, including the number of CD8+ intra-tumor T cells, tumor mutation burden, and PD-1/PD-L1 expression. As FAP expression can vary among lesions in individual patients, a per-patient and per-lesion analysis is needed.

SUMMARY

FAPI-PET imaging holds great promise for improving the clinical management of CRC. High FAP expression is particularly observed in lymph node metastases, in the aggressive CMS4, in PM, and in tumors that respond poorly to immunotherapy. We have defined six clinical dilemmas in the diagnosis and treatment of CRC, which FAPI-PET may help solve. Future clinical trials should include patients undergoing tumor resection, allowing correlation of FAPI-PET signals with in-depth histopathological, cellular, and molecular tissue analyses.

CLINICS CARE POINTS

- Fibroblast activation protein inhibitor (FAPI)-PET imaging shows high sensitivity and specificity for imaging primary colorectal cancer (CRC), lymph node metastases, and peritoneal metastases compared with conventional imaging.

- Fibroblast activation protein is highly expressed by cancer-associated fibroblasts in CRC lymph node metastases, the Consensus Molecular Subtype 4, peritoneal metastases and tumors that show a poor response to immunotherapy.

- To assess the true sensitivity and specificity of FAPI-PET imaging for various indications, prospective studies comparing in vivo FAPI signal and ex vivo tissue analyses are needed.

DISCLOSURE

All authors declare that they have no relevant conflict of interest.

REFERENCES

1. Sung H, Ferlay J, Siegel RL, et al. Global cancer statistics 2020: GLOBOCAN estimates of incidence

and mortality Worldwide for 36 cancers in 185 Countries. CA Cancer J Clin 2021;71(3):209–49.

2. Biller LH, Schrag D. Diagnosis and treatment of metastatic colorectal cancer: a review. JAMA 2021; 325(7):669–85.

3. American cancer society. 2022. Available at: https://www.cancer.org/research/cancer-facts-statistics/all-cancer-facts-figures/cancer-facts-figures-2022.html.

4. Baghban R, Roshangar L, Jahanban-Esfahlan R, et al. Tumor microenvironment complexity and therapeutic implications at a glance. Cell Commun Signal 2020;18(1):1–19.

5. Deng L, Jiang N, Zeng J, et al. The versatile roles of cancer-associated fibroblasts in colorectal cancer and therapeutic implications. Front Cell Dev Biol 2021;9(October):1–16.

6. Xin L, Gao J, Zheng Z, et al. Fibroblast activation protein-α as a target in the bench-to-bedside diagnosis and treatment of tumors: a narrative review. Front Oncol 2021;11(August). https://doi.org/10.3389/fonc.2021.648187.

7. Niedermeyer J, Garin-Chesa P, Kriz M, et al. Expression of the fibroblast activation protein during mouse embryo development. Int J Dev Biol 2001;45(2):445–7.

8. Jacob M, Chang L, Puré E. Fibroblast activation protein in remodeling tissues. Curr Mol Med 2012; 12(10):1220–43.

9. Liu F, Qi L, Liu B, et al. Fibroblast activation protein overexpression and clinical implications in solid tumors: a meta-analysis. PLoS One 2015;10(3):1–18.

10. Altmann A, Haberkorn U, Siveke J. The latest developments in imaging of fibroblast activation protein. J Nucl Med 2021;62(2):160–7.

11. Puré E, Blomberg R. Pro-tumorigenic roles of fibroblast activation protein in cancer: back to the basics. Oncogene 2018;37(32):4343–57.

12. Elboga U, Sahin E, Kus T, et al. Comparison of 68Ga-FAPI PET/CT and 18FDG PET/CT modalities in gastrointestinal system malignancies with peritoneal involvement. Mol Imaging Biol 2022. https://doi.org/10.1007/s11307-022-01729-x. 0123456789.

13. Kömek H, Can C, Kaplan İ, et al. Comparison of [68 Ga]Ga-DOTA-FAPI-04 PET/CT and [18F]FDG PET/CT in colorectal cancer. Eur J Nucl Med Mol Imag 2022;49(11):3898–909.

14. Zhao L, Pang Y, Luo Z, et al. Role of [68Ga]Ga-DOTA-FAPI-04 PET/CT in the evaluation of peritoneal carcinomatosis and comparison with [18F]-FDG PET/CT. Eur J Nucl Med Mol Imag 2021. https://doi.org/10.1007/s00259-020-05146-6.

15. Şahin E, Elboğa U, Çelen YZ, et al. Comparison of (68)Ga-DOTA-FAPI and (18)FDG PET/CT imaging modalities in the detection of liver metastases in patients with gastrointestinal system cancer. Eur J Radiol 2021;142:109867.

16. Koerber SA, Staudinger F, Kratochwil C, et al. The role of FAPI-PET/CT for patients with malignancies of the lower gastrointestinal tract – first clinical experience. J Nucl Med 2020. https://doi.org/10.2967/jnumed.119.237016. jnumed.119.237016.

17. Pang Y, Zhao L, Luo Z, et al. Comparison of 68 Ga-FAPI and 18 F-FDG uptake in gastric, duodenal, and colorectal cancers. Radiology 2020;(13):203275.

18. Qin C, Song Y, Gai Y, et al. Gallium-68-labeled fibroblast activation protein inhibitor PET in gastrointestinal cancer: insights into diagnosis and management. Eur J Nucl Med Mol Imag 2022;4228–40.

19. Cheng Z, Wang S, Xu S, et al. FAPI PET/CT in diagnostic and treatment management of colorectal cancer : review of current research status. J Clin Med 2023;12(2):577.

20. Kratochwil C, Flechsig P, Lindner T, et al. 68Ga-FAPI PET/CT: tracer uptake in 28 different kinds of cancer. J Nucl Med 2019;60(6):801–5.

21. Ichimasa K, Kudo SE, Miyachi H, et al. Risk stratification of T1 colorectal cancer metastasis to Lymph nodes: current status and perspective. Gut Liver 2021;15(6):818–26.

22. Backes Y, Elias SG, Groen JN, et al. Histologic factors associated with need for surgery in patients with pedunculated T1 colorectal Carcinomas. Gastroenterology 2018;154(6):1647–59.

23. Body A, Prenen H, Latham S, et al. The role of neoadjuvant chemotherapy in locally advanced colon cancer. Cancer Manag Res 2021;13:2567–79.

24. Seligmann JF. FOxTROT: neoadjuvant FOLFOX chemotherapy with or without panitumumab (Pan) for patients (pts) with locally advanced colon cancer (CC). J Clin Oncol 2020;38(15_suppl):4013.

25. Glynne-Jones R, Wyrwicz L, Tiret E, et al. Rectal cancer: ESMO Clinical Practice Guidelines for diagnosis, treatment and follow-up. Ann Oncol 2017; 28(Supplement 4):iv22–40.

26. Brouwer NPM, Stijns RCH, Lemmens VEPP, et al. Clinical lymph node staging in colorectal cancer; a flip of the coin? Eur J Surg Oncol 2018;44(8): 1241–6.

27. Polack M, Hagenaars SC, Couwenberg A, et al. Characteristics of tumour stroma in regional lymph node metastases in colorectal cancer patients: a theoretical framework for future diagnostic imaging with FAPI PET/CT. Clin Transl Oncol 2022;24(9): 1776–84.

28. Solano-iturri JD, Beitia M, Errarte P, et al. Altered expression of fibroblast activation protein- α (FAP) in colorectal adenoma-carcinoma sequence and in lymph node and liver metastases. Aging (Albany NY) 2020;12:1–22.

29. Henry LR, Lee HO, Lee JS, et al. Clinical implications of fibroblast activation protein in patients with colon cancer. Clin Cancer Res 2007;13(6):1736–41.

30. Guinney J, Dienstmann R, Wang X, et al. The consensus molecular subtypes of colorectal cancer. Nat Med 2015;21(11):1350–6.

31. Hoorn S Ten, De Back TR, Sommeijer DW, et al. Clinical value of consensus molecular subtypes in colorectal cancer: a systematic review and meta-analysis. J Natl Cancer Inst 2022;114(4):503–16.

32. Eide PW, Moosavi SH, Eilertsen IA, et al. Metastatic heterogeneity of the consensus molecular subtypes of colorectal cancer. npj Genomic Med 2021;6(1):59.

33. Strating E, Wassenaar E, Verhagen M, et al. Fibroblast activation protein identifies Consensus Molecular Subtype 4 in colorectal cancer and allows its detection by 68Ga-FAPI-PET imaging. Br J Cancer 2022;(February):1–11. https://doi.org/10.1038/s41416-022-01748-z.

34. Peters NA, Constantinides A, Ubink I, et al. Consensus molecular subtype 4 (CMS4)-targeted therapy in primary colon cancer: a proof-of-concept study. Front Oncol 2022;12:969855.

35. Trumpi K, Ubink I, Trinh A, et al. Neoadjuvant chemotherapy affects molecular classification of colorectal tumors. Oncogenesis 2017;6(7):e357.

36. Wei Y, Cheng K, Fu Z, et al. [(18)F]AlF-NOTA-FAPI-04 PET/CT uptake in metastatic lesions on PET/CT imaging might distinguish different pathological types of lung cancer. Eur J Nucl Med Mol Imag 2021. https://doi.org/10.1007/s00259-021-05638-z.

37. Mona CE, Benz MR, Hikmat F, et al. Correlation of (68)Ga-FAPi-46 PET biodistribution with FAP expression by immunohistochemistry in patients with solid cancers: interim analysis of a prospective translational exploratory study. J Nucl Med 2022;63(7):1021–6.

38. Kessler L, Ferdinandus J, Hirmas N, et al. 68)Ga-FAPI as a diagnostic tool in sarcoma: data from the (68)Ga-FAPI PET prospective observational trial. J Nucl Med 2022;63(1):89–95.

39. Segelman J, Granath F, Holm T, et al. Incidence, prevalence and risk factors for peritoneal carcinomatosis from colorectal cancer. Br J Surg 2012;99(5):699–705.

40. Elias D, Faron M, Iuga BS, et al. Prognostic similarities and differences in optimally resected liver metastases and peritoneal metastases from colorectal cancers. Ann Surg 2015;261(1):157–63.

41. Huang Y, Alzahrani NA, Chua TC, et al. Impacts of low peritoneal cancer index on the survival outcomes of patient with peritoneal carcinomatosis of colorectal origin. Int J Surg 2015;23(Pt A):181–5.

42. Dromain C, Leboulleux S, Auperin A, et al. Staging of peritoneal carcinomatosis: enhanced CT vs. PET/CT. Abdom Imaging 2008;33(1):87–93.

43. Sugarbaker PH. Laparoscopy in the diagnosis and treatment of peritoneal metastases. Ann Laparosc Endosc Surg 2019;4(42). https://doi.org/10.21037/ales.2019.04.04.

44. Sugarbaker PH, Zhu BW, Sese GB, et al. Peritoneal carcinomatosis from appendiceal cancer: results in 69 patients treated by cytoreductive surgery and intraperitoneal chemotherapy. Dis Colon Rectum 1993;36(4):323–9.

45. Sugarbaker PH. Intraperitoneal chemotherapy and cytoreductive surgery for the prevention and treatment of peritoneal carcinomatosis and sarcomatosis. Semin Surg Oncol 1998;14(3):254–61.

46. Goéré D, Souadka A, Faron M, et al. Extent of colorectal peritoneal carcinomatosis: attempt to define a threshold above which HIPEC does not offer survival benefit: a comparative study. Ann Surg Oncol 2015;22(9):2958–64.

47. van Oudheusden TR, Braam HJ, Luyer MDP, et al. Peritoneal cancer patients not suitable for cytoreductive surgery and HIPEC during explorative surgery: risk factors, treatment options, and prognosis. Ann Surg Oncol 2015;22(4):1236–42.

48. Laoukili J, Constantinides A, Wassenaar ECE, et al. Peritoneal metastases from colorectal cancer belong to Consensus Molecular Subtype 4 and are sensitised to oxaliplatin by inhibiting reducing capacity. Br J Cancer 2022;126(12):1824–33.

49. Lenos KJ, Bach S, Ferreira Moreno L, et al. Molecular characterization of colorectal cancer related peritoneal metastatic disease. Nat Commun 2022;13(1):4443.

50. van 't Sant I, van Eden WJ, Engbersen MP, et al. Diffusion-weighted MRI assessment of the peritoneal cancer index before cytoreductive surgery. Br J Surg 2019;106(4):491–8.

51. van Gestel YRBM, Thomassen I, Lemmens VEPP, et al. Metachronous peritoneal carcinomatosis after curative treatment of colorectal cancer. Eur J Surg Oncol J Eur Soc Surg Oncol Br Assoc Surg Oncol 2014;40(8):963–9.

52. Bastiaenen VP, Klaver CEL, Kok NFM, et al. Second and third look laparoscopy in pT4 colon cancer patients for early detection of peritoneal metastases; the COLOPEC 2 randomized multicentre trial. BMC Cancer 2019;19(1):1–12.

53. Franko J, Shi Q, Goldman CD, et al. Treatment of colorectal peritoneal carcinomatosis with systemic chemotherapy: a pooled analysis of north central cancer treatment group phase III trials N9741 and N9841. J Clin Oncol Off J Am Soc Clin Oncol 2012;30(3):263–7.

54. Tseng J, Bryan DS, Poli E, et al. Under-representation of peritoneal metastases in published clinical trials of metastatic colorectal cancer. Lancet Oncol 2017;18(6):711–2.

55. Heger U, Mack C, Schillings L, et al. FAPI-PET imaging for assessment of response to induction chemotherapy for locally advanced pancreatic cancer. HPB 2021;23(3):S888–9.

56. Lee IK, Noguera-Ortega E, Xiao Z, et al. Monitoring therapeutic response to anti-fibroblast activation protein (FAP) CAR T cells using [18F]AlF-FAPI-74.

Clin Cancer Res 2022. https://doi.org/10.1158/1078-0432.CCR-22-1379.

57. O'Neil M, Damjanov I. Histopathology of colorectal cancer after neoadjuvant Chemoradiation therapy. Open Pathol J 2009;3(2):91–8.

58. Chen H, Zhao L, Ruan D, et al. Usefulness of [(68) Ga]Ga-DOTA-FAPI-04 PET/CT in patients presenting with inconclusive [(18)F]FDG PET/CT findings. Eur J Nucl Med Mol Imag 2021;48(1):73–86.

59. Rovers KP, Bakkers C, Simkens GAAM, et al. Perioperative systemic therapy and cytoreductive surgery with HIPEC versus upfront cytoreductive surgery with HIPEC alone for isolated resectable colorectal peritoneal metastases: protocol of a multicentre, open-label, parallel-group, phase II-III, rando. BMC Cancer 2019;19(1):390.

60. Rovers KP, Wassenaar ECE, Lurvink RJ, et al. Pressurized intraperitoneal aerosol chemotherapy (oxaliplatin) for unresectable colorectal peritoneal metastases: a multicenter, single-arm, phase II trial (CRC-PIPAC). Ann Surg Oncol 2021;28(9):5311–26.

61. Sahin IH, Akce M, Alese O, et al. Immune checkpoint inhibitors for the treatment of MSI-H/MMR-D colorectal cancer and a perspective on resistance mechanisms. Br J Cancer 2019;121(10):809–18.

62. André T, Shiu K-K, Kim TW, et al. Pembrolizumab in microsatellite-instability-high advanced colorectal cancer. N Engl J Med 2020;383(23):2207–18.

63. Hanley CJ, Thomas GJ. Targeting cancer associated fibroblasts to enhance immunotherapy: emerging strategies and future perspectives. Oncotarget 2021;12(14):1427–33.

64. Kieffer Y, Hocine HR, Gentric G, et al. Single-cell analysis reveals fibroblast Clusters linked to immunotherapy resistance in cancer. Cancer Discov 2020;10(9):1330–51.

65. Chen L, Qiu X, Wang X, et al. FAP positive fibroblasts induce immune checkpoint blockade resistance in colorectal cancer via promoting immunosuppression. Biochem Biophys Res Commun 2017;487(1):8–14.

66. Qi J, Sun H, Zhang Y, et al. Single-cell and spatial analysis reveal interaction of FAP + fibroblasts and SPP1 + macrophages in colorectal cancer. Nat Commun 2022;13(1):1–20.

67. Khaliq AM, Erdogan C, Kurt Z, et al. Refining colorectal cancer classification and clinical stratification through a single-cell atlas. Genome Biol 2022; 23(1):1–30.

68. Rong X, Lv J, Liu Y, et al. PET/CT imaging of activated cancer-associated fibroblasts predict response to PD-1 blockade in gastric cancer patients. Front Oncol 2022;11(January):1–10.

69. Tauriello F, Palomo-ponce S, Stork D, et al. TGF β drives immune evasion in genetically reconstituted colon cancer metastasis. Nature 2018;554(7693): 538–43.

70. Mariathasan S, Turley SJ, Nickles D, et al. TGFβ attenuates tumour response to PD-L1 blockade by contributing to exclusion of T cells. Nature 2018; 554(7693):544–8.

71. Ford K, Hanley CJ, Mellone M, et al. NOX4 inhibition potentiates immunotherapy by overcoming cancer-associated fibroblast-mediated CD8 T-cell exclusion from tumors. Cancer Res 2020;80(9):1846–60.

72. Kleinendorst SC, Oosterwijk E, Bussink J, et al. Combining targeted radionuclide therapy and immune checkpoint inhibition for cancer treatment. Clin Cancer Res 2022;28(17):3652–7.

73. Eiber M, Kratochwil C, Lapa C, et al. Nuklearmedizinische Theranostik. Der Onkol. 2021;27(8):809–19.

Fibroblast Activation Protein Inhibitor PET/CT in Gastric Cancer

Tadashi Watabe, MD, PhD[a,b,]*, Frederik L. Giesel, MD, MBA[b,c]

KEYWORDS

• Fibroblast activation protein • Positron emission tomography • Gastric cancer

KEY POINTS

- The utility of [18F]fluorodeoxyglucose (FDG)-PET is rather limited in gastric cancer owing to the physiologic accumulation and existence of cases with low uptake.
- Fibroblast activation protein inhibitor (FAPI)-PET shows higher accumulation in the primary site and metastatic lesions than does FDG-PET, especially in detection of peritoneal carcinomatosis.
- In the case of gastric signet ring cell carcinoma, FAPI-PET showed excellent performance as uptake is usually weak on FDG-PET in this cohort.

INTRODUCTION

The tumor microenvironment is closely related to cancer invasion and metastasis. Cancer-associated fibroblasts (CAFs) are major component of the cancer stroma and play an important role in cancer growth and progression.[1] CAFs express fibroblast activation protein (FAP), and FAP expression levels have been reported to correlate with prognosis in patients with cancer.[1] In addition, FAP expression has been confirmed in various cancer types, with minimal expression in normal organs.[2,3] FAP inhibitor (FAPI), a ligand of FAP, is attracting attention as an excellent PET probe that can accurately detect many types of cancer compared with the conventional glucose analog of [18F]fluorodeoxyglucose (FDG). 68Ga-labeled FAPI ([68Ga]FAPI-04 or [68Ga]FAPI-46) and 18F-labeled FAPI ([18F]FAPI-74) are mainly available for clinical use.[4–6] Recently, the number of published papers reporting the usefulness of FAPI-PET has increased, and clinical trials are being conducted in Europe, the United States, China, and elsewhere. It is expected that FAPI-PET will be used more commonly in cancer diagnosis and treatment in the future.

In this article, the authors focus on FAPI-PET imaging of gastric cancer based on recent reports and our experience.

CURRENT STATUS OF [18F] FLUORODEOXYGLUCOSE-PET IMAGING IN GASTRIC CANCER

In current clinical practice, [18F]FDG PET is the standard of care for the diagnosis of initial staging, evaluation of treatment response, and detection of recurrent lesions in patients with cancer. However, the utility of [18F]FDG PET is limited in gastric cancer compared with that in other malignancies. The disadvantages of FDG-PET in gastric cancers are as follows: (1) physiologic accumulation is often observed in the stomach, (2) gastric cancer lesions sometimes show faint uptake, and (3) thickening of the stomach wall is difficult to detect on computed tomography (CT) unless gastric distension protocols are used, which leads to difficulty in identifying matched lesions on PET/CT.[7] In particular,

[a] Department of Nuclear Medicine and Tracer Kinetics, Graduate School of Medicine, Osaka University, 2-2 Yamadaoka, Suita, Osaka 565-0871, Japan; [b] Institute for Radiation Sciences, Osaka University; [c] Department of Nuclear Medicine, University Hosptial Duesseldorf (UKD), Geb. 13.52.01.50, Moorenstrasse 5D-40225 Düsseldorf, Germany
* Corresponding author.
E-mail address: watabe@tracer.med.osaka-u.ac.jp

PET Clin 18 (2023) 337–344
https://doi.org/10.1016/j.cpet.2023.02.009
1556-8598/23/© 2023 Elsevier Inc. All rights reserved.

Table 1
Summary of recent papers that reported the utility and superiority of fibroblast activation protein inhibitor (FAPI)-PET in gastric cancers compared with [18F]fluorodeoxyglucose (FDG)-PET

Reference No	Year	Author	Journal	Total	Primary Staging	PET Probe	Primary Tumor		
							Detection	SUVmax (FDG vs FAPI)	Number (FDG vs FAPI)
Pang et al,[12] 2021	2021	Pang Y, et al	Radiology	35	19	[68Ga]FAPI-04	FDG < FAPI	3.7 vs 12.7 (median)	4 vs 11
Qin et al,[13] 2022	2022	Qin C, et al	J Nucl Med	20	14	[68Ga]FAPI-04	FDG < FAPI	6.2 vs 11.3 (mean)	10 vs 14
Kuten et al,[14] 2022	2022	Kuten J, et al	Eur J Nucl Med Mol Imaging	13	10	[68Ga]FAPI-04	FDG < FAPI	4.5 vs 12.9 (mean)	10 vs 10
Jiang et al,[15] 2022	2022	Jiang D, et al	Eur J Nucl Med Mol Imaging	38	38	[68Ga]FAPI-04	FDG < FAPI	4.5 vs 11.0[a] (mean)	12 vs 17[a]
Fu et al,[16] 2022	2022	Fu L, et al	European Radiology	61	61	[68Ga]FAPI-04 and [18F]FAPI-42	FDG < FAPI	4.4 vs 14.6 (mean)	45 vs 58
Lin et al,[17] 2022	2022	Lin R, et al	Eur J Nucl Med Mol Imaging	56	45	[68Ga]FAPI-04	FDG < FAPI	8.1 vs 10.3 (mean)	44 vs 45
Chen et al,[18] 2022	2022	Chen H, et al	European Radiology	34	22	[68Ga]FAPI-04	FDG < FAPI	2.2 vs 5.2 (median)	4 vs 16

Reference No	LN Metastasis			Other Metastasis		
	Detection	SUVmax (FDG vs FAPI)	Number (FDG vs FAPI)	Detection	SUVmax of Peritoneal Metastases (FDG vs FAPI)	Number of Peritoneal Metastases (FDG vs FAPI)
Pang et al,[12] 2021	FDG < FAPI[b]	2.4 vs 6.7 (median)	48 vs 96	FDG < FAPI[b]	3.6 vs 8.4 (median)	51 vs 93
Qin et al,[13] 2022	FDG < FAPI	6.6 vs 9.9 (mean)	33 vs 45	FDG < FAPI	7.6 vs 8.4 (mean)	14 vs 42
Kuten et al,[14] 2022	FDG = FAPI	4.9 vs 6.5 (mean)	16 vs 17	FDG < FAPI	2.0 vs 10.7 (mean)	2 vs 2
Jiang et al,[15] 2022	FDG = FAPI	NA	5 vs 6	NA		
Fu et al,[16] 2022	FDG < FAPI	2.8 vs 8.7 (mean)	407 vs 637	FDG < FAPI	2.5 vs 9.9 (mean)	14 vs 24
Lin et al,[17] 2022	FDG = FAPI	7.6 vs 7.4 (mean)	16 vs 20	FDG < FAPI	6.0 vs 8.2 (mean)	47 vs 159
Chen et al,[18] 2022	FDG < FAPI	2.5 vs 6.8 (median)	38 vs 83	FDG < FAPI	2.3 vs 6.3 (median)	20 vs 59

a In primary tumors >4 cm.
b Including duodenal and colorectal cancers.

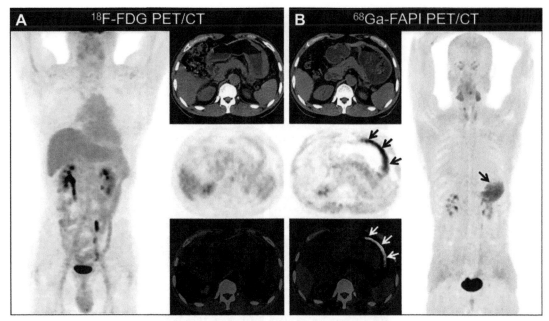

Fig. 1. A 55-year-old man with known gastric signet ring cell carcinoma who underwent [18F]FDG PET/CT for initial staging. (*A*) [18F]FDG PET/CT demonstrating normal findings (left image: anterior maximum intensity projection image obtained using [18F]FDG PET; right upper image: axial unenhanced CT image; right middle image: axial PET image; right lower image: axial fused PET/CT image). (*B*) Images obtained during [68Ga]FAPI PET/CT performed for further evaluation revealed intense [68Ga]FAPI uptake along the gastric wall (*arrows*) (maximum standardized uptake value, 11) (right image: anterior maximum intensity projection image obtained using [18F]FDG PET; left upper image: axial unenhanced CT image; left middle image: axial PET image; left lower image: axial fused PET/CT image). No distant metastasis was observed. (*From* Pang Y, Zhao L, Luo Z, et al. Comparison of 68Ga-FAPI and 18F-FDG Uptake in Gastric, Duodenal, and Colorectal Cancers. Radiology 2021;298:393-402.)

gastric signet ring cell carcinoma (SRCC) shows low FDG uptake and low sensitivity for its detection on [18F]FDG PET/CT.[8] Owing to the above background, the use of FDG-PET in gastric cancer is relatively limited compared with other cancers in oncology.

FIBROBLAST ACTIVATION PROTEIN EXPRESSION IN GASTRIC CANCER

FAP is reported to be expressed in the CAFs of more than 90% of human epithelial cancers.[9] FAP has also been identified as a novel biomarker that significantly contributes to the poor prognosis of stomach adenocarcinoma, and increased FAP expression is related to a more advanced tumor stage.[10] It has been suggested that there is a close relationship between FAP expression and the state of the tumor microenvironment. According to the Human Protein Atlas Web site, among major cancers, gastric cancer exhibits mid-level FAP RNA expression and the second highest FAP protein expression, followed by breast cancer and pancreatic cancer.[11] Considering these reports and atlas information, gastric cancer can be a good indication for FAPI-PET imaging.

CLINICAL APPLICATIONS OF FIBROBLAST ACTIVATION PROTEIN INHIBITOR-PET IN GASTRIC CANCER

Many recent studies have reported the utility and superiority of FAPI-PET in gastric cancers compared with FDG-PET (**Table 1**). For example, Pang and colleagues reported the superiority of [68Ga]FAPI-04 in 20 patients with gastric cancer (11 patients for initial staging and 9 for recurrence detection: moderately or poorly differentiated adenocarcinoma [$n = 11$] and SRCC [$n = 9$]) (**Figs. 1** and **2**).[12] Moreover, FAPI uptake was higher with [68Ga]FAPI-04 PET/CT than with [18F]FDG PET/CT in primary lesions (gastric cancer: 12.7 vs 3.7, respectively, $P = .003$). In addition, [68Ga]FAPI-04 PET also detected more lymph node (LN) and peritoneal metastases, particularly in SRCC cases.

Furthermore, Qin and colleagues evaluated 20 patients with histologically proven gastric carcinomas (14 patients for initial staging and 6 for recurrence detection: poorly differentiated adenocarcinoma [$n = 10$], SRCC [$n = 4$], and so forth). They reported that [68Ga]FAPI-04 PET was superior to [18F]FDG PET in the detection of primary

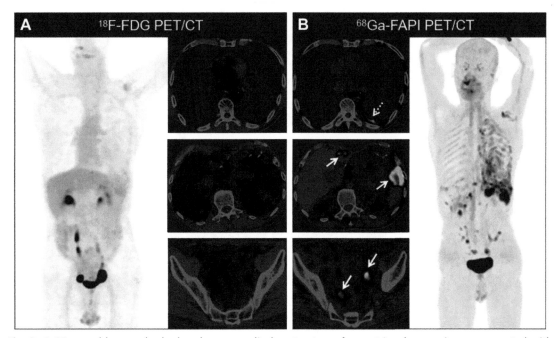

Fig. 2. A 66-year-old man who had undergone radical gastrectomy for gastric adenocarcinoma presented with abdominal pain and elevated tumor marker levels. (*A*) Images from [^{18}F]FDG PET/CT show thickened pleura and multiple nodules in the peritoneum and mesentery, with low-to-moderate [^{18}F]FDG activity in these lesions (left image: anterior maximum intensity projection image from [^{18}F]FDG PET; right images: axial fused PET/CT images). (*B*) Images from [^{68}Ga]FAPI PET/CT show much higher tracer uptake in the thickened pleura (*dashed arrow*) and peritoneal nodules (*solid arrows*) (right image: anterior maximum intensity projection image from [^{18}F]FDG PET; left images: axial fused PET/CT images). A subsequent biopsy of the pleura and peritoneal nodules revealed metastatic gastric adenocarcinoma (poorly differentiated). (*From* Pang Y, Zhao L, Luo Z, et al. Comparison of ^{68}Ga-FAPI and ^{18}F-FDG Uptake in Gastric, Duodenal, and Colorectal Cancers. Radiology 2021;298:393-402.)

tumors with higher uptake (100% [14/14] vs 71.4% [10/14]; $P = .034$) and metastases in the peritoneum, abdominal LNs, liver, and bones (**Fig. 3**).[13] However, the detection ability of [^{68}Ga]FAPI-04 PET for ovarian metastases was not better than that of [^{18}F]FDG.

Kuten and colleagues performed a head-to-head prospective comparison between [^{68}Ga] FAPI-04 PET and [^{18}F]FDG PET in 13 patients with gastric adenocarcinoma (most of them were poorly differentiated adenocarcinomas) who presented for either initial staging ($n = 10$) or restaging ($n = 3$).[14] All ten primary gastric tumors were FAPI-positive (100% detection rate), whereas only five were also FDG-positive (50%). The tumor-to-background ratio (TBR) was significantly higher for FAPI (mean: 12.9 [range: 2.2–23.9]) than for FDG (4.5 [0.8–9.7]). Although the detection rates of regional LN involvement were comparable, FAPI showed a superior detection rate for peritoneal carcinomatosis (100% vs none).

Jiang and colleagues evaluated 38 patients with therapy-naive gastric cancer with histopathologic confirmation (31 with adenocarcinoma and 7 with SRCC). For detection of the primary lesion, the sensitivities of [^{68}Ga]FAPI-04 PET and [^{18}F] FDG PET were 100% (38/38) and 82% (31/38), respectively ($P = .016$).[15] Four cases of adenocarcinoma and three cases of SRCC were missed on [^{18}F]FDG PET. The mean maximum standardized uptake value (SUVmax) of FAPI was higher in T2–4 tumors (9.7 $\pm$ 4.4) than in T1 tumors (3.1 $\pm$ 1.5) ($P = .0002$). For the detection of metastatic lesions, the sensitivities of [^{68}Ga]FAPI-04 PET and [^{18}F]FDG PET in the 10 patients with regional LN metastasis and distant metastasis were 6/10 and 5/10, respectively. These data suggested that it is essential to improve the detection rate of metastatic lesion by FAPI-PET to avoid invasive staging, such as diagnostic laparoscopy.

Fu and colleagues retrospectively compared [^{68}Ga]Ga-FAPI-04/[^{18}F]FAPI-42 PET/CT with [^{18}F] FDG PET/CT in 61 patients with an initial gastric cancer.[16] The pathologic types of the disease were highly and/or moderately differentiated adenocarcinoma ($n = 10$), moderately and poorly differentiated adenocarcinoma ($n = 8$), poorly

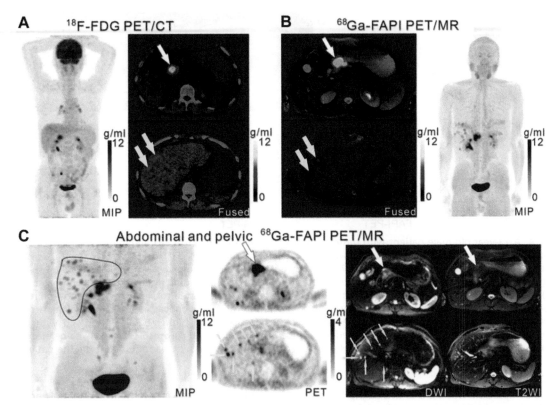

Fig. 3. A 61-year-old man with moderately differentiated gastric adenocarcinoma. In addition to the primary tumor (*A: white arrow*, SUVmax = 11.0), two foci of elevated activity in the liver were noted on the [18F]FDG PET/CT images (*A*: yellow *arrows*, SUVmax = 5.8). On the [68Ga]FAPI PET/MR images, the primary tumor had more intense uptake (*B* and *C: white arrows*, SUVmax = 14.2), and the two hepatic lesions had more prominent [68Ga]FAPI accumulation (*B: yellow arrows*, SUVmax = 7.6). In addition, multiple foci of increased [68Ga]FAPI activity were also revealed in the liver (*C: red outline, yellow arrows*), which corresponded to multiple high signals on DWI (*yellow arrows*), suggesting multiple hepatic metastases. DWI, diffusion weighted imaging. This research was originally published in JNM. Qin C, Shao F, Gai Y, et al., 68Ga-DOTA-FAPI-04 PET/MR in the Evaluation of Gastric Carcinomas: Comparison with 18F-FDG PET/CT. J Nucl Med 2022 Jan;63(1):81-88. © SNMMI.

differentiated adenocarcinoma without SRCC ($n = 13$), poorly differentiated adenocarcinoma containing SRCC ($n = 21$), SRCC ($n = 7$), and other types ($n = 2$). Lesions containing SRCC occurred in 45.9% (28/61) of patients. For primary lesions, higher uptake of FAPI than of FDG was observed (median SUVmax, 14.60 vs 4.35, $P < .001$), resulting in higher positive detection using FAPI-PET than FDG-PET (95.1% vs 73.8%, $P < .001$), particularly for tumors with SRCC (96.4% vs 57.1%, $P < .001$). FAPI PET/CT detected more positive LNs than did FDG PET/CT (637 vs 407). However, both modalities underestimated N staging compared with pathologic N staging. FAPI PET/CT showed a higher sensitivity (92.3% vs 53.8%, $P = .002$) and peritoneal cancer index score (18 vs 3, $P < .001$) in peritoneum metastasis and other suspected metastases than did FDG PET/CT.

Lin and colleagues evaluated 56 patients with histologically proven gastric carcinomas, including 45 patients for staging and 11 patients for restaging after surgery, of which 17 (37.8%) contained SRCC.[17] [68Ga]FAPI-04 PET/CT was comparable with [18F]FDG in detecting primary tumors and LN metastases, whereas FAPI outperformed FDG in detecting peritoneal (159 vs 47, $P < .001$) and bone metastases (64 vs 55, $P = .003$) on lesion-based analysis. Compared with [18F]FDG PET, FAPI-PET showed higher SUVmax (10.3 vs 8.1, $P = .004$) and TBR (11.6 vs 5.8, $P < .001$) in the primary tumor, and higher TBR in LN involvement (8.0 vs 3.7, $P < .001$) and peritoneal metastases (8.1 vs 3.2, $P < .001$). The specificity and positive predictive value of FAPI were significantly higher than those of FDG (100.0% vs 97.7%, $P < .001$; 100.0% vs 57.1%, $P = .001$, respectively) in determining LN status. The excellent specificity and positive predictive value of FAPI-PET indicated that it can lead to the proper staging and appropriate patient management. The FAPI

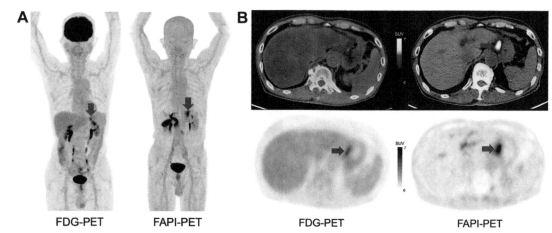

Fig. 4. A 73-year old male patient with gastric cancer underwent [^{18}F]FAPI-74 PET and [^{18}F]FDG PET after three courses of preoperative chemotherapy (docetaxel, oxaliplatin, and S-1). [^{18}F]FDG PET showed mild uptake in the stomach (SUVmax = 5.5), and [^{18}F]FAPI-74 PET showed more intense and extensive uptake in the corresponding area (SUVmax = 8.2) (*red arrows*) without metastatic lesions: (*A*) Maximum intensity projection images and (*B*) axial PET/CT fusion and PET images. The patient underwent a robot-assisted total gastrectomy and lymphadenectomy. The pathologic diagnosis was residual poorly differentiated adenocarcinoma without lymph node metastasis. [^{18}F]FAPI-74 PET clearly detected residual active lesions with higher uptake compared with [^{18}F]FDG-PET. [^{18}F]FAPI-74 PET scan was performed in a clinical research. The study protocol was approved by the institutional review board of Osaka University Hospital. Written informed consent was obtained from the patient.

was comparable with FDG in evaluating N staging (47.1% vs 23.5%, P = .282). FAPI PET/CT detected more positive recurrent lesions in all restaging patients and showed clearer tumor delineation.

Chen and colleagues evaluated 34 patients with histologically confirmed SRCCs and showed excellent performance of [^{68}Ga]FAPI-04 PET compared with [^{18}F]FDG PET.[18] [^{68}Ga]FAPI-04 PET showed higher SUVmax and TBR values than did [^{18}F]FDG PET in the primary tumors (SUVmax: 5.2 vs 2.2, P = .001; TBR: 7.6 vs 1.3, P < .001), involved LNs (SUVmax: 6.8 vs 2.5, P < .001; TBR: 5.8 vs 1.3, P < .001), and bone and visceral metastases (SUVmax: 6.5 vs 2.4, P < .001; TBR: 6.3 vs 1.3, P < .001). In diagnostic performance, [^{68}Ga]FAPI-04 PET exhibited higher sensitivity than [^{18}F]FDG PET for detecting primary tumors (73% [16/22] vs 18% [4/22], P < .001), local recurrence (100% [7/7] vs 29% [2/7], P = .071), LN metastases (77% [59/77] vs 23% [18/77], P < .001), and distant metastases (93% [207/222] vs 39% [86/222], P < .001).

Kratochwil and colleagues reported FAPI uptake in 28 different kinds of cancer, with an SUVmax value of approximately 5.0 in gastric cancer (n = 3); which belongs to the relatively low uptake group compared with many other types of cancer.[3] However, the reported value in the other studies was approximately 10 to 15 in SUVmax on average, which is also higher than FDG uptake.

Previous reports by Kratochwil and colleagues might have underestimated the FAPI uptake in gastric cancer due to the limited number of included patients. In addition, a pretest selection bias may have also be in operation here with many clinicians not using FDG PET/CT for other than intestinal type adenocarcinoma because of recognized limitations in diffuse gastric cancer (SRCC).

In the interpretation of FAPI-PET images, there is a need to be careful about specificity. There are several pitfalls of noncancer uptake in benign lesions. A previous study reported that benign uptake occurs in bone degeneration, wound healing, the endometrium, and inflammation including pancreatitis and pneumonia.[19,20] Benign tumors sometimes showed high FAPI uptakes in renal angiomyolipoma, thyroid adenoma, necrotizing granuloma, and splenic hemangioma.[20]

In one study, the specificity of [^{68}Ga]FAPI PET/CT was not higher than that of [^{18}F]FDG (82% [46 of 56] vs 89% [50 of 56], respectively; P = .50).[12] In another, the specificity of FAPI-PET was lower than that of [^{18}F]FDG PET (46% vs 71%) for bone and visceral metastases because more false-positive lesions were observed on [^{68}Ga]FAPI PET (including myelofibrosis [n = 6/24], arthritis [n = 2/24], granulomatous disease [n = 2/24], uterine fibroid [n = 1/24], pneumonia [n = 1/24], and esophagitis [n = 1/24]).[18] However, in the study of Lin and colleagues, the specificity for metastatic disease was superior.[17] Therefore, there is a need for careful interpretation regarding the possibility of benign or inflammatory uptake on FAPI-PET to maintain a high positive predictive value, particularly if avoidance of invasive staging or curative treatment would be considered based on PET/CT findings.

Regarding the labeling radionuclide for FAPI, the short half-life of ^{68}Ga (68 minute) can be a limitation for its production and delivery. ^{18}F-labeling (half-life = 110 minute) will enable large-scale production such as [^{18}F]FDG and will have wider availability. Evaluation using [^{18}F]FAPI-74 also shows excellent performance in gastric cancer.[21] A case study presentation using [^{18}F]FAPI-74 is shown in **Fig. 4**.

SUMMARY

The utility of FAPI-PET imaging in gastric cancer is summarized in this article. FAPI-PET shows higher accumulation in primary sites and metastatic lesions than does FDG-PET, especially for the detection of peritoneal carcinomatosis. In the case of gastric SRCC, FAPI-PET showed excellent performance because uptake is usually weak on FDG-PET in this cohort of patients. It is highly expected that FAPI-PET will be increasingly used in the diagnosis and treatment planning of gastric cancer.

CLINICS CARE POINTS

- Fibroblast activation protein inhibitor (FAPI)-PET should be considered for pretreatment evaluation of gastric cancers if [^{18}F]fluorodeoxyglucose (FDG)-PET shows weak uptake.
- If the histologic type is gastric signet ring cell carcinoma, FAPI-PET is strongly recommended.
- FAPI-PET is useful for the detection of peritoneal carcinomatosis in gastric cancer.

FUNDING

This study was funded by the QiSS program of OPERA (Grant Number: JPMJOP1721) from the Japan Science and Technology Agency. The authors declare no potential conflicts of interest relevant to this study. FLG is advisor at ABX Radiopharmaceuticals, SOFIE Biosciences, Telix pharma 301 and Alpha Fusion. FLG has also shares in a consultancy group for iTheranostics. The precursor of FAPI was provided by SOFIE Biosciences, which holds a license to the FAPI family of compounds for diagnostic use.

DISCLOSURE

FLG is advisor at ABX Radiopharmaceuticals, SOFIE Biosciences, Telix pharma 301 and Alpha Fusion. FLG has also shares in a consultancy group for iTheranostics.

REFERENCES

1. Kobayashi H, Enomoto A, Woods SL, et al. Cancer-associated fibroblasts in gastrointestinal cancer. Nat Rev Gastroenterol Hepatol 2019;16:282–95.
2. Giesel FL, Kratochwil C, Lindner T, et al. 68Ga-FAPI PET/CT: biodistribution and preliminary dosimetry estimate of 2 DOTA-containing FAP-targeting agents in patients with various cancers. J Nucl Med 2019; 60:386–92.
3. Kratochwil C, Flechsig P, Lindner T, et al. 68Ga-FAPI PET/CT: tracer uptake in 28 different kinds of cancer. J Nucl Med 2019;60:801–5.
4. Loktev A, Lindner T, Burger EM, et al. Development of fibroblast activation protein-targeted radiotracers with improved tumor retention. J Nucl Med 2019; 60:1421–9.
5. Giesel FL, Adeberg S, Syed M, et al. FAPI-74 PET/CT using either ^{18}F-AlF or cold-kit ^{68}Ga labeling: biodistribution, radiation dosimetry, and tumor delineation in lung cancer patients. J Nucl Med 2021;62:201–7.
6. Naka S, Watabe T, Lindner T, et al. One-pot and one-step automated radio-synthesis of [18F]AlF-FAPI-74 using a multi purpose synthesizer: a proof-of-concept experiment. EJNMMI Radiopharm Chem 2021;6:28.
7. Le Roux PY, Duong CP, Cabalag CS, et al. Incremental diagnostic utility of gastric distension FDG PET/CT. Eur J Nucl Med Mol Imaging 2016;43(4): 644–53.
8. Dondi F, Albano D, Giubbini R, et al. 18F-FDG PET and PET/CT for the evaluation of gastric signet ring cell carcinoma: a systematic review. Nucl Med Commun 2021;42:1293–300.
9. Zhi K, Shen X, Zhang H, et al. Cancer-associated fibroblasts are positively correlated with metastatic potential of human gastric cancers. J Exp Clin Cancer Res 2010;29(1):66.
10. Lyu Z, Li Y, Zhu D, et al. Fibroblast activation protein-alpha is a prognostic biomarker associated with ferroptosis in stomach adenocarcinoma. Front Cell Dev Biol 2022;10:859999.
11. The human protein atlas, Available at: https://www.proteinatlas.org/ENSG00000078098-FAP/pathology. Accessed March 18, 2023.
12. Pang Y, Zhao L, Luo Z, et al. Comparison of ^{68}Ga-FAPI and ^{18}F-FDG uptake in gastric, duodenal,

and colorectal cancers. Radiology 2021;298: 393–402.

13. Qin C, Shao F, Gai Y, et al. ^{68}Ga-DOTA-FAPI-04 PET/MR in the evaluation of gastric carcinomas: comparison with ^{18}F-FDG PET/CT. J Nucl Med 2022;63(1): 81–8.

14. Kuten J, Levine C, Shamni O, et al. Head-to-head comparison of [68Ga]Ga-FAPI-04 and [18F]-FDG PET/CT in evaluating the extent of disease in gastric adenocarcinoma. Eur J Nucl Med Mol Imaging 2022;49:743–50.

15. Jiang D, Chen X, You Z, et al. Comparison of [68 Ga]Ga-FAPI-04 and [18F]-FDG for the detection of primary and metastatic lesions in patients with gastric cancer: a bicentric retrospective study. Eur J Nucl Med Mol Imaging 2022;49:732–42.

16. Fu L, Huang S, Wu H, et al. Superiority of [68Ga]Ga-FAPI-04/[18F]FAPI-42 PET/CT to [18F]FDG PET/CT in delineating the primary tumor and peritoneal metastasis in initial gastric cancer. Eur Radiol 2022;32:6281–90.

17. Lin R, Lin Z, Chen Z, et al. [68Ga]Ga-DOTA-FAPI-04 PET/CT in the evaluation of gastric cancer: comparison with [18F]FDG PET/CT. Eur J Nucl Med Mol Imaging 2022;49:2960–71.

18. Chen H, Pang Y, Li J, et al. Comparison of [68Ga]Ga-FAPI and [18F]FDG uptake in patients with gastric signet-ring-cell carcinoma: a multicenter retrospective study. Eur Radiol 2022;33(2):1329–41.

19. Kessler L, Ferdinandus J, Hirmas N, et al. Pitfalls and common findings in ^{68}Ga-FAPI PET: a pictorial analysis. J Nucl Med 2022;63:890–6.

20. Hotta M, Rieger AC, Jafarvand MG, et al. Non-oncologic incidental uptake on FAPI PET/CT imaging. Br J Radiol 2022;20220463.

21. Watabe T, Naka S, Tatsumi M. et al. Initial evaluation of [18F]FAPI-74 PET for various histopathologically confirmed cancers and benign lesions. J Nucl Med. 2023 (in press).

Current Status of Fibroblast Activation Protein Imaging in Gynecologic Malignancy and Breast Cancer

Katharina Dendl, Can.Med[a,b,*], Stefan A. Koerber, MD, PD Dr[c,d],
Tadashi Watabe, MD, PhD, Prof[e], Uwe Haberkorn, Prof. Dr., MD[a],
Frederik L. Giesel, Prof. Dr. MD[a,b]

KEYWORDS

- Fibroblast activation protein inhibitor (FAPI) • PET/CT • Gynecological malignancies • Breast cancer
- FAP

KEY POINTS

- FAPI-PET/computed tomography demonstrated encouraging results in gynecologic malignancies urging more extensive and prospective studies to follow.
- FAPI seems to be equal or even superior compared with fluordesoxyglucose (FDG) in most included gynecologic malignancies.
- Hormone-sensitive organs supposedly present varying ^{68}Ga-FAPI uptake, requiring cautious interpretation.

INTRODUCTION

^{68}Ga-FAPI-PET/computed tomography (CT) targets specific cells within the tumor stroma. These are cancer-associated fibroblasts, which overexpress the fibroblast activation protein (FAP). FAP is a membrane-anchored serine protease with both dipeptidyl peptidase and endopeptidase activities.[1] Through stromal modification, FAP can promote tumorigenesis.[2] ^{68}Ga-FAPI-PET/CT has recently emerged as an intriguing imaging tool, particularly in cases where ^{18}F-FDG, the conventional oncologic PET tracer, faces challenges. The rather low expression of FAP in normal tissue as well as the rapid elimination from the circulation contribute to a high sensitivity through the excellent image contrast achieved.[3,4] ^{68}Ga-FAPI has already been evaluated in numerous patients suffering from a range of tumor types.[5–7]

Breast cancer, known to be the most common tumor entity in women worldwide,[8] might profit from ^{68}Ga-FAPI-PET/CT as it abundantly overexpresses FAP in the surrounding stroma, and sometimes in cancer cells themselves,[9] potentially ensuring a strong signal. In particular, some variants of breast cancer, lobular carcinoma in particular, can have low FDG-avidity, limiting the utility of conventional PET/CT.[10] Furthermore, other female-sex-associated cancers like ovarian cancer, currently lack reliable early detection and might benefit enormously from alternative imaging strategies.[11] Thus, in this review, we aim to elucidate the current state of the art of FAPI-PET/CT in imaging breast cancer and the dominant gynecologic tumor types.

[a] Department of Nuclear Medicine, INF 400, University Hospital Heidelberg, Heidelberg, Germany; [b] Deaprtment of Nuclear medicine, Geb. 13.55, Moorenstraße 5, 40225 Düsseldorf; [c] Department of Radioncology and Radiation Therapy, Krankenhaus Barmherzige Brüder, Prüfeninger Str. 86 93049 Regensburg, Germany; [d] Department of Radiooncology and Radiation Therapy, University Hospital Heidelberg; [e] Department of Nuclear Medicine, 2-15 Yamadaoka, Suita, Osaka 565-0871, Japan
* Corresponding author. Department of Nuclear Medicine, INF 400, University Hospital Heidelberg, Heidelberg, Germany.
E-mail address: Katharina_11@icloud.com

PET Clin 18 (2023) 345–351
https://doi.org/10.1016/j.cpet.2023.03.005
1556-8598/23/© 2023 Elsevier Inc. All rights reserved.

Breast Cancer

Breast cancer is responsible for approximately 30% of all registered cancer cases worldwide and, thereby, ranks as the most common malignancy in women. In 2020, roughly 2.3 million new cases of breast cancer and about 685,000 breast cancer-related deaths were reported globally.[8] These numbers underline the enormous impact of breast cancer on society. Interestingly, developed countries reveal 88% higher incidence rates than developing countries (55.9 vs 29.7 per 100.000), which is most likely due to an increased prevalence of risk factors (eg, higher age at first birth, and greater use of oral contraceptives), lifestyle factors (eg, alcohol, obesity), but also earlier and more regular screenings (mammography) that impact prevalence data.[8] By contrast, developing countries demonstrated higher death rates compared with developed countries, suggesting a positive influence of access to good health systems on outcomes.[8] Thus, early detection apparently represents a key approach to improving survival.

Limitations of ^{18}F-FDG-PET/Computed Tomography

The clinical routine for local tumor staging includes ultrasonography, mammography, and MR imaging. Whole-body staging, focused on detection of distant metastatic disease, has traditionally been performed with CT or MR imaging, but more recently ^{18}F-FDG-PET/CT or PET/MR imaging have been shown to improve sensitivity for this purpose.[12] The studies conducted thus far indicate the standard oncologic PET tracer ^{18}F-FDG to be useful for the initial staging of breast cancer across all tumor phenotypes and grades.[13] However, in patients with stage 1 (T1N0) no incremental information seems to be provided by hybrid FDG-PET/CT imaging.

On the contrary, patients with suspected or proven locoregional and/or distant recurrence benefit more from ^{18}F-FDG-PET/CT than conventional imaging, even in the absence of elevated tumor markers.[13] Nevertheless, ^{18}F-FDG is also known to have limitations related to its inextricable linkage to glycolytic metabolism, which varies in breast cancer, and represents an exceptionally heterogeneous tumor entity with various histologic and molecular subtypes. The underlying mechanism behind the differing level of glucose metabolism is, as yet, not fully elucidated. Some studies have indicated a positive correlation between higher proliferative rates as well as certain tumor types, for example, triple-negative breast cancer has elevated FDG levels as reflected by high standardized uptake values.[14,15] Beyond the heterogeneity of breast cancer, benign diseases demonstrating elevated standardized uptake values (SUVs) may also mimic cancerous processes, and thereby, produce false positive results. For example, mastitis, trauma, inflammatory changes, and other malignancies must be considered as differential diagnoses when interpreting ^{18}F-FDG-PET/CT scans.[16]

FAPI versus FDG

^{68}Ga-FAPI, a newly developed PET tracer, may overcome some of the limitations associated with ^{18}F-FDG while still offering the advantages of hybrid imaging. Unlike ^{18}F-FDG, FAPI agents do not depend on glucose metabolism, but rather on the presence of elevated FAP levels in the tumor stroma or, possibly, in the cancer cells themselves[9,17] Based on preliminary studies, ^{68}Ga-FAPI-PET/CT seems to hold great potential in patients with breast cancer, particularly when compared with ^{18}F-FDG. Kömek and colleagues analyzed the sensitivity and specificity of ^{68}Ga-FAPI and ^{18}F-FDG-PET/CT in 20 patients with primary or recurrent breast cancer in a prospective pilot study.[18] Their research revealed significantly higher SUVmax values with ^{68}Ga-FAPI than ^{18}F-FDG in primary breast tumors, lymph nodes, lung metastases, and bone metastases, whereas no significant difference was detected for hepatic metastases. In terms of better delineation of tumor extent, ^{68}Ga-FAPI also seems favorable in comparison to ^{18}F-FDG with significantly higher tumor-to-background-ratios (TBRs) in breast lesions, and hepatic, bone, brain, and lung metastases. A study, conducted by Elboga and colleagues,[19] supports these first findings, demonstrating a higher accuracy with ^{68}Ga-FAPI than with ^{18}F-FDG based on more detected lesions and higher uptake. Moreover, an analysis of various female-sex-related malignancies including breast cancer once more proved beneficial features for ^{68}Ga-FAPI with respect to tumor uptake, and tumor-to-background ratios.[20] In addition to the ^{68}Ga-FAPI agents, an ^{18}F-labeled FAPI, [^{18}F]FAPI-74, has been developed with the benefit of a higher synthetic yield and delivery from centralized large-scale production,[21] but has not been extensively evaluated in breast cancer. In summary, in comparison to ^{18}F-FDG, FAPI agents seem to provide lower background activity and higher uptake in most identified lesions, as demonstrated in **Fig. 1**, which is likely due to a combination of uptake primarily in the stroma but, in some cases, also in the cancerous cells themselves as visualized in **Fig. 2**. This enables a high sensitivity for the detection of disease sites.

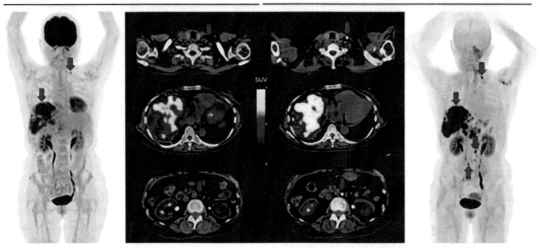

Fig. 1. Visualization of a patient diagnosed with breast cancer receiving ^{18}F-FAPI-74 and ^{18}F-FDG-PET/CT before therapy (from clinical research in Osaka University Hospital). FAPI achieves better contrasts and higher SUV metrics compared with FDG once more showing its potential.

^{68}Ga-FAPI-PET/MR Imaging in Breast Cancer

MR imaging serves a key role in imaging breast cancer as it has proven to be the most sensitive imaging technique ranging from 90% to 99% depending on the study.[22–26] However, the specificity of MR imaging represents a limiting factor (72%–89%) due to false positive findings.[22–26] Thus, additional information provided by the synergy of combining PET and MR imaging might improve the overall accuracy. The first study by Backhaus and colleagues assessed 19 women, with histologically confirmed invasive breast cancer.[27] Their study included one patient for restaging after completion of therapy and 18 patients in

whom it was performed as a complement to standard initial staging. All 18 patients analyzed in the context of primary staging demonstrated strong accumulation in the confirmed primary lesion (mean SUVmax 13.9). No differences in tracer uptake were found, regardless of histologic subtype, receptor status, or tumor grade. Proven lymph nodes, present in 13 women, all demonstrated strong ^{68}Ga-FAPI uptake. Furthermore, no false positive lymph node findings were reported, supporting the hypothesis of an enhanced specificity with hybrid imaging. A subsequent study by Backhaus and colleagues evaluated the response to neoadjuvant chemotherapy by ^{68}Ga-FAPI-PET/

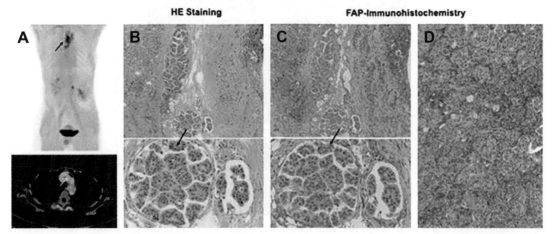

Fig. 2. Staining with HE and anti-FAP α monoclonal antibody of a pleural biopsy induced by breast cancer. The pleural metastasis in the mediastinum demonstrated a SUVmax of 7.46 with FAPI-PET/CT 8 months before the biopsy (A). The stroma showed markedly strong FAP expression (D), and high-to-moderate expression was observed in neoplastic cells (B,C). The arrows are showing the magnified pictures.

MR imaging in 13 patients with breast cancer. However, the results of this small population rather endorsed the use of solely MR imaging over combined PET/MR imaging.[28] In summary, larger and prospective analyses are warranted to clarify the potential of ^{68}Ga-FAPI-PET/MR imaging in patients with breast cancer.

Theranostic Approach

As opposed to ^{18}F-FDG, FAPI agents offer the possibility of a theranostic approach by providing patients not only with improved diagnostic assessment but also therapeutic options. Rathke and colleagues reported a patient diagnosed with breast cancer and colorectal cancer receiving experimental therapy after a positive ^{68}Ga-FAPI scan with ^{90}Y-FAPI46.[29] This therapeutic approach led to a mixed response with peritoneal metastases being eliminated, while metastases from the breast cancer showed hardly any response. Further results of therapy for metastatic are lacking and conclusions based on this single case study must be reserved.

^{68}Ga-FAPI in Gynecologic Malignancies

An investigation of ^{68}Ga-FAPI in female-sex malignancies including breast cancer (n = 14), ovarian cancer (n = 9), cervical cancer (n = 4), endometrial cancer (n = 2), leiomyosarcoma of the uterus (n = 1), and tubal cancer (n = 1) has indicated that this novel tracer can be used successfully in a broad spectrum of tumor entities.[20] In this series,

SUV metrics and TBRs were impressive, even when compared with ^{18}F-FDG. In addition, immunohistochemical staining has indicated a significant expression of FAP in ovarian cancer, breast cancer, and leiomyosarcoma of the uterus,[20] which is consistent with the findings of these imaging results particularly for ovarian cancer ^{68}Ga-FAPI-PET/CT might provide a valuable diagnostic contribution as prior studies have established a presence of FAP in 97% of all analyzed samples. Moreover, there seems to be a correlation between high FAP levels and a poor clinical prognosis, resistance to chemotherapy, and shorter time until recurrence.[17,30–34]

Mona and colleagues also confirmed strong FAP presence in ovarian cancer in a prospective exploratory study.[35] These results suggest that ^{68}Ga-FAPI- PET/CT might be able to complement conventional imaging and maybe even facilitate much-needed therapeutic approaches as treatment options in platinum-resistant ovarian cancer remain limited. Furthermore, one case report by Siripongsatian and colleagues described a patient with recurrent ovarian cancer who presented with rising CA-125 levels 7 months after surgical resection.[36] Only the PET/CT scan performed with ^{68}Ga-FAPI could reveal recurrent intra-abdominal node and distant metastases based on higher TBR values compared with ^{18}F-FDG. Thus, therapeutic patient management was impacted according to these new findings.

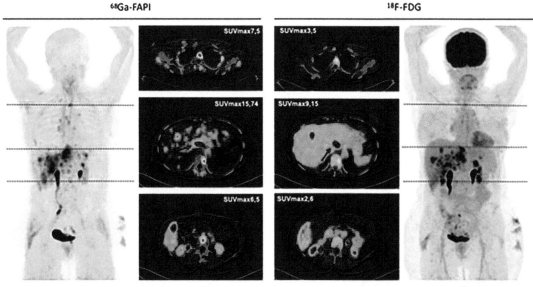

Fig. 3. Visualization of a woman diagnosed with metastasized ovarian cancer undergoing both ^{68}Ga-FAPI-PET/CT and ^{18}F-FDG-PET/CT 4 weeks later. FAPI was able to impress with higher uptake in one liver and two bone metastases compared with FDG. (*Adapted from* Dendl K, Koerber SA, Finck R, Mokoala KMG, Staudinger F, Schillings L, Heger U, Röhrich M, Kratochwil C, Sathekge M, Jäger D, Debus J, Haberkorn U, Giesel FL. 68Ga-FAPI-PET/CT in patients with various gynecological malignancies. Eur J Nucl Med Mol Imaging. 2021a Nov;48(12):4089-4100.)

Data related to cervical cancer are currently limited, but Zhang and colleagues retrospectively analyzed 77 gynecology patients, including 10 patients with cervical cancer.[37] This study found higher SUV values in patients diagnosed with cancer than in those with no disease. In conclusion, a variety of gynecologic cancers express FAP; hence, it is possible that FAPI-PET/CT will prove to be an effective diagnostic tool (**Fig. 3**), and possibly even a theranostic one in the future. That is why, further, particularly larger, and prospective studies are urgently required.

Benign Uptake in Hormone-Sensitive Organs

Non-malignant uptake in hormone-responsive organs needs to be recognized to accurately interpret ^{68}Ga-FAPI scans. Previous studies have indicated a correlation between elevated FAP levels in the uterus of women of reproductive age as well as a possible negative association with age and particularly with post-menopausal status.[20,38,39] The intensity of FAPI uptake in the breast, ovary, and uterus was found to be higher uptake in pre-menopausal (n = 12) than post-menopausal (n = 68) women, and was significantly different for both breast and uterine tissue.[20] Zang and colleagues further elaborated on this topic by conducting a study with 77 patients, which included 67 women without a cancer diagnosis and 10 with cervical cancer who underwent ^{68}Ga-FAPI-PET/MR imaging. They analyzed the uptake of the uterus in premenopausal, perimenopausal, and women of reproductive age and found higher SUV metrics in those who were defined as having reproductive potential.[37] This hypothesis is supported by two individual case reports noting increased uptake in breasts and uterus due to hormonal stimulation and post-partum status.[39–41] The varying uptake in hormone-sensitive organs might represent a challenging fact and must be interpreted with caution as it may also be induced by physiologic or benign conditions. Whether FAPI would overcome the assessment of potential cancer involving lactating breast, which is severely constrained on FDG-PET, is unknown.[42]

SUMMARY

Preliminary studies in female-sex-related malignancies, including breast and various gynecologic cancers, have revealed encouraging results but are mostly of retrospective nature and require validation in larger and preferably prospective studies.

CLINICS CARE POINTS

- First highly promising results in breast cancer and several other gynecologic malignancies
- Hormone-sensitive organs must be interpreted with caution, as uptake may vary not only due to malignant processes but also based on the hormonal influence
- FAPI seems to provide advantages over the standard oncological tracer FDG, and therefore, may add additional value in a clinical setting

DISCLOSURES

F.L. Giesel is an adviser at ABX Radiopharmaceuticals, SOFIE Biosciences, Telix pharma 301, and Alpha Fusion. F.L. Giesel has also shares in a consultancy group for iTheranostics. U. Haberkorn Royalties from iTheranostics and SOFIE Biosciences; patent for FAPI tracers licensed to SOFIE Biosciences.

REFERENCES

1. Gascard P, Tlsty TD. Carcinoma-associated fibroblasts: orchestrating the composition of malignancy. Genes Dev 2016;30(9):1002–19.
2. Barbazán J, Matic Vignjevic D. Cancer associated fibroblasts: is the force the path to the dark side? Curr Opin Cell Biol 2019;56:71–9.
3. Lindner T, Loktev A, Altmann A, et al. Development of quinoline-based theranostic ligands for the targeting of fibroblast activation protein. J Nucl Med 2018;59(9):1415–22.
4. Loktev A, Lindner T, Mier W, et al. A tumor-imaging method targeting cancer-associated fibroblasts. J Nucl Med 2018;59(9):1423–9.
5. Kratochwil C, Flechsig P, Lindner T, et al. ^{68}Ga-FAPI PET/CT: tracer uptake in 28 different Kinds of cancer. J Nucl Med 2019;60(6):801–5.
6. Dendl K, Koerber SA, Kratochwil C, et al. FAP and FAPI-PET/CT in malignant and non-malignant diseases: a perfect symbiosis? Cancers 2021;13(19):4946.
7. Dendl K, Finck R, Giesel FL, et al. FAP imaging in rare cancer entities-first clinical experience in a broad spectrum of malignancies. Eur J Nucl Med Mol Imaging 2022a;49(2):721–31.
8. Sung H, Ferlay J, Siegel RL, et al. Global cancer Statistics 2020: GLOBOCAN Estimates of incidence and mortality worldwide for 36 cancers in 185 countries. CA Cancer J Clin 2021;71(3):209–49.

9. Goodman JD, Rozypal TL, Kelly T. Seprase, a membrane-bound protease, alleviates the serum growth requirement of human breast cancer cells. Clin Exp Metastasis 2003;20(5):459–70.

10. Fujii T, Yajima R, Kurozumi S, et al. Clinical significance of 18F-FDG-PET in invasive lobular carcinoma. Anticancer Res 2016;36(10):5481–5.

11. Dendl K, Koerber SA, Tamburini K, et al. Advancement and future perspective of FAPI PET/CT in gynecological malignancies. Semin Nucl Med 2022b; 52(5):628–34.

12. Balma M, Liberini V, Racca M, et al. Non-conventional and investigational PET radiotracers for breast cancer: a Systematic review. Front Med 2022;9: 881551.

13. Groheux D. FDG-PET/CT for primary staging and detection of recurrence of breast cancer. Semin Nucl Med 2022;52(5):508–19.

14. Kikano EG, Avril S, Marshall H, et al. PET/CT variants and Pitfalls in breast cancers. Semin Nucl Med 2021;51(5):474–84.

15. Tchou J, Sonnad SS, Bergey MR, et al. Degree of tumor FDG uptake correlates with proliferation index in triple negative breast cancer. Mol Imaging Biol 2010;12(6):657–62.

16. Hofman MS, Hicks RJ. How We Read oncologic FDG PET/CT. Cancer Imag 2016;16(1):35.

17. Garin-Chesa P, Old LJ, Rettig WJ. Cell surface glycoprotein of reactive stromal fibroblasts as a potential antibody target in human epithelial cancers. Proc Natl Acad Sci U S A 1990;87(18): 7235–9.

18. Kömek H, Can C, Güzel Y, et al. 68Ga-FAPI-04 PET/CT, a new step in breast cancer imaging: a comparative pilot study with the 18F-FDG PET/CT. Ann Nucl Med 2021;35(6):744–52.

19. Elboga U, Sahin E, Kus T, et al. Superiority of 68Ga-FAPI PET/CT scan in detecting additional lesions compared to 18FDG PET/CT scan in breast cancer. Ann Nucl Med 2021;35(12):1321–31.

20. Dendl K, Koerber SA, Finck R, et al. 68Ga-FAPI-PET/CT in patients with various gynecological malignancies. Eur J Nucl Med Mol Imaging 2021a; 48(12):4089–100.

21. Giesel FL, Adeberg S, Syed M, et al. FAPI-74 PET/CT using Either 18F-AlF or Cold-Kit 68Ga labeling: biodistribution, radiation dosimetry, and tumor delineation in lung cancer patients. J Nucl Med 2021; 62(2):201–7.

22. Peters NH, Borel Rinkes IH, Zuithoff NP, et al. Meta-analysis of MR imaging in the diagnosis of breast lesions. Radiology 2008;246(1):116–24.

23. Bennani-Baiti B, Bennani-Baiti N, Baltzer PA. Diagnostic performance of breast magnetic resonance imaging in non-calcified equivocal breast findings: results from a systematic review and Meta-analysis. PLoS One 2016;11(8):e0160346.

24. Mann RM, Kuhl CK, Kinkel K, et al. Breast MRI: guidelines from the European society of breast imaging. Eur Radiol 2008;18(7):1307–18.

25. Mann RM, Balleyguier C, Baltzer PA, et al. Breast MRI: EUSOBI recommendations for women's information. Eur Radiol 2015;25(12):3669–78.

26. Mann RM, Cho N, Moy L. Breast MRI: state of the art. Radiology 2019;292(3):520–36.

27. Backhaus P, Burg MC, Roll W, et al. Simultaneous FAPI PET/MRI targeting the fibroblast-activation protein for breast cancer. Radiology 2022;302(1):39–47.

28. Backhaus P, Burg MC, Asmus I, et al. Initial results of FAPI-PET/MRI to assess response to neoadjuvant chemotherapy in breast cancer [published online ahead of print, 2022 Nov 17]. J Nucl Med 2022; 122:264871. jnumed.

29. Rathke H, Fuxius S, Giesel FL, et al. Two tumors, one target: preliminary experience with 90Y-FAPI therapy in a patient with metastasized breast and colorectal cancer. Clin Nucl Med 2021;46(10):842–4.

30. Jin X, Iwasa S, Okada K, et al. Expression patterns of seprase, a membrane serine protease, in cervical carcinoma and cervical intraepithelial neoplasm [published correction appears in Anticancer Res. 2003;23:5371-2]. Anticancer Res 2003;23(4): 3195–8.

31. Lai D, Ma L, Wang F. Fibroblast activation protein regulates tumor-associated fibroblasts and epithelial ovarian cancer cells. Int J Oncol 2012;41(2):541–50.

32. Hussain A, Voisin V, Poon S, et al. Distinct fibroblast functional states drive clinical outcomes in ovarian cancer and are regulated by TCF21. J Exp Med 2020;217(8):e20191094.

33. Mhawech-Fauceglia P, Yan L, Sharifian M, et al. Stromal expression of fibroblast activation protein Alpha (FAP) Predicts platinum resistance and shorter recurrence in patients with epithelial ovarian cancer. Cancer Microenviron 2015;8(1):23–31.

34. Zhang Y, Tang H, Cai J, et al. Ovarian cancer-associated fibroblasts contribute to epithelial ovarian carcinoma metastasis by promoting angiogenesis, lymphangiogenesis and tumor cell invasion. Cancer Lett 2011;303(1):47–55.

35. Mona CE, Benz MR, Hikmat F, et al. Correlation of 68Ga-FAPi-46 PET Biodistribution with FAP expression by Immunohistochemistry in patients with Solid cancers: interim analysis of a prospective Translational exploratory study. J Nucl Med 2022;63(7): 1021–6.

36. Siripongsatian D, Promteangtrong C, Kunawudhi A, et al. Intense 68Ga-FAPI-46 activity in lesions of recurrent ovarian Clear cell carcinoma that were negative on FDG PET/CT study. Clin Nucl Med 2022;47(2):e210–2.

37. Zhang X, Song W, Qin C, et al. Uterine uptake of 68Ga-FAPI-04 in uterine Pathology and Physiology. Clin Nucl Med 2022;47(1):7–13.

38. Kessler L, Ferdinandus J, Hirmas N, et al. Pitfalls and common findings in ^{68}Ga-FAPI PET: a Pictorial analysis. J Nucl Med 2022;63(6):890–6.

39. Dendl K, Koerber SA, Adeberg S, et al. Physiological FAP-activation in a postpartum woman observed in oncological FAPI-PET/CT. Eur J Nucl Med Mol Imaging 2021;48(6):2059–61.

40. Sonni I, Lee-Felker S, Memarzadeh S, et al. ^{68}Ga-FAPi-46 diffuse bilateral breast uptake in a patient with cervical cancer after hormonal stimulation. Eur J Nucl Med Mol Imaging 2021;48(3):924–6.

41. Wang LJ, Zhang Y, Wu HB. Intense diffuse uptake of 68Ga-FAPI-04 in the breasts found by PET/CT in a patient with Advanced Nasopharyngeal carcinoma. Clin Nucl Med 2021;46(5):e293–5.

42. Hicks RJ, Binns D, Stabin MG. Pattern of uptake and excretion of (18)F-FDG in the lactating breast. J Nucl Med 2001;42(8):1238–42.

Fibroblast Activation Protein Inhibitor (FAPI)-PET Imaging in Sarcoma

Lukas Kessler, MD[a,b],*

KEYWORDS

• Sarcoma • Cancer imaging • FAPI • Fibroblast activation protein

KEY POINTS

- Soft tissue and bone sarcoma are rare tumor entities that show high expression of fibroblast activation protein alpha (FAP) in tumor cells.
- FAP expression in sarcomas is linked to cancer prognosis, metastasis, and affects sensitivity to chemotherapy.
- Novel ^{68}Ga-FAPI radiotracers show high average tracer uptake in patients with sarcoma, but uptake values have high ranges depending on the sarcoma subtype.
- High-grade sarcomas, such as pleomorphic sarcomas, high-grade liposarcomas, and osteosarcomas, and the generally benign solitary fibrous tumors show the highest average uptake values.
- Theranostic approaches with FAPI sarcoma show promising results in preliminary evaluation.

INTRODUCTION

Sarcoma represents a wide spectrum of individually rare neoplasms arising from mesenchymal cells. Sarcomas can arise in various connective tissues, such as bone, cartilage, fat, muscle, and blood vessels. More than 100 different histopathologic and molecular genetic subtypes have been described so far and classifications are updated regularly to meet novel molecular findings in rare sarcoma entities. These advances will potentially allow identification of novel diagnostic and therapeutic targets for specific subtypes, but there is a pressing need for a "pan-sarcoma" target. This article provides an overview of one potential candidate, fibroblast activation protein (FAP), and discusses current data on ^{68}Ga-FAPI radiotracers as a novel diagnostic modality for soft tissue and bone sarcomas with potential translation into the therapeutic domain.

BACKGROUND

In general, sarcomas are divided into two main groups: soft tissue sarcoma and bone sarcoma. Soft tissue sarcomas can occur anywhere in the body and originate from any type of connective tissue, including cartilage, fat, muscle, and blood vessels. Most common subtypes in adults are liposarcoma, leiomyosarcoma, angiosarcoma, and not-other-specified sarcomas. The overall incidence of all soft tissue sarcomas is low with 7.1 cases per 100,000 people in North America between 2002 and 2014, but has been apparently increasing over recent decades from 6.8 in 2002 to 7.7 in 2014.[1] Although bone sarcomas have a lower overall incidence of about 0.9 cases per 100,000 people per year in the United States, these tumors occur most often in children and teenagers and manifest commonly in the long bones of the arms and legs.[2] Sarcoma is a difficult

[a] Department of Nuclear Medicine, University Hospital Essen, University of Duisburg-Essen, Essen, Germany;
[b] German Cancer Consortium (DKTK), Partner Site University Hospital Essen, and German Cancer Research Center (DKFZ), Essen, Germany
* Hufelandstraße 55, Essen 45147, Germany.
E-mail address: lukas.kessler@uk-essen.de

PET Clin 18 (2023) 353–359
https://doi.org/10.1016/j.cpet.2023.03.001
1556-8598/23/© 2023 Elsevier Inc. All rights reserved.

disease to diagnose and treat and treatment varies depending on the type, grading, and stage of the cancer.[3] If possible surgical resection is preferred in most cases, but multidisciplinary approaches are needed for adequate treatment and systemic treatments are limited for most entities and in some cases nonexistent. Therefore, development of novel therapeutic drugs is urgently needed.

FIBROBLAST ACTIVATION PROTEIN

FAP was named after its expression in activated fibroblast and it was independently identified by multiple researchers in the 1980s and 1990s.[4,5] FAP is a serine protease, which has very low expression levels in most tissues and is not expressed in normal fibroblasts, which have been found to express dipeptidyl-peptidase-IV (DPP-IV or CD26), a similar serine integral membrane proteinase. Nonetheless, physiologic FAP expression has been observed in multiple human tissue (uterus, pancreas), bone marrow stem cells, and during embryonic stages. Still, mostly reactive or activated stromal fibroblasts show high expression levels of FAP; these are found in various physiologic and pathophysiologic processes, such as wound healing or solid tumors. In solid tumors, carcinoma-associated fibroblasts have been described, which are fibroblasts in the tumor stroma but not tumor cells.[6] These carcinoma-associated fibroblasts have been shown to influence the cancer microenvironment and secrete various growth factors and extracellular matrix proteins that promote tumor growth and metastasis. A meta-analysis by Liu and colleagues[7] showed that FAP overexpression in tumor tissue is associated with poor overall survival, tumor progression, and metastasis. This makes FAP a promising target for cancer therapy and several FAP-targeting therapies are currently in development, including small molecule inhibitors, monoclonal antibodies, and FAP-CAR-T cells.[8–10] Despite these data, activated fibroblasts and FAP expression have been observed in benign/physiologic and carcinoma-associated fibroblasts alike, which leaves many unanswered questions regarding the tumor specificity of FAP.

FIBROBLAST ACTIVATION PROTEIN AND SARCOMA

Because of their mesenchymal origin, sarcomas are not just rare tumor entities but rather unique in terms of FAP expression compared with other solid tumors. First in vitro evidence was published in 1994, showing FAP expression in a sarcoma tumor cell line.[11] Still, it took many years to follow up

on these data. Eventually Dohi and colleagues[12] analyzed 41 specimens of various bone and soft tissue tumors and investigated the FAP and DPP-IV expression levels. Their study showed strong FAP and DPP-IV expression in fibroblast-like tumor cells in low-grade myofibroblastic sarcoma and fibroblastic areas of osteosarcoma comparable with activated fibroblasts and myofibroblasts.[12] But in contrast to known data, round or oval cells of Ewing sarcoma or rhabdomyosarcoma did not express FAP in their specimen cohort.[12] FAP and DPP-IV expression was independent of the malignant potential of the analyzed tumors and the authors postulated a relationship between the histogenesis (eg, fibroblast-like phenotype) and positive tumor cells.[12]

Following this, researchers found that in the HT1080, an aggressive fibrosarcoma cell line, in vitro FAP expression was strongly linked to cell migration, adhesion, and invasion increasing the metastatic potential of these sarcoma cells.[13] Similar findings were observed in osteosarcoma cells, which exhibit not just FAP expression but additionally show markedly decreased in vitro growth, adhesion, migration, and invasion if FAP was knocked out in these sarcoma cells.[14] Furthermore, in vitro data suggest variable therapy responses to chemotherapeutic drugs depending on FAP expression levels.[15] Therefore, in vitro data of recent decades identified FAP as an important player in tumoral behavior and proved it to be a highly promising target not just for carcinoma-associated fibroblasts but sarcoma cells as well. Ultimately this initiated the development of new diagnostic and therapeutic probes for FAP.

[68]GA-FAPI FROM BENCH TO BEDSIDE IN PATIENTS WITH SARCOMA

In 2013 Jansen and colleagues[16] laid the foundation for a novel group of FAP inhibitors (FAPI). Based on these data Loktev and colleagues[17] developed a set of radiolabeled FAPIs (FAPI-01 and FAPI-02) with high FAP affinity. They could show that FAPI bind to FAP in the known FAP-positive HT1080 fibrosarcoma cell line but not to the closely related protein CD26 (DPP-IV).[17] Furthermore, the authors could show in vivo tumor uptake of ^{68}Ga-FAPI-02 in murine HT1080 xenografts leading to the conclusion that those novel radiolabeled FAPIs are specific diagnostic and therapeutic probes for FAP-positive tumors including sarcomas. Compared with FAPI-01, FAPI-02 showed better pharmacokinetic and biochemical properties and 10-fold higher retention after 24 hours of incubation.[17,18] This led to further development of other probes in the following years and evaluation of their pharmaco-kinetic and biochemical properties. From these studies, FAPI-04 and FAPI-46 emerged as the most promising tracers for therapeutic clinical application, with the latter having higher tumor uptake, retention, and decreased uptake in normal organs compared with FAPI-04.[19–21]

Kratochwil and colleagues[22] were the first to evaluate tracer uptake values in 80 patients with cancer with 28 different tumor entities. In their cohort, sarcomas showed one the highest average SUVmax (>12) compared with other tumor entities, but with a high standard deviation that is likely explained by the heterogeneity of sarcoma entities.[22] Data from Hirmas and colleagues[23] on 324 patients with 21 tumor entities confirmed sarcomas as a cancer group with highest average FAPI-uptake values.

PET IMAGING IN SARCOMA AND IMPACT OF [68]GA-FAPI

PET imaging is not the modality of choice in early stages or diagnosis of sarcomas. However, ^{18}F-fluorodeoxyglucose (FDG)-PET/computed tomography has been proven to be a useful tool in the assessment of soft tissue and bone sarcomas in early and metastatic stages and for the assessment of therapeutic responses. FDG-avidity is highly variable in these tumors but, depending on the sarcoma entity, has been demonstrated to be correlated with proliferation rates and grade.[24,25] Furthermore, high metabolic activity of sarcomas has been shown to be related to an adverse overall prognosis[26–28] and a decrease in metabolic activity is a marker of therapy response.[29] Many studies align in the differentiation between high-grade and benign tumors in FDG-PET, but there is lack of evidence of its ability to differentiate between low-grade and benign soft tissue lesions.[30] Low-grade sarcomas were found to have low FDG uptake related to their metabolic activity, whereas false-positive results of benign lesions were often the result of inflammation.[31]

^{68}Ga-FAPI could potentially close this gap and offers a novel imaging approach for sarcomas, because of known in vitro/in vivo FAP expression in tumor cells of high- and low-grade sarcomas. ^{68}Ga-FAPI has been introduced only recently to the clinical arena and, because of this, data on patients with sarcoma are scarce so far. **Table 1** provides common imaging parameters.

In 2021, our research group published the first large registered observational trial of ^{68}Ga-FAPI-PET in patients with sarcoma (NCT04571086).[32] In this trial, 47 patients with bone or soft tissue sarcomas were imaged with ^{68}Ga-FAPI-04 and

Table 1
Common imaging parameters in sarcoma studies based on current imaging data with ^{68}Ga-FAPI in patients with sarcoma[32–34,48]

Common Imaging Parameters	
Radioisotope	Gallium-68
FAPI	FAPI-04, FAPI-46
Acquisition delay	10–60 min post injection
Injected activity	Approximately 150–200 MBq, or bodyweight-based (2–3 MBq per kg)[33]

FAPI-46 independent of tumor stage and previous therapies. Key findings in this study were a significant correlation between FAPI-PET uptake intensity and histopathologic FAP-expression, a high positive predictive value and sensitivity of 100% and 96%, respectively, on a per patient basis.[32] Detection rates of ^{68}Ga-FAPI and ^{18}F-FDG were comparable in this cohort. The comparison of low- to high-grade sarcomas was limited because of small number of patients in the low-grade sarcoma group, but did not show a difference.[32] To date, this is the only prospective data available on the diagnostic performance of ^{68}Ga-FAPI in bone and soft tissue sarcoma.

In recent years, only a few studies and cases reports have additionally provided data in this field. Nevertheless, these studies mostly align in respect of the overall high FAPI tracer uptake.[32–41] A difficulty of all sarcoma studies compared with other solid tumors is the heterogeneity of this tumors and the great differences in molecular phenotypes. Therefore, FAPI uptake values differ between the sarcoma entities but without reliable data so far. **Fig. 1** shows a case example with tracer uptake in fibroblastic areas of an osteosarcoma but no uptake in osteoblastic areas, which aligns with immunohistologic data from Dohi and colleagues.[12]

So far, multiple studies have shown that FAPI tracer uptake is generally high compared with uptake in other solid tumors. In particular, undifferentiated pleomorphic sarcoma, high-grade osteosarcoma, high-grade liposarcomas, and the rare solitary fibrous tumors (SFT) show increased FAPI uptake.[32–34] **Table 2** summarizes some of the highest measured uptake values and the respective sarcoma subtypes. **Fig. 2** provides 12 representative ^{68}Ga-FAPI images of various local and metastatic bone and soft tissue sarcomas. Some entities are of particular interest.

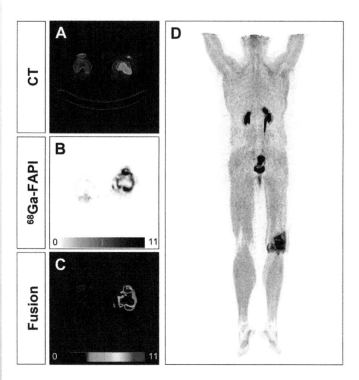

Fig. 1. Case presentation: a 23-year-old female patient with an osteosarcoma of the left knee. (*A*) Computed tomography (CT) shows an osteoblastic lesion in the distal femur. (*B–D*) ^{68}Ga-FAPI-PET shows a high tracer uptake (SUVmax 79.0) of the surrounding soft tissue with almost no tracer uptake of the osteoblastic lesion indicating tracer uptake in fibroblastic areas of the tumor or associated desmoplastic reaction.

Solitary Fibrous Tumors

Although generally benign in their natural history, malignant SFT have shown very high tumor uptake values.[34,42,43] Our institution reported some SFTs with SUVmax less than 200 (Hamacher et al., 2023, unpublished data), and these tumors have very low metabolic activity, which leads to low uptake on ^{18}F-FDG PET.[42,43] Among sarcomas, SFT are rare with unknown prevalence in most countries and there are no Food and Drug Administration–approved therapies in metastatic or advanced stages.

Chordoma

Chordoma are another rare bone sarcoma entity with destructive growth that have been found to show increased ^{68}Ga-FAPI uptake in multiple studies. These tumors have a high resistance to chemotherapy and therefore therapeutic options are limited and, similar to SFT, no therapeutic drugs have been Food and Drug Administration–approved so far.[44,45] Therefore, FAP-targeting could open new possibilities for affected patients of these rare malignant tumors.

Fibrosarcoma/Myxofibrosarcoma

Most fibroblast-like sarcoma entities, such as fibrosarcoma or myxofibrosarcoma, vary in their FAPI uptake intensity but have overall moderate uptake values, which partially contradicts the high in vitro FAP expression.[33,34] A reasons for this might be variability of tumor and stromal tissue, especially in the ratio of extracellular matrix to sarcoma cells in these tumors, which could lead to a dilution of the signal in PET imaging.[46] Nonetheless, high uptake values were observed

Table 2
Sarcoma subtypes

Sarcoma Subtype	Highest SUVmax
Malignant solitary fibrous tumor	223.0[a], 78.5,[34] 40.0,[43] 30.9[42]
Interdigitating dendritic cell sarcoma	119.3[34]
Osteosarcoma	89.6,[32] 44.3[33]
Liposarcoma	47.5,[34] 33.6[33]
Undifferentiated soft tissue sarcoma (not-other-specified, round cell, undifferentiated pleomorphic sarcoma)	44.3,[33] 37.9,[34] 31.2[32]
Endometrial stromal sarcoma	30.2[32]
Chordoma	23.0,[32] 9.0[22]

Some subtypes with the highest reported uptake values in current literature.
[a] Unpublished data by our research group.

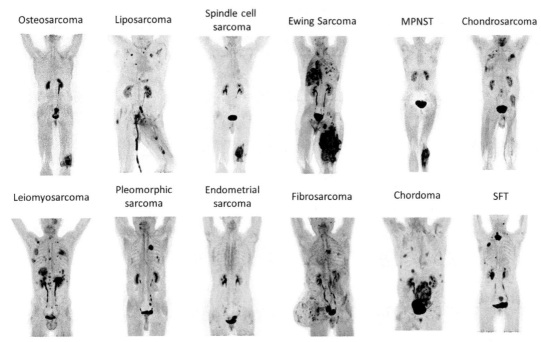

Osteosarcoma   Liposarcoma   Spindle cell sarcoma   Ewing Sarcoma   MPNST   Chondrosarcoma

Leiomyosarcoma   Pleomorphic sarcoma   Endometrial sarcoma   Fibrosarcoma   Chordoma   SFT

Fig. 2. MIP images of ^{68}Ga-FAPI-PET/CT of 12 representative patients with different types of soft tissue and bone sarcoma. The cases show patients with local primary tumor and metastatic stages. Of note: physiologic FAP expression of the endometrium can mimic and mask tumors in ^{68}Ga-FAPI-PET/CT as seen in the patient with endometrial sarcoma. MPNST, malignant peripheral nerve sheath tumor; SFT, solitary fibrous tumor.

in high- and low-grade sarcoma, independently. This leads to the conclusion that ^{68}Ga-FAPI provides a different angle on imaged-based characterization and might show better performance in the detection of low-grade sarcomas with low metabolic activity compared with ^{18}F-FDG.

In summary, based on the existing in vitro/in vivo and clinical data, ^{68}Ga-FAPI is a promising tool for evaluation of soft tissue and bone sarcoma. However, there are multiple limitations to this method that need to be understood before drawing firm conclusions.

LIMITATIONS OF CURRENT DATA AND FUTURE PERSPECTIVES

Current studies are significantly limited by small, heterogeneous cohorts of patients, which include low- and high-grade sarcomas of various entities and heavily pretreated patients. To overcome these shortcomings, studies recruiting selective sarcoma entities are needed, or at least involving large numbers of patients with sarcoma to allow subgroup analyses. In some sarcoma entities it has been shown that not just the tumor cells are expressing FAP but the neighboring desmoplastic reaction as well, and therefore high FAPI uptake should not be misunderstood as a surrogate for tumoral FAP expression.

All uncertainties aside, ^{68}Ga-FAPI opens new diagnostic paths for patients with sarcoma, which could impact clinical management. Currently there are multiple clinical trials ongoing to gain a better understanding of ^{68}Ga-FAPI in various tumor entities including sarcoma (eg, NCT05160051 and NCT04457258), which could provide prospective evidence on diagnostic performance of ^{68}Ga-FAPI over other imaging modalities in sarcoma. Additionally, ^{68}Ga-FAPI might be a great tool to measure in situ FAP expression for FAP-targeted therapies, such as antibodies, FAP-CAR-T cell therapy, or ^{90}Y-FAPI-radioligand therapy. The latter already has shown partial responses in a small cohort of patients with sarcoma with a low toxicity profile.[10,47]

SUMMARY

^{68}Ga-FAPI-PET/computed tomography could potentially offer important complementary information that can be used in the diagnostic work-up, assessment of therapy response, and prognostication of soft tissue and bone sarcomas. Especially low-grade sarcoma and rare subtypes of these tumor are of interest for theranostic use of FAPIs because of low metabolic activity and limited therapeutic options. Further data are needed to increase knowledge on this novel imaging modality

and to evaluate the impact on clinical management and enhance patient care, particularly for rare sarcoma subtypes.

CLINICS CARE POINTS

- Early data show high positive predictive values (100%) and sensitivity (96%) of ^{68}Ga-FAPI for various sarcomas.
- ^{68}Ga-FAPI tracer uptake shows association with immunohistologic FAP-expression levels.
- ^{68}Ga-FAPI tracer uptake is observed in low- and high-grade sarcomas but with high variability of the uptake intensity depending on the entity.
- Pitfall: physiologic FAP expression of the endometrium can mask endometrial sarcomas.

DISCLOSURE

L. Kessler is consultant for BTG and AAA and received fees from Sanofi outside of the submitted work.

REFERENCES

1. Gage MM, Nagarajan N, Ruck JM, et al. Sarcomas in the United States: recent trends and a call for improved staging. Oncotarget 2019;10(25):2462–74.
2. Ottaviani G, Jaffe N. The epidemiology of osteosarcoma. Cancer Treat Res 2009;152:3–13.
3. Gamboa AC, Gronchi A, Cardona K. Soft-tissue sarcoma in adults: an update on the current state of histiotype-specific management in an era of personalized medicine. CA Cancer J Clin 2020;70(3):200–29.
4. Rettig WJ, Chesa PG, Beresford HR, et al. Differential expression of cell surface antigens and glial fibrillary acidic protein in human astrocytoma subsets. Cancer Res 1986;46(12 Pt 1):6406–12. Available at: http://www.ncbi.nlm.nih.gov/pubmed/2877731.
5. Aoyama A, Chen WT. A 170-kDa membrane-bound protease is associated with the expression of invasiveness by human malignant melanoma cells. Proc Natl Acad Sci U S A 1990;87(21):8296–300.
6. Kalluri R. The biology and function of fibroblasts in cancer. Nat Rev Cancer 2016;16(9):582–98.
7. Liu F, Qi L, Liu B, et al. Fibroblast activation protein overexpression and clinical implications in solid tumors: a meta-analysis. PLoS One 2015;10(3):1–18.
8. Scott AM, Lee F-T, Hopkins W, et al. A phase I dose-escalation study of sibrotuzumab in patients with advanced or metastatic fibroblast activation protein-positive cancer. Clin Cancer Res 2003;9(5):1639–47.
9. Bughda R, Dimou P, D'Souza RR, et al. Fibroblast activation protein (FAP)-Targeted CAR-T cells: launching an attack on tumor stroma. ImmunoTargets Ther 2021;10:313–23.
10. Ferdinandus J, Fragoso Costa P, Kessler L, et al. Initial clinical experience with 90 Y-FAPI-46 radioligand therapy for advanced stage solid tumors: a case series of nine patients. J Nucl Med 2021. https://doi.org/10.2967/jnumed.121.262468. jnumed.121.262468.
11. Scanlan MJ, Raj BKM, Calvo B, et al. Molecular cloning of fibroblast activation protein α, a member of the serine protease family selectively expressed in stromal fibroblasts of epithelial cancers. Proc Natl Acad Sci U S A 1994;91(12):5657–61.
12. Dohi O, Ohtani H, Hatori M, et al. Histogenesis-specific expression of fibroblast activation protein and dipeptidylpeptidase-IV in human bone and soft tissue tumours. Histopathology 2009;55(4):432–40.
13. Baird SK, Allan L, Renner C, et al. Fibroblast activation protein increases metastatic potential of fibrosarcoma line HT1080 through upregulation of integrin-mediated signaling pathways. Clin Exp Metastasis 2015;32(5):507–16.
14. Ding L, Ye L, Xu J, et al. Impact of fibroblast activation protein on osteosarcoma cell lines in vitro. Oncol Lett 2014;7(3):699–704.
15. Baird SK, Rigopoulos A, Cao D, et al. Integral membrane protease fibroblast activation protein sensitizes fibrosarcoma to chemotherapy and alters cell death mechanisms. Apoptosis 2015;20(11):1483–98.
16. Jansen K, De Winter H, Heirbaut L, et al. Selective inhibitors of fibroblast activation protein (FAP) with a xanthine scaffold. Med Chem Commun 2014;5(11):1700–7.
17. Loktev A, Lindner T, Mier W, et al. A tumor-imaging method targeting cancer-associated fibroblasts. J Nucl Med 2018;59(9):1423–9.
18. Lindner T, Loktev A, Giesel F, et al. Targeting of activated fibroblasts for imaging and therapy. EJNMMI Radiopharm Chem 2019. https://doi.org/10.1186/s41181-019-0069-0.
19. Loktev A, Lindner T, Burger E-M, et al. Development of fibroblast activation protein–targeted radiotracers with improved tumor retention. J Nucl Med 2019;60(10):1421–9.
20. Lindner T, Loktev A, Altmann A, et al. Development of Quinoline-based theranostic ligands for the targeting of fibroblast activation protein. J Nucl Med 2018;59(9):1415–22.
21. Meyer C, Dahlbom M, Lindner T, et al. Radiation dosimetry and biodistribution of 68ga-fapi-46 pet

imaging in cancer patients. J Nucl Med 2020;61(8): 1171–7.

22. Kratochwil C, Flechsig P, Lindner T, et al. 68 Ga-FAPI PET/CT: tracer uptake in 28 different kinds of cancer. J Nucl Med 2019;60(6):801–5.

23. Hirmas N, Hamacher R, Sraieb M, et al. Fibroblast activation protein positron emission tomography and histopathology in a single-center database of 324 patients and 21 tumor entities. J Nucl Med 2022. https://doi.org/10.2967/jnumed.122.264689.

24. Rakheja R, Makis W, Skamene S, et al. Correlating metabolic activity on 18F-FDG PET/CT with histopathologic characteristics of osseous and soft-tissue sarcomas: a retrospective review of 136 patients. Am J Roentgenol 2012;198(6):1409–16.

25. Charest M, Hickeson M, Lisbona R, et al. FDG PET/CT imaging in primary osseous and soft tissue sarcomas: a retrospective review of 212 cases. Eur J Nucl Med Mol Imaging 2009;36(12):1944–51.

26. Fuglø HM, Jørgensen SM, Loft A, et al. The diagnostic and prognostic value of 18F-FDG PET/CT in the initial assessment of high-grade bone and soft tissue sarcoma. A retrospective study of 89 patients. Eur J Nucl Med Mol Imaging 2012;39(9):1416–24.

27. Ioannidis JPA, Lau J. 18F-FDG PET for the diagnosis and grading of soft-tissue sarcoma: a meta-analysis. J Nucl Med 2003;44(5):717–24.

28. Herrmann K, Benz MR, Czernin J, et al. 18F-FDG-PET/CT imaging as an early survival predictor in patients with primary high-grade soft tissue sarcomas undergoing neoadjuvant therapy. Clin Cancer Res 2012;18(7):2024–31.

29. Evilevitch V, Weber WA, Tap WD, et al. Reduction of glucose metabolic activity is more accurate than change in size at predicting histopathologic response to neoadjuvant therapy in high-grade soft-tissue sarcomas. Clin Cancer Res 2008;14(3): 715–20.

30. Katal S, Gholamrezanezhad A, Kessler M, et al. PET in the diagnostic management of soft tissue sarcomas of musculoskeletal origin. Pet Clin 2018; 13(4):609–21.

31. Bastiaannet E, Groen H, Jager PL, et al. The value of FDG-PET in the detection, grading and response to therapy of soft tissue and bone sarcomas; a systematic review and meta-analysis. Cancer Treat Rev 2004;30(1):83–101.

32. Kessler L, Ferdinandus J, Hirmas N, et al. 68 Ga-FAPI as a diagnostic tool in sarcoma: data from the 68 Ga-FAPI PET prospective observational trial. J Nucl Med 2022;63(1):89–95.

33. Koerber SA, Finck R, Dendl K, et al. Novel FAP ligands enable improved imaging contrast in sarcoma patients due to FAPI-PET/CT. Eur J Nucl Med Mol Imaging 2021;48(12):3918–24.

34. Gu B, Liu X, Wang S, et al. Head-to-head evaluation of [(18)F]FDG and [(68) Ga]Ga-DOTA-FAPI-04 PET/CT in recurrent soft tissue sarcoma. Eur J Nucl Med Mol Imaging 2022;49(8):2889–901.

35. Wu S, Lin Z, Shang Q, et al. Use of 68Ga-FAPI PET/CT for detecting myeloid sarcoma of the breast and assessing early response to chemotherapy. Clin Nucl Med 2022;47(6):549–50.

36. Zhang L, Liu Z, Jiang S, et al. 68 Ga-FAPI versus 18 F-FDG PET/CT in recurrent undifferentiated pleomorphic sarcoma of colon mesentery. Clin Nucl Med 2022;47(10):e651–3.

37. Dong A, Zhang Z, Yang Q, et al. 68 Ga-FAPI-04 versus 18 F-FDG PET/CT in a case with intimal sarcoma of the pulmonary artery. Clin Nucl Med 2022; 47(8):748–50.

38. Xu T, Ding H, Ban H, et al. 68 Ga-DOTA-FAPI-04 PET/CT imaging in a case of cardiac angiosarcoma. Clin Nucl Med 2022;47(9):834–5.

39. Wu J, Zhang S, Rao Z, et al. Comparison of 68Ga-FAPI and 18F-FDG PET/CT in dermatofibrosarcoma protuberans. Clin Nucl Med 2022;47(7):629–31.

40. Yang X, Chen H, Li M, et al. Increased 68 Ga-FAPI uptake in dermatofibrosarcoma protuberans. Clin Nucl Med 2022;47(8):710–1.

41. Qiu S, Zou S, Cheng S, et al. Positive FAPI PET/CT in a bilateral mammary angiosarcoma patient with less impressive FDG PET/CT images. Clin Nucl Med 2022;47(7):648–50.

42. Zhang Y, Cai J, Wu Z, et al. Intense [68Ga]Ga-FAPI-04 uptake in solitary fibrous tumor/hemangiopericytoma of the central nervous system. Eur J Nucl Med Mol Imaging 2021;48(12):4103–4.

43. Wang R, Liu Q, Sui H, et al. 68Ga-FAPI outperforms 18F-FDG PET/CT in identifying solitary fibrous tumor. Eur J Nucl Med Mol Imaging 2021;48(6):2055–6.

44. Schwab JH, Boland PJ, Agaram NP, et al. Chordoma and chondrosarcoma gene profile: implications for immunotherapy. Cancer Immunol Immunother 2009;58(3):339–49.

45. Walcott BP, Nahed BV, Mohyeldin A, et al. Chordoma: current concepts, management, and future directions. Lancet Oncol 2012;13(2):e69–76.

46. Pankova V, Thway K, Jones RL, et al. The extracellular matrix in soft tissue sarcomas: pathobiology and cellular signalling. Front Cell Dev Biol 2021;9: 1–17.

47. Fendler WP, Pabst KM, Kessler L, et al. Safety and efficacy of 90Y-FAPI-46 radioligand therapy in patients with advanced sarcoma and other cancer entities. Clin Cancer Res 2022. https://doi.org/10.1158/1078-0432.CCR-22-1432.

48. Ferdinandus J, Kessler L, Hirmas N, et al. Equivalent tumor detection for early and late FAPI-46 PET acquisition. Eur J Nucl Med Mol Imaging 2021; 48(10):3221–7.

Fibroblast Activation Protein Inhibitor Theranostics
The Case for Use in Sarcoma

Rainer Hamacher, MD[a,b,*], Helena Lanzafame, MD[b,c],
Ilektra A. Mavroeidi, MD[a,b], Kim M. Pabst, MD[b,c], Lukas Kessler, MD[b,c],
Phyllis F. Cheung, PhD[d,e], Sebastian Bauer, MD[a,b], Ken Herrmann, MD[b,c],
Hans-Ulrich Schildhaus, MD[b,f], Jens T. Siveke, MD[a,b,d,e],
Wolfgang P. Fendler, MD[b,c]

KEYWORDS

• FAPI • FAP-Alpha • Sarcoma • PET • Radioligand • Therapy • Oncology

KEY POINTS

• Fibroblast activation protein inhibitors (FAPIs) represent a novel theranostic approach in oncology.
• High medical need of novel and more effective treatments in advanced/metastatic sarcoma.
• Sarcoma show high in vivo uptake of FAPI in PET.
• Case reports and case series demonstrate feasibility and preliminary signs for efficacy of FAPI radioligand therapy in sarcoma.

INTRODUCTION

Sarcoma is the umbrella term for rare and heterogenous malignant diseases of the connective tissues with more than 150 different histological subtypes compromising soft tissue and bone sarcoma.[1] The overall incidence of sarcoma is reported with $95.1/10^6$/y but ranging between less than 0.1 to $10/10^6$/y depending on the histological subtype.[2] For patients with localized disease, the aim is to achieve complete resection of the tumor. Depending on histological subtype, tumor size, grading and location of the tumor patients might receive additional perioperative chemotherapy and radiation therapy. The tumor staging is, in general, performed with MR imaging scan for the assessment of the primary lesion complemented by computed tomography (CT) for the exclusion of distant metastases, particularly in the lungs, and with ^{18}F-FDG-PET in selected cases.[3,4] In advanced/metastatic disease, the treatment decision is mainly based on the histological subtype, grading, and resectability. For nonresectable disease, systemic treatment is proposed with palliative intention. In the latter situation, anthracycline-based chemotherapy is the standard first-line treatment of soft tissue sarcoma, whereas high-grade bone sarcomas typically receive multiagent chemotherapy.[3,4] However, many subtypes do not respond to standard

a Department of Medical Oncology, West German Cancer Center, University Hospital Essen, Hufelandstr. 55, Essen, 45122 Germany; b German Cancer Consortium (DKTK), Partner Site University Hospital Essen, Hufelandstr. 55, Essen, 45122 Germany; c Department of Nuclear Medicine, West German Cancer Center, University Hospital Essen, Hufelandstr. 55, Essen, 45122 Germany; d Bridge Institute of Experimental Tumor Therapy, West German Cancer Center, University Hospital Essen, Hufelandstr. 55, Essen, 45122 Germany; e Division of Solid Tumor Translational Oncology, German Cancer Consortium (DKTK, Partner Site Essen) and German Cancer Research Center, DKFZ, Heidelberg, Germany; f Institute of Pathology, West German Cancer Center, University Hospital Essen, Hufelandstr. 55, Essen, 45122 Germany
* Corresponding author. Sarcoma Center.
E-mail address: rainer.hamacher@uk-essen.de

PET Clin 18 (2023) 361–367
https://doi.org/10.1016/j.cpet.2023.02.008
1556-8598/23/© 2023 Elsevier Inc. All rights reserved.

chemotherapy and limited evidence-based data are available for histology-driven systemic therapies. Beyond the first-line setting, several systemic agents are approved for soft tissue sarcoma with modest improvements in the overall survival.[5,6]

The fibroblast activation protein alpha (FAPα) is gaining an emerging interest as novel theranostic target in several malignant diseases due to the high expression on cancer-associated (stromal) fibroblasts (CAFs) infiltrating the tumor microenvironment (TME) but absence in normal adult tissues.[7–9] It is a type II membrane-bound glycoprotein, belonging to the dipeptidyl peptidase 4 family, found in activated stromal fibroblasts. It is expressed in several fetal mesenchymal tissues, during wound healing, fibrosis, or in the microenvironment of a majority of malignant tumors.[7,10,11] In normal adult tissue, the expression of FAPα is restricted to occasional fibroblasts and to alpha cells in the pancreas, which are a glucagon-secreting subset of pancreatic neuroendocrine cells.[11]

The discovery of abundant expression of FAPα in a wide range of malignant tumors raised interest in it as a target for diagnosis and therapy. However, early clinical studies in epithelial cancers, using the approach of FAPα-specific antibodies with iodine 131-labeled monoclonal antibody F19 (^{131}I-mAbF19) or 131-labeled humanized antibody sibrotuzumab, failed due to low efficacy.[12–14] Another approach of FAPα-targeted therapy investigated the use of chimeric antigen receptor-T cell therapy. Although mainly in preclinical studies, results from ongoing clinical studies are pending.[15]

A new and emerging interest in FAPα as a diagnostic and therapeutic target came up with a recently developed series of theranostic FAP inhibitors (FAPIs) that have shown favorable pharmacokinetic properties and high tumor uptake in vivo.[16–24] Here, sarcoma revealed particularly high uptake of the ligand ^{68}Ga-FAPI on PET (**Fig. 1**).[19,25–27] Moreover, we could recently demonstrate that the tumoral uptake intensity to ^{68}Ga-FAPI-46 PET in sarcoma correlates with histopathological FAPα expression (**Fig. 2**) in biopsy/surgical specimens.[26] These findings make sarcoma particularly interesting for FAPI theranostics, which will be addressed in this review article.

Clinical Relevance

Management of sarcoma is challenging due to its rarity, which limits robust randomized control trial data, and the clinical and biological heterogeneity of the disease. Although there has been progress in local therapy through standardized approaches in expert centers, the prognosis of advanced/metastatic disease remains poor with 2-year survival rates of only 20% to 30% in soft tissue sarcoma and 5-year survival rates of 10% to 30% in bone sarcoma.[28,29] Consequently, there is a high need for novel and more effective treatments.

Although sarcoma is a group of heterogeneous malignancies, they share a common origin from connective tissue of mesenchymal or ectodermal origin.[30,31] Already in 1988, Rettig and colleagues analyzed more than 200 malignant tumors, where they showed that most sarcoma were positive for FAPα, whereas carcinoma, lymphoma, and neuroectodermal tumors were negative but the surrounding reactive stroma of these tumors showed a high FAPα expression.[11] An in silico analysis based on RNA expression data of more than 1700 human cancer specimens combined with immunohistochemistry of selected cases similarly showed that FAPα expression in epithelial cancers was restricted to the reactive stromal fibroblasts of the cancer stroma, whereas in sarcoma it could be regularly localized to the malignant cell components.[32] In sarcoma, the expression seems to be independent of their malignancy because low-grade as well as high-grade subtypes express FAPα.[32,33] Recently, our group reported that the tumoral uptake intensity on ^{68}Ga-FAPI-46 PET correlated with histopathological FAPα expression in sarcoma, and the uptake was independent of grading.[26] The high in vivo uptake of FAPI in a variety of different sarcoma subtypes and the expression of FAPα on the tumor cell surface[19,25–27] make sarcoma an attractive candidate for FAPI theranostics. In contradistinction to epithelial cancers, FAPI radioligand therapy (RLT) targets tumor cells directly in many sarcoma entities. Therefore, FAPI RLT in sarcoma might demonstrate efficacy similar to established RLTs, such as ^{177}Lu-Dotatate in neuroendocrine tumors (NET) or ^{177}Lu-PSMA-617 in prostate cancer[34,35] because the target of RLT is highly expressed directly on the tumor cells themselves and allows crossfire effects when aggregated into mass lesions. FAPI RLT has a high potential to become a novel targeted therapeutic approach for a variety of different sarcoma subtypes in advanced/metastatic disease, where patients who might benefit from RLT are identified by diagnostic FAPI PET, which serves as noninvasive tool to screen patients.

Current Evidence

The evidence for FAP-targeted RLT is currently only based on an emerging number of case reports and case series in a plethora of different tumor entities, mainly epithelial cancers.[24,36–41] Most of these studies and reports primarily focused on

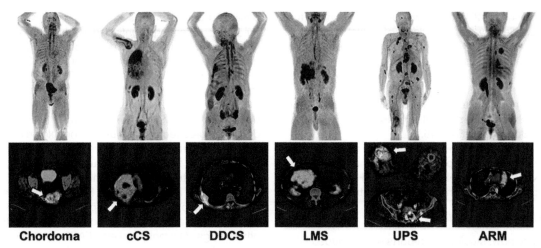

Fig. 1. ^{68}Ga-FAPI-46 PET of different low-grade and high-grade sarcoma subtypes. Maximum intensity projection (MIP) and sagittal PET/CT fusion of low-grade (chordoma and conventional chondrosarcoma [cCS]) and high-grade sarcoma subtypes (dedifferentiated chondrosarcoma [DDCS], leiomyosarcoma [LMS], undifferentiated pleomorphic sarcoma [UPS], and alveolar rhabdomyosarcoma [ARM]). *Arrows* indicate tumor lesions.

feasibility, biodistribution, dosimetry, and safety with preliminary signs for efficacy. Investigated were different FAPI compounds, FAPI-46, FAP-2286, DOTA.SA.FAPi or DOTAGA.(SA.FAPi)2, linked with different radioisotopes, mainly Lutetium-177 (^{177}Lu) and Yttrium-90 (^{90}Y). These studies could demonstrate that repeated application of FAPI RLT is feasible and safe. Notably, in these studies clinical efficacy was observed with mostly disease stabilization in a variety of different tumor types, although, as previously noted, mainly in epithelial cancers. The majority were breast cancer, pancreatic cancer, and thyroid cancer.[24,36–41]

However, our group recently reported on the safety and efficacy of ^{90}Y-FAPI-46 RLT in a cohort of 21 patients with advanced sarcoma and other cancer entities, who received up to 4 cycles RLT.

We could demonstrate that ^{90}Y-FAPI-46-RLT was safe and led to disease control in 8 of 16 evaluable patients, which was associated with improved overall survival.[39] In this cohort of 21 patients, 16 patients had the diagnosis sarcoma, which is so far the largest cohort of patients who received FAPI-RLT. Included were different subtypes, including fibrosarcoma, solitary fibrous tumor, chondrosarcoma, spindle cell sarcoma, osteosarcoma, chordoma, and gastrointestinal neuroectodermal tumor. Patients with sarcoma showed the highest uptake in diagnostic ^{68}Ga-FAPI-46 PET with median standardized uptake value (SUV)$_{max}$ of 25.4. The response evaluation in the cohort of 12 evaluable sarcoma patients showed partial response in 1 (8%) and stable disease in 6 patients (50%).[39] In another cohort published by Assadi and

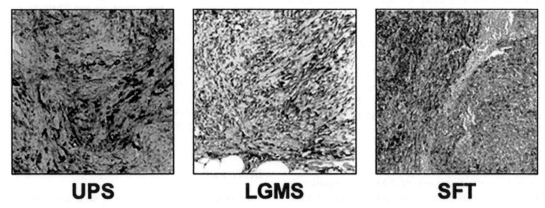

Fig. 2. Immunohistochemistry fibroblast activation protein alpha (FAPα). FAPα immunohistochemical staining in undifferentiated pleomorphic sarcoma [UPS], low-grade myofibroblastic sarcoma [LGMS], and solitary fibrous tumor [SFT].

colleagues, 2 patients with sarcoma, not further classified, were included, of which 1 patient showed insufficient uptake and the other had progressive disease after 4 cycles.[36] Kratochwil and colleagues report a patient with advanced spindle cell sarcoma (NOS) who achieved stable disease for 8 months after 3 cycles of RLT with a cumulative administered activity of 20 GBq with ^{153}Sm- and 8GBq with ^{90}Y-FAPI-46.[41]

According to clinicalTrials.gov at the time of this review, 2 phase 1 trials are recruiting (NCT04849247, NCT05432193). However, prospective results on FAPI RLT are still pending.

Therapeutic Options

Up to now, studies and reports have included FAPI RLT performed with palliative intent in patients with FAPα-positive tumors, as defined by FAPI uptake on PET/CT.[24,36–41] At our center, we offer clinical FAPI RLT to patients after exhaustion of all other treatment options under compassionate-use dispensations available in Germany. Therefore, we have defined the following clinical inclusion criteria[39,40]: (1) progressive metastatic solid tumor, (2) exhaustion of approved therapies based on multidisciplinary tumor board decision, (3) high FAP expression, defined as ^{68}Ga-FAPI-46 PET $SUV_{max} \geq 10$ in more than 50% of tumor lesions, and (4) adequate hematopoiesis (ie, leukocytes >2.5/nL, hemoglobin >7.0 mg/dL, thrombocytes >75/nL) with exceptions for patients who are stable on transfusion. Thus far, we have screened 119 patients, with 21 (18%) found to be eligible for FAPI RLT. The main reason for not performing RLT was insufficient FAPI uptake in tumor lesions.[39] The treatment protocol was published previously.[39,40] In brief, patients at our center receive a first activity of approximately 3.7 GBq ^{90}Y-FAPI-46 *i.v.* followed by dosimetry and approximately 7.4 GBq for up to 4 subsequent RLT cycles with time interval between cycles of 4 to 8 weeks. Noteworthy, based on the recently published safety and efficacy data for patients with sarcoma,[39] we achieved a consensus agreement for partial reimbursement of FAPI RLT in patients with sarcoma fulfilling the above-mentioned inclusion criteria with the medical advisory service of the German association of statutory health insurance funds in the district of North Rhine.

FUTURE DIRECTIONS

For further development of FAPI theranostics in cancer and sarcoma, prospective clinical trials are now required on safety, dosage, and efficacy. An ongoing prospective trial at our site assesses the positive predictive value on a per-region-basis and per-patient-basis of ^{68}Ga-FAPI-46 PET for tumor detection, confirmed by histopathology/biopsy, with additional data about impact on management and reproducibility (NCT05160051).

Current studies indicate that FAPI RLT is well tolerated with a low-rate of severe adverse events, even after multiple cycles.[24,36–41] Nevertheless, optimal activity and treatment regimen has to be defined in prospective studies with oncologic endpoints. Importantly, the low rate of partial responses so far observed under FAPI RLT requires a future improvement. This might be addressed by improvement of FAPI compounds, choice of radioisotopes and approaches to investigate combination therapies of FAPI RLT with other drugs. Currently several FAPI compounds are used, whereas up to now most case series and reports are on FAPI-02, FAPI-04, or FAPI-46. Although having the longest tissue retention of these radiopharmaceuticals, FAPI-46 still has a relatively short retention in tumor tissue and, therefore, contributes to suboptimal tumor radiation. This might be overcome by improvement of radioligand design. For example, promising results have been observed with cyclic peptide-based FAPIs (eg, FAP-2286), squaramide-based FAPIs (eg, DOTAGA.(SA.FAPi)2), Evans blue-modified FAPIs, or FAPI dimeric radiotracers.[23,24,37,42–44] Another promising approach will be combining FAPI RLT with other systemic treatments, especially with radiosensitizing drugs, such as chemotherapy and PARP inhibitors, or with immune checkpoint inhibitors.[45]

These clinical trials have to be accompanied with comprehensive translational research programs for a better understanding which cells are targeted by FAPI RLT and to gain insights into the central impact on tumor progression, adaptive remodeling, and immunoregulation, especially in the context of directly targeting tumor cells in sarcoma, CAFs, and the effect on the TME. In sarcoma, we need a better understanding of which cells express FAPα and particularly how the regularly observed expression on tumor cells themselves is regulated. We do not know, if this might be a subtype specific phenotype or might also be regulated by the TME. This will help to better identify patients who might benefit from FAPI RLT, to understand possible mechanisms of resistance and potential combination therapies.

DISCUSSION

Theranostics are an emerging safe and effective therapeutic approach in precision oncology, as shown for thyroid cancer, NETs, and recently prostate cancer.[34,35,46] However, for many tumor types specific targets are missing. Here, FAPI theranostics are promising pan-cancer radioligands because the target FAPα is expressed at high levels on tumor-associated fibroblasts in a variety of tumor types but almost absent in normal adult tissue.[7–9,11] Several studies showed that FAPI radioligands have a high tumor-to-background ratio[16–24] and, in addition, the feasibility of FAPI RLT could already be shown for different tumor types.[24,36–40] Here, we discussed the specific role of the rare malignant disease sarcoma as an important potential candidate for FAPI theranostics. The rationale for this rests in the high expression of FAPα in the tumor tissue of several sarcoma subtypes, which is particularly observed to be expressed on tumor cells,[11,32,33] and consequently associated with high uptake of the ligand ^{68}Ga-FAPI.[19,25–27] Due to the rarity of sarcoma, it is not surprising that the majority of reports on FAPI RLT are on epithelial cancers. We report our experience from an expert sarcoma center from which we recently analyzed and published the largest cohort of patients with sarcoma who have received FAPI RLT.[39] The high proportion of sarcoma in our cohort (16 of 21 patients), might be explained with the high rate of patients suffering of advanced/metastasized disease and exhaustion of evidence-based therapies at a specialist sarcoma center but also the higher uptake of FAPI in sarcoma compared with epithelial cancers[19,25,26,39,47] (not published NCT04571086).

SUMMARY

The heterogenous disease of sarcoma offers unique opportunities for the implementation of FAPI theranostics. Several studies reported high uptake of the ligand ^{68}Ga-FAPI on PET.[19,25–27] Moreover, studies showed a high expression not only on tumor-associated fibroblasts but also regularly on tumor cells themselves.[11,32,33]

An increasing number of case reports and case series demonstrated feasibility, safety, and preliminary signs for efficacy for FAPI RLT in cancer, including a significant number of patients with different sarcoma subtypes.[24,36–41] Further investigations are needed, to systematically and prospectively address the role of FAPI in sarcoma.

CLINICS CARE POINTS

- Several studies demonstrated high expression of FAPα in different sarcoma subtypes, particularly on tumor cells themselves but systematic and mechanistic studies are missing.

- Retrospective studies showed promising results for theranostic use of FAPIs in sarcoma but prospective studies are required.
- For improvement of FAPI RLT, studies investigating different FAPI compounds and isotopes as well as combinations therapies are necessary.

DECLARATION OF INTERESTS

R. Hamacher reports travel grants from Lilly, Novartis, Switzerland, and PharmaMar, Spain as well as personal fees from Lilly and PharmaMar outside of the submitted work. S. Bauer reports personal fees from Bayer, Eli Lilly, Novartis, Pfizer, and PharmaMar; serves in an advisory/consultancy role for ADC Therapeutics, Bayer, Blueprint Medicines, Daiichi Sankyo, Deciphera, Eli Lilly, Exelixis, Janssen-Cilag, Nanobiotix, Novartis, PharmaMar, Plexxikon, Roche; receives research funding from Novartis; serves as a member of the External Advisory Board of the Federal Ministry of Health for "Off-label use in oncology", all outside of the submitted work. K. Herrmann reports personal fees from Bayer, Sofie Biosciences, SIRTEX, Adacap, Curium, Endocyte, IPSEN, Siemens Healthineers, GE Healthcare, Amgen, Novartis, ymabs, Aktis, Oncology, Pharma15; nonfinancial support from ABX; grants and personal fees from BTG. J.T. Siveke receives honoraria as consultant or for continuing medical education presentations from AstraZeneca, Bayer, Immunocore, Roche, Servier. His institution receives research funding from Bristol-Myers Squibb, Celgene, Roche. He holds ownership and serves on the Board of Directors of Pharma15, all outside the submitted work. W.P. Fendler reports fees from SOFIE Bioscience (research funding), Janssen (consultant, speakers bureau), Calyx (consultant), Bayer (consultant, speakers bureau), and Parexel (image review) outside of the submitted work.

REFERENCES

1. Board WCoTE. Soft Tissue and Bone Tumours International Agency for Research on Cancer. 2020;3(5th Edition).
2. de Pinieux G, Karanian M, Le Loarer F, et al. Nationwide incidence of sarcomas and connective tissue tumors of intermediate malignancy over four years using an expert pathology review network. PLoS One 2021;16(2):e0246958.
3. Gronchi A, Miah AB, Dei Tos AP, et al. Soft tissue and visceral sarcomas: ESMO-EURACAN-GENTURIS Clinical Practice Guidelines for

diagnosis, treatment and follow-up(☆). Ann Oncol 2021;32(11):1348–65.

4. Strauss SJ, Frezza AM, Abecassis N, et al. Bone sarcomas: ESMO-EURACAN-GENTURIS-ERN Paed-Can clinical practice guideline for diagnosis, treatment and follow-up. Ann Oncol 2021;32(12):1520–36.

5. Le Cesne A, Blay JY, Cupissol D, et al. A randomized phase III trial comparing trabectedin to best supportive care in patients with pre-treated soft tissue sarcoma: T-SAR, a French Sarcoma Group trial. Ann Oncol 2021;32(8):1034–44.

6. van der Graaf WT, Blay JY, Chawla SP, et al. Pazopanib for metastatic soft-tissue sarcoma (PALETTE): a randomised, double-blind, placebo-controlled phase 3 trial. Lancet 2012;379(9829):1879–86.

7. Garin-Chesa P, Old LJ, Rettig WJ. Cell surface glycoprotein of reactive stromal fibroblasts as a potential antibody target in human epithelial cancers. Proc Natl Acad Sci U S A 1990;87(18):7235–9.

8. Hamson EJ, Keane FM, Tholen S, et al. Understanding fibroblast activation protein (FAP): substrates, activities, expression and targeting for cancer therapy. Proteomics Clin Appl 2014;8(5–6):454–63.

9. Liu F, Qi L, Liu B, et al. Fibroblast activation protein overexpression and clinical implications in solid tumors: a meta-analysis. PLoS One 2015;10(3):e0116683.

10. Kelly T, Huang Y, Simms AE, et al. Fibroblast activation protein-α: a key modulator of the microenvironment in multiple pathologies. Int Rev Cell Mol Biol 2012;297:83–116.

11. Rettig WJ, Garin-Chesa P, Beresford HR, et al. Cell-surface glycoproteins of human sarcomas: differential expression in normal and malignant tissues and cultured cells. Proc Natl Acad Sci U S A 1988;85(9):3110–4.

12. Hofheinz RD, al-Batran SE, Hartmann F, et al. Stromal antigen targeting by a humanised monoclonal antibody: an early phase II trial of sibrotuzumab in patients with metastatic colorectal cancer. Onkologie 2003;26(1):44–8.

13. Scott AM, Wiseman G, Welt S, et al. A Phase I dose-escalation study of sibrotuzumab in patients with advanced or metastatic fibroblast activation protein-positive cancer. Clin Cancer Res 2003;9(5):1639–47.

14. Welt S, Divgi CR, Scott AM, et al. Antibody targeting in metastatic colon cancer: a phase I study of monoclonal antibody F19 against a cell-surface protein of reactive tumor stromal fibroblasts. J Clin Oncol 1994;12(6):1193–203.

15. Zi F, He J, He D, et al. Fibroblast activation protein α in tumor microenvironment: recent progression and implications (review). Mol Med Rep 2015;11(5):3203–11.

16. Altmann A, Haberkorn U, Siveke J. The latest developments in imaging of fibroblast activation protein. J Nucl Med 2021;62(2):160–7.

17. Ballal S, Yadav MP, Moon ES, et al. Biodistribution, pharmacokinetics, dosimetry of [(68)Ga]Ga-DOTA.SA.FAPi, and the head-to-head comparison with [(18)F]F-FDG PET/CT in patients with various cancers. Eur J Nucl Med Mol Imag 2021;48(6):1915–31.

18. Giesel FL, Kratochwil C, Lindner T, et al. 68)Ga-FAPI PET/CT: biodistribution and preliminary dosimetry estimate of 2 DOTA-containing FAP-targeting agents in patients with various cancers. J Nucl Med 2019;60(3):386–92.

19. Kratochwil C, Flechsig P, Lindner T, et al. 68)Ga-FAPI PET/CT: tracer uptake in 28 different kinds of cancer. J Nucl Med 2019;60(6):801–5.

20. Lindner T, Loktev A, Altmann A, et al. Development of quinoline-based theranostic ligands for the targeting of fibroblast activation protein. J Nucl Med 2018;59(9):1415–22.

21. Loktev A, Lindner T, Burger EM, et al. Development of fibroblast activation protein-targeted radiotracers with improved tumor retention. J Nucl Med 2019;60(10):1421–9.

22. Loktev A, Lindner T, Mier W, et al. A tumor-imaging method targeting cancer-associated fibroblasts. J Nucl Med 2018;59(9):1423–9.

23. Moon ES, Elvas F, Vliegen G, et al. Targeting fibroblast activation protein (FAP): next generation PET radiotracers using squaramide coupled bifunctional DOTA and DATA(5m) chelators. EJNMMI Radiopharm Chem 2020;5(1):19.

24. Baum RP, Schuchardt C, Singh A, et al. Feasibility, biodistribution, and preliminary dosimetry in peptide-targeted radionuclide therapy of diverse adenocarcinomas using (177)Lu-FAP-2286: first-in-humans results. J Nucl Med 2022;63(3):415–23.

25. Gu B, Liu X, Wang S, et al. Head-to-head evaluation of [(18)F]FDG and [(68) Ga]Ga-DOTA-FAPI-04 PET/CT in recurrent soft tissue sarcoma. Eur J Nucl Med Mol Imag 2022;49(8):2889–901.

26. Kessler L, Ferdinandus J, Hirmas N, et al. 68)Ga-FAPI as a diagnostic tool in sarcoma: data from the (68)Ga-FAPI PET prospective observational trial. J Nucl Med 2022;63(1):89–95.

27. Koerber SA, Finck R, Dendl K, et al. Novel FAP ligands enable improved imaging contrast in sarcoma patients due to FAPI-PET/CT. Eur J Nucl Med Mol Imag 2021;48(12):3918–24.

28. Brown HK, Schiavone K, Gouin F, et al. Biology of bone sarcomas and new therapeutic developments. Calcif Tissue Int 2018;102(2):174–95.

29. Tap WD, Wagner AJ, Schöffski P, et al. Effect of doxorubicin plus olaratumab vs doxorubicin plus placebo on survival in patients with advanced soft

tissue sarcomas: the ANNOUNCE randomized clinical trial. JAMA 2020;323(13):1266–76.

30. Taylor BS, Barretina J, Maki RG, et al. Advances in sarcoma genomics and new therapeutic targets. Nat Rev Cancer 2011;11(8):541–57.

31. Yang J, Ren Z, Du X, et al. The role of mesenchymal stem/progenitor cells in sarcoma: update and dispute. Stem Cell Invest 2014;1:18.

32. Dolznig H, Schweifer N, Puri C, et al. Characterization of cancer stroma markers: in silico analysis of an mRNA expression database for fibroblast activation protein and endosialin. Cancer Immun 2005;5: 10.

33. Dohi O, Ohtani H, Hatori M, et al. Histogenesis-specific expression of fibroblast activation protein and dipeptidylpeptidase-IV in human bone and soft tissue tumours. Histopathology 2009;55(4):432–40.

34. Sartor O, de Bono J, Chi KN, et al. Lutetium-177-PSMA-617 for metastatic castration-resistant prostate cancer. N Engl J Med 2021;385(12):1091–103.

35. Strosberg J, El-Haddad G, Wolin E, et al. Phase 3 trial of (177)Lu-dotatate for midgut neuroendocrine tumors. N Engl J Med 2017;376(2):125–35.

36. Assadi M, Rekabpour SJ, Jafari E, et al. Feasibility and therapeutic potential of 177Lu-fibroblast activation protein inhibitor-46 for patients with relapsed or refractory cancers: a preliminary study. Clin Nucl Med 2021;46(11):e523–30.

37. Ballal S, Yadav MP, Moon ES, et al. First-in-human results on the biodistribution, pharmacokinetics, and dosimetry of [(177)Lu]Lu-DOTA.SA.FAPi and [(177)Lu]Lu-DOTAGA.(SA.FAPi)(2). Pharmaceuticals 2021;14(12):1212.

38. Ballal S, Yadav MP, Moon ES, et al. Novel fibroblast activation protein inhibitor-based targeted theranostics for radioiodine-refractory differentiated thyroid cancer patients: a pilot study. Thyroid 2022;32(1): 65–77.

39. Fendler WP, Pabst KM, Kessler L, et al. Safety and efficacy of 90Y-FAPI-46 radioligand therapy in patients with advanced sarcoma and other cancer entities. Clin Cancer Res 2022;28(19):4346–53.

40. Ferdinandus J, Costa PF, Kessler L, et al. Initial clinical experience with (90)Y-FAPI-46 radioligand therapy for advanced-stage solid tumors: a case series of 9 patients. J Nucl Med 2022;63(5):727–34.

41. Kratochwil C, Giesel FL, Rathke H, et al. [(153)Sm] Samarium-labeled FAPI-46 radioligand therapy in a patient with lung metastases of a sarcoma. Eur J Nucl Med Mol Imag 2021;48(9):3011–3.

42. Wen X, Xu P, Shi M, et al. Evans blue-modified radiolabeled fibroblast activation protein inhibitor as long-acting cancer therapeutics. Theranostics 2022; 12(1):422–33.

43. Zboralski D, Hoehne A, Bredenbeck A, et al. Preclinical evaluation of FAP-2286 for fibroblast activation protein targeted radionuclide imaging and therapy. Eur J Nucl Med Mol Imag 2022;49(11):3651–67.

44. Zhao L, Chen J, Pang Y, et al. Development of fibroblast activation protein inhibitor-based dimeric radiotracers with improved tumor retention and antitumor efficacy. Mol Pharm 2022;19(10):3640–51.

45. Chan TG, O'Neill E, Habjan C, et al. Combination strategies to improve targeted radionuclide therapy. J Nucl Med 2020;61(11):1544–52.

46. Sgouros G, Bodei L, McDevitt MR, et al. Radiopharmaceutical therapy in cancer: clinical advances and challenges. Nat Rev Drug Discov 2020;19(9): 589–608.

47. Hicks RJ, Roselt PJ, Kallur KG, et al. Fapi PET/CT: will it end the hegemony of (18)F-fdg in oncology? J Nucl Med 2021;62(3):296–302.

Radiation Therapy Planning Using Fibroblast Activation Protein Inhibitor

Stefan A. Koerber, MD[a,b,c],*

KEYWORDS

- FAPI-PET/CT • Radiation oncology • Treatment planning • Oncologic management

KEY POINTS

- Computed tomography (CT), MR imaging, and PET with fluorodeoxyglucose F18/CT are commonly used for radiation therapy planning; however, issues including precise nodal staging on CT or false positive results on PET/CT limit the usability of these imaging techniques.
- Several clinical trials using fibroblast activation protein ligands for additional imaging have provided promising results regarding staging and target volume delineation—particularly suitable for sarcoma, some gastrointestinal tumors, head and neck tumors, and lung and pancreatic cancer.
- Although further prospective trials are necessary to identify clinical settings for its application in radiation oncology, fibroblast activation protein inhibitor PET/CT indisputably represents an excellent opportunity for assisting radiotherapy planning, particularly among tumor types less suitable for conventional PET imaging.

INTRODUCTION

The use of high-energy rays, alone or in combination with further treatment modalities such as chemotherapy, has been a very effective tool for treating cancer for more than 120 years. After the discovery of X rays by German physicist W.C. Roentgen in 1895, the first efforts were made to irradiate patients just 1 year later.[1,2] In November 1896, the Austrian radiologist Leopold Freund performed the first successful x-ray treatment in a clinical setting (fractionated radiation therapy of a hairy nevus) and provided the first scientific proof of the biological effectiveness of x rays marking the inauguration of radiation oncology as a new discipline.[3] Since that time, the field of radiation oncology has dramatically changed. Substantial progress has been made owing to technical innovations leading to a more precise treatment approach. Advances in imaging techniques, radiotherapy equipment, and linacs enable irradiation of complex and irregularly shaped tumor volumes while excluding the surrounding healthy tissue. Moreover, modern techniques like radiosurgery, high linear energy transfer therapy, and recent developments, such as MR-guided irradiation, contribute to the success of the oncologic treatment approach.[4] However, because of absent histopathologic verification in the field of radiation oncology, reliable and precise imaging tools for treatment planning are tremendously important for an effective and well-tolerated irradiation. Progress in conventional imaging (ie, computed tomography [CT] and MR imaging) has resulted in an improvement in tumor localization. However, accurate target volume delineation often remains challenging.

The author has nothing to disclose.
[a] Department of Radiation Oncology, Heidelberg University Hospital, Heidelberg, Germany; [b] Clinical Cooperation Unit Radiation Oncology, German Cancer Research Center, Heidelberg, Germany; [c] Department of Radiation Oncology, Barmherzige Brueder Hospital Regensburgh, Regensburg, Germany
* Department of Radiation Oncology, Heidelberg University Hospital, Heidelberg, Germany.
E-mail addresses: stefan.koerber@med.uni-heidelberg.de; stefan.koerber@barmherzige-regensburg.de

STANDARD IMAGING TECHNIQUES FOR RADIATION ONCOLOGY

Regarding dose calculation, CT imaging provides the basis for radiation therapy in general. Thus, a CT scan with or without contrast is performed for almost every patient and is used for gross tumor volume (GTV) delineation, which is used as the starting point for detailed radiotherapy planning. Although CT for treatment planning might be sufficient for several radiooncologic indications issues, such as palliative irradiation of bone metastases or a whole-brain radiation therapy, there is a lack of relevant information when performing CT-only–based radiation planning for sophisticated target volumes, such as brain tumors, sarcoma, and head and neck cancers (**Fig. 1**).

Therefore, the use of additional MR imaging with a superior soft tissue contrast is noticeably increasing and adds a significant value in delineation of many tumor entities involving head and neck, prostate, and brain lesions.[5–10] State-of-the-art MR protocols often provide excellent imaging data and support complex target volume delineation for both external beam radiotherapy and brachytherapy.[11] However, MR imaging also has several limitations. These include identification of small nodal metastases, precise GTV delineation for some cancers, or distinguishing the primary tumor from adjacent atelectasis. PET scan has proven exceptionally useful in such cases. Different tracers are used for target volume delineation and are often integrated in the radiooncologic planning workflow by default (**Table 1**).

For radiotherapy planning, PET/CT is commonly used for lung,[12–14] prostate,[15–17] head and neck cancers,[18–20] brain tumors,[21–23] and several gastrointestinal (GI) tumors, such as esophageal and anal cancer.[24–26] Nevertheless, apart from technical features influencing imaging evaluation and complicating standardization, cautious image interpretation should be given with regard to non-tumor sources of false positive findings on PET scan. Physiologic brown fat uptake, inflammation, or patient movement artifacts may obscure or simulate tumor activity influencing target volume delineation.[27] Moreover, low glucose transporter and hexokinase activity in certain tumor types and a lack of specificity limit the validity of fluorodeoxyglucose F 18 (^{18}F-FDG)—the most frequently used tracer for oncologic PET imaging.[28] Thus, innovative tracers allowing precise tumor staging before irradiation as well as assisting with individual radiotherapy planning are of great interest.

CLINICAL APPLICATIONS OF FIBROBLAST ACTIVATION PROTEIN INHIBITOR FOR RADIATION ONCOLOGY

Since the introduction of PET imaging of the fibroblast activation protein (FAP), which is overexpressed by stromal fibroblasts in more than 90% of epithelial cancers, promising tracers with high diagnostic performance for tumor staging and demarcation of malignant tissue were born.[28] First clinical results demonstrated remarkably high uptake and image contrast in several cancers, such as sarcoma and lung cancer.[29] This diagnostic value may grant new applications for fibroblast activation protein inhibitors (FAPIs) as a PET tracer in radiotherapy planning. The following section takes a closer look at the potential of these novel PET tracers in the field of radiation oncology.

Sarcoma

Although clinical data on FAPI-PET/CT and radiation therapy are generally limited, the use of FAPIs appears promising, especially for cancers less suitable for FDG imaging. First clinical data on sarcoma from 2021 demonstrated excellent tumor-to-background ratios (>7), suggesting a high potential for the clinical use of FAPI-PET/CT (**Fig. 2**).[30] Compared with conventional ^{18}F-FDG tracer, ^{68}Ga-DOTA-FAPI-04 PET/CT proved to be a promising new imaging modality.[31,32] In a cohort of 45 patients with recurrent soft tissue sarcoma, FAPI-04 detected more lesions compared with FDG and outperformed in sensitivity, specificity, positive predictive value (PPV), negative predictive value, and accuracy.[32] These data were confirmed by a prospective observational trial resulting in a high PPV and sensitivity in sarcoma staging.[33] The investigators observed almost 20% of all patients with an upstaging and 30% with changes in oncologic management after ^{68}Ga-FAPI-PET/CT.[33] Thus, the use of FAP tracers may add relevant clinical information before starting radiation therapy also compared with conventional PET staging and allows individual treatment approaches. Future trials must focus on the clinical role of FAPI for target delineation considering MR imaging is still a crucial part of radiotherapy planning.[34–36]

Gastrointestinal Tumors (Esophageal and Gastric Carcinoma, Colorectal and Anal Cancer)

The first clinical experience with FAPI and lower GI tumors was published in 2020.[37] Although the cohort was small (22 patients), a change in tumor stage after ^{68}Ga-FAPI-PET/CT was found in

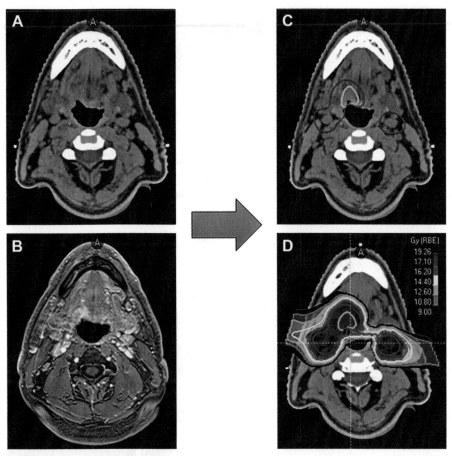

Fig. 1. A 55-year-old male patient with cT2 cN2c adenoid cystic carcinoma of the tongue in CT (*A*). MR imaging (*B*) was particularly helpful for boost delineation (*C*), which was performed with carbon ions (*D*).

Table 1 Common PET tracers used for radiotherapy planning		
Tracer	**Radiopharmaceutical**	**Clinical Application**
Choline	^{11}C	Prostate cancer, hepatocellular carcinoma
Dihydroxyphenylalanine (DOPA)	^{18}F	Glioma
DOTATOC	^{18}F	Meningioma, neuroendocrine tumors
Fluoroethyl-L-tyrosine (FET)	^{18}F	Glioma
Fluorodeoxyglucose (FDG)	^{18}F	Many tumor types (eg, lung, esophageal cancer)
Misonidazole (MISO)	^{18}F	For identification of hypoxic regions for a radiation boost in several tumor types (eg, head & neck)
Prostate-specific membrane antigen (PSMA)	$^{68}Ga, {}^{18}F$	Prostate cancer

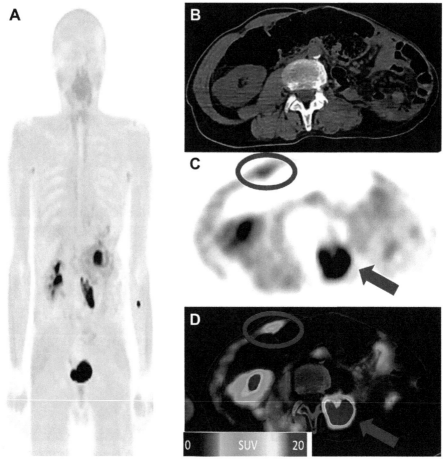

Fig. 2. A patient with a relapse of a liposarcoma (*arrows*). ⁶⁸Ga-FAPI-PET/CT (*A*: MIP; *B*: CT Dx; *C*: FAPI-PET Dx; *D*: FAPI-PET/CT Dx) before local radiation therapy showed tracer uptake suspicious of peritoneal carcinomatosis (*circles*).

almost half the study population.[37] Thus, there is a promising role for FAP tracers as a staging tool before radiation therapy. Although improved nodal detection in colorectal cancer (CRC) was suggested, FAPI-PET/CT is also highly suitable for detecting peritoneal involvement.[38,39] Elboga and colleagues[39] reported a high efficacy regarding the detection of peritoneal involvement as well as for definition of primary tumor and metastatic lesions—all superior to ¹⁸F-FDG-PET/CT. These observations were confirmed by a comparison of ⁶⁸Ga-FAPI-PET/CT and ¹⁸F-FDG-PET/CT for patients with CRC. ⁶⁸Ga-FAPI-PET/CT resulted in a much higher sensitivity and specificity regarding the detection of primary lesions, nodal involvement, and peritoneal lesions[40] (**Fig. 3**).

Similar results were obtained for upper GI tumors. Again, the use of FAP tracer suggested a high potential for increasing the diagnostic accuracy for esophageal as well as gastric cancer

outperforming FDG-PET/CT.[41–46] Several trials reported a superior detection for both primary tumor and peritoneal carcinomatosis, thereby providing better diagnostic performance.[41,42] For patients with esophageal cancer undergoing radiation therapy, the use of FAPI-PET/CT may adapt simultaneous integrated boost concepts and assist tumor volume delineation owing to excellent radiotracer uptake.[45,47] Regarding GTV delineation, ⁶⁸Ga-FAPI-PET/CT imaging data were comparable with findings obtained from endoscopic examination, suggesting a potential benefit of this novel tracer for target volume delineation and avoidance of tumor geographic misses, which are defined by the percentage of tumor not receiving the planned treatment dose.[47]

Head and Neck Cancer

Because of complex anatomy, reliable staging tools and imaging allowing accurate identification

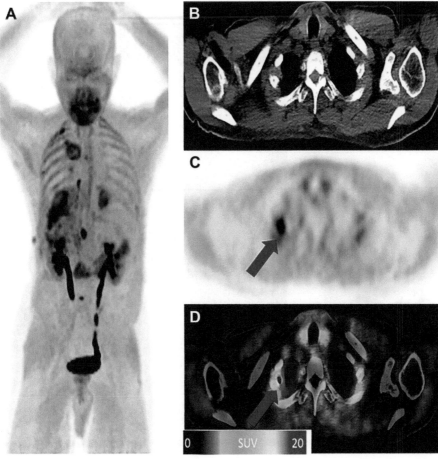

Fig. 3. A 65-year-old patient with M1 CRC and severe pain of the right upper thorax. ^{68}Ga-FAPI-PET/CT (*A*: MIP; *B*: CT Dx; *C*: FAPI-PET Dx; *D*: FAPI-PET/CT Dx) demonstrated a pleural lesion (*arrows*) leading to local irradiation.

of tumor tissue and its relation to radiation-sensitive normal tissues are essential for radiation therapy. ^{18}F-FDG-PET/CT is often used for staging and radiotherapy planning but has several limitations. Although peritumoral inflammation or surgery may lead to false positive uptake, a high FDG uptake is also observed in normal tissues, such as lymphoid tissue and salivary glands.[48,49] For head and neck squamous cell carcinoma, FAP imaging seems to be a promising tool for pretherapeutic staging and appears to reduce false positive results obtained by ^{18}F-FDG with respect to nodal metastases located in the neck region.[49–51] Moreover, ^{68}Ga-FAPI-PET/CT resulted in an improved detection rate of the primary tumor location also for cancers of unknown primary undetected by ^{18}F-FDG findings.[52,53] For numerous patients with head and neck tumors, the use of FAPI tracers proved helpful for precise staging before radiation therapy and enhanced the accuracy of radiotherapy planning volumes—compared with conventional imaging like CT or

MR imaging as well as ^{18}F-FDG-PET/CT (**Fig. 4**).[54–58] In one of the largest trials, which included 45 patients with nasopharyngeal carcinoma, FAPI-PET/CT was found highly suitable for target volume delineation, especially for patients with tumor relapse. However, T stage was underestimated in 2 patients compared with MR imaging.[58] Therefore, forgoing MR imaging in the context of radiotherapy planning of head and neck tumors should be done with the utmost caution owing to the potential loss of clinically relevant information.

Lung Cancer

Although lung tumors were found to have among the highest uptake of ^{68}Ga-FAPI ligand of tumors evaluated thus far (average maximum standardized uptake value >12), clinical data remain limited. One possible reason may lie in the well-established use of ^{18}F-FDG-PET/CT in this oncologic setting. However, first results of several

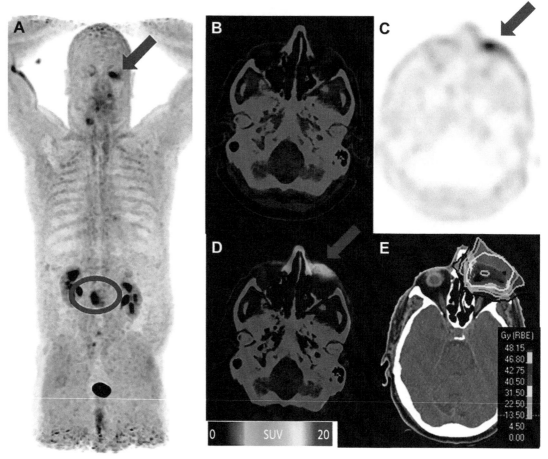

Fig. 4. ⁶⁸Ga-FAPI-PET/CT (*A*: MIP; *B*: CT Dx; *C*: FAPI-PET Dx; *D*: FAPI-PET/CT Dx) of a patient with a cancer of unknown primary and a resected lymph node. Imaging provided a second lesion in the left orbit (*arrows*) treated with irradiation (*E*) and the potential primary tumor within the duodenum (*circle*).

clinical studies, including FAPI-PET/CT imaging for lung cancer, provided promising results regarding its accuracy and detection rate.[59–62] A prospective trial with 134 diagnosed or suspected patients with non–small cell lung cancer (NSCLC) reported an improved diagnostic performance of ⁶⁸Ga-DOTA-FAPI-04 PET/CT with respect to T, N, and M staging compared with conventional ¹⁸F-FDG-PET imaging (**Fig. 5**). Considering false positive uptake of ¹⁸F-FDG in reactive nodes in the mediastinum and hilum, the novel tracer was able to accurately differentiate nonmetastatic and metastatic nodes, allowing avoidance of histologic verification.[62]

For radiotherapy planning, reliable information regarding N as well as T stage is tremendously important owing to its influence on target volume delineation and hence treatment toxicity, especially for adjacent lung and esophagus. Thus, precise staging may reduce target volume and treatment-related side effects, improving the

tolerance of irradiation as well as patients' compliance. Although first clinical data attribute a potential value to FAPI-PET/CT for clinical routine evaluation of patients with NSCLC, a larger prospective trial will be necessary to confirm its role.

Pancreatic Cancer

For pancreatic cancer, conventional PET/CT using ¹⁸F-FDG is challenging. Although FDG-avidity in pancreatic tumors is only marginally higher compared with healthy parenchyma itself, the detection rate of nodal metastases is variable, and false positive findings may occur with inflammation.[63–65] Moreover, FDG-PET/CT provided false negative results in about 10% of patients with pancreatic cancer.[66] Therefore, FAPI-PET/CT may add relevant diagnostic value with regard to tumor identification, staging, and target volume delineation (**Fig. 6**). Several trials concluded that ⁶⁸Ga-FAPI-PET/CT is a promising imaging tracer

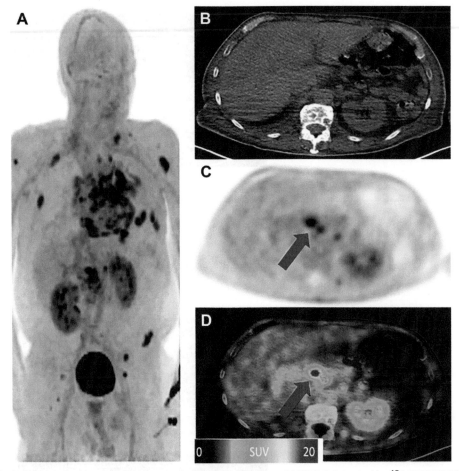

Fig. 5. Cholestasis caused by a nodal metastasis (*arrows*) of a stage IV NSCLC detected by ^{18}F-FAPI-PET/CT (*A*: MIP; *B*: CT Dx; *C*: FAPI-PET Dx; *D*: FAPI-PET/CT Dx). Palliative radiation therapy was initiated after imaging.

outperforming conventional imaging owing to its high tumor-to-background contrast.[67–70] The novel tracer was highly efficient regarding nodal metastases and influenced target volume definition.[65,70] Although the cohort was small and consisted of patients with local relapse, even automatic GTV contouring was achieved based on the FAPI signal with convincing results suggesting a high potential as an additional imaging modality for patients with pancreatic cancer.[65] However, also nonmalignant findings in patients with fibroplasia or fibrotic activity will be detected by FAPI and should be kept in mind during image evaluation and radiotherapy planning. Delayed imaging or the use of multisequence MR imaging may help to distinguish between malignant and benign findings[71]

DISCUSSION

Since the development of FAPIs as appealing radiopharmaceuticals for molecular imaging

applications and therapeutic treatment approaches, numerous trials have highlighted their promising role as a reliable staging tool and pointed out multiple applications also for radiation oncology. For several cancers, ^{68}Ga-FAPI seems to be superior compared with ^{18}F-FDG owing to a lower background uptake in most healthy organs, resulting in an equal or higher tumor-to-background contrast.[28,72] Moreover, interobserver agreement rates on FAPI imaging demonstrated a fair to good concordance rate, which in principle enables clinical use.[73] Although several trials already strengthen FAPI-PET/CT as an additional diagnostic tool for radiotherapy planning, several aspects should currently be considered. First, the number of prospective and histologically confirmed clinical trials remains limited. Thus, routine application of these novel tracers should be implemented with caution. Considering some pitfalls also for FAPI-PET/CT, image interpretation and target volume delineation must be performed painstakingly—similar to other PET tracers. Only

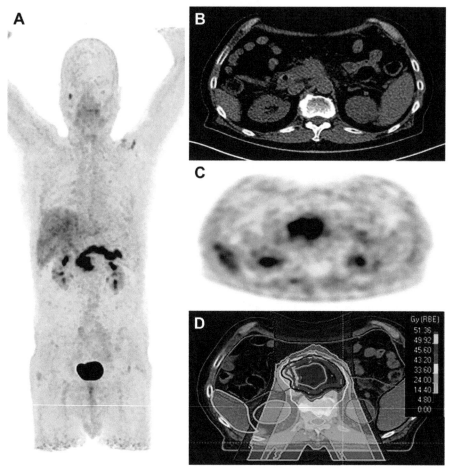

Fig. 6. A 72-year-old patient with cT4 pancreatic cancer not suitable for surgery. Target volume delineation for definitive chemoradiation with carbon ions (*D*) was performed after ⁶⁸Ga-FAPI-PET/CT (*A*: MIP; *B*: CT Dx; *C*: FAPI-PET Dx).

a multiprofessional and interdisciplinary team may avoid misinterpretation of false positive FAPI uptake in, for example, muscles, uterus, or wound healing, resulting in erroneous changes in oncologic management (worst case: palliative instead of curative treatment) or incorrect adaptation of radiation treatment plans.[74,75] Finally, to achieve optimal conditions for radiotherapy planning, FAPI-PET/CT should be performed in radiation treatment position. Similar conditions (eg, with regard to individual positioning of the patient or location of organs) considerably influence the precision in treatment planning and are the prerequisite for hypofractionation, radiosurgery, or particle therapy within critical anatomical regions.[76]

However, FAP ligands are highly promising novel tracers offering a new diagnostic potential for radiation oncology in a variety of diseases. Some reasons for a potential success story of FAPI-PET/CT include a low uptake in almost all normal tissue, the ability to provide also prognostic information adapting oncologic management, and a high expression in many different cancers (including several with typically low ¹⁸F-FDG-avidity) leading to a perfect diagnostic candidate for precise and individual radiation oncology treatment planning.[77] There are numerous ongoing and planned studies that will provide further clinical data and closely evaluate the role of FAPI-PET/CT in clinical routine in the near future.

SUMMARY

First clinical trials on FAPI-PET/CT for radiation therapy and treatment planning demonstrated promising results particularly among cancers, such as pancreatic cancer, which are less suitable for conventional PET imaging owing to either low FDG-avidity or high adjacent physiologic activity.

Nevertheless, further prospective trials, including histopathologic verification, a comparison with standard imaging modalities, and—as an optimum—randomization, are mandatorily required to confirm the increasing importance of the novel tracer and finally assess the impact on radiation oncology. Improved radiation planning should ideally increase local control rates and have similar or lower toxicity to conventional planning strategies.

CLINICS CARE POINTS

- Promising results particularly among cancers which are less suitable for conventional imaging (e.g. pancreatic cancer), be aware of the detection of also nonmalignant finding, large prospective trials are highly awaited.

REFERENCES

1. Foray N. Victor Despeignes, the forgotten pioneer of radiation oncology. Int J Radiat Oncol Biol Phys 2016;96(4):717–21.
2. Mould RF. Emil Herman Grubbé (1875–1960) with special reference to priority for X-ray cancer therapy. Nowotwory 2018;68(5–6):286–9.
3. Kogelnik HD. Inauguration of radiotherapy as a new scientific speciality by Leopold Freund 100 years ago. Radiother Oncol 1997;42(3):203–11.
4. Holsti LR. Development of clinical radiotherapy since 1896. Acta Oncol 1995;34(8):995–1003.
5. Westphalen AC, McKenna DA, Kurhanewicz J, et al. Role of magnetic resonance imaging and magnetic resonance spectroscopic imaging before and after radiotherapy for prostate cancer. J Endourol 2008; 22(4):789–94.
6. Parker CC, Damyanovich A, Haycocks T, et al. Magnetic resonance imaging in the radiation treatment planning of localized prostate cancer using intraprostatic fiducial markers for computed tomography co-registration. Radiother Oncol 2003;66(2):217–24.
7. Lemort M, Canizares AC, Kampouridis S. Advances in imaging head and neck tumours. Curr Opin Oncol 2006;18(3):234–9.
8. Chauhan D, Rawat S, Sharma MK, et al. Improving the accuracy of target volume delineation by combined use of computed tomography, magnetic resonance imaging and positron emission tomography in head and neck carcinomas. J Cancer Res Ther 2015;11(4):746–51.
9. Prabhakar R, Haresh KP, Ganesh T, et al. Comparison of computed tomography and magnetic resonance based target volume in brain tumors. J Cancer Res Ther 2007;3(2):121–3.
10. Datta NR, David R, Gupta RK, et al. Implications of contrast-enhanced CT-based and MRI-based target volume delineations in radiotherapy treatment planning for brain tumors. J Cancer Res Ther 2008; 4(1):9–13.
11. Pötter R, Tanderup K, Schmid MP, et al. MRI-guided adaptive brachytherapy in locally advanced cervical cancer (EMBRACE-I): a multicentre prospective cohort study. Lancet Oncol 2021;22(4):538–47.
12. van Tinteren H, Hoekstra OS, Smit EF, et al. Effectiveness of positron emission tomography in the preoperative assessment of patients with suspected non-small-cell lung cancer: the PLUS multicentre randomised trial. Lancet 2002;359(9315): 1388–92.
13. Fischer B, Lassen U, Mortensen J, et al. Preoperative staging of lung cancer with combined PET–CT. N Engl J Med 2009;361(1):32–9.
14. Nestle U, Schimek-Jasch T, Kremp S, et al. Imaging-based target volume reduction in chemoradiotherapy for locally advanced non-small-cell lung cancer (PET-Plan): a multicentre, open-label, randomised, controlled trial. Lancet Oncol 2020;21(4): 581–92.
15. Hope TA, Goodman JZ, Allen IE, et al. Metaanalysis of 68Ga-PSMA-11 PET accuracy for the detection of prostate Cancer validated by histopathology. J Nucl Med 2019;60(6):786–93.
16. Perera M, Papa N, Roberts M, et al. Gallium-68 prostate-specific membrane antigen positron emission tomography in advanced prostate cancer-updated diagnostic utility, sensitivity, specificity, and distribution of prostate-specific membrane antigen-avid lesions: a systematic review and meta-analysis. Eur Urol 2020;77(4):403–17.
17. Hofman MS, Lawrentschuk N, Francis RJ, et al. Prostate-specific membrane antigen PET-CT in patients with high-risk prostate cancer before curative-intent surgery or radiotherapy (proPSMA): a prospective, randomised, multicentre study. Lancet 2020;395(10231):1208–16.
18. Pedraza S, Ruiz-Alonso A, Hernández-Martínez AC, et al. 18F-FDG PET/CT in staging and delineation of radiotherapy volume for head and neck cancer. Rev Esp Med Nucl 2019;38(3):154–9.
19. Wright CL, Washington IR, Bhatt AD, et al. Emerging opportunities for digital PET/CT to advance locoregional therapy in head and neck cancer. Semin Radiat Oncol 2019;29(2):93–101.
20. Samołyk-Kogaczewska N, Sierko E, Zuzda K, et al. PET/MRI-guided GTV delineation during radiotherapy planning in patients with squamous cell carcinoma of the tongue. Strahlenther Onkol 2019; 195(9):780–91.
21. Niyazi M, Geisler J, Siefert A, et al. FET-PET for malignant glioma treatment planning. Radiother Oncol 2011;99(1):44–8.

22. Pafundi DH, Laack NN, Youland RS, et al. Biopsy validation of 18F-DOPA PET and biodistribution in gliomas for neurosurgical planning and radiotherapy target delineation: results of a prospective pilot study. Neuro Oncol 2013;15(8):1058–67.

23. Galldiks N, Langen KJ, Albert NL, et al. PET imaging in patients with brain metastasis-report of the RANO/PET group. Neuro Oncol 2019;21(5):585–95.

24. Jimenez-Jimenez E, Mateos P, Aymar N, et al. Radiotherapy volume delineation using 18F-FDG-PET/CT modifies gross node volume in patients with oesophageal cancer. Clin Transl Oncol 2018; 20(11):1460–6.

25. Münch S, Marr L, Feuerecker B, et al. Impact of 18 F-FDG-PET/CT on the identification of regional lymph node metastases and delineation of the primary tumor in esophageal squamous cell carcinoma patients. Strahlenther Onkol 2020;196(9): 787–94.

26. Albertsson P, Alverbratt C, Liljegren A, et al. Positron emission tomography and computed tomographic (PET/CT) imaging for radiation therapy planning in anal cancer: a systematic review and meta-analysis. Crit Rev Oncol Hematol 2018;126:6–12.

27. McKay MJ, Taubman KL, Foroudi F, et al. Molecular imaging using PET/CT for radiation therapy planning for adult cancers: current status and expanding applications. Int J Radiat Oncol Biol Phys 2018;102(4): 783–91.

28. Giesel FL, Kratochwil C, Schlittenhardt J, et al. Head-to-head intra-individual comparison of biodistribution and tumor uptake of 68 Ga-FAPI and 18 F-FDG PET/CT in cancer patients. Eur J Nucl Med Mol Imaging 2021;48(13):4377–85.

29. Kratochwil C, Flechsig P, Lindner T, et al. 68 Ga-FAPI PET/CT: tracer uptake in 28 different kinds of cancer. J Nucl Med 2019;60(6):801–5.

30. Koerber SA, Finck R, Dendl K, et al. Novel FAP ligands enable improved imaging contrast in sarcoma patients due to FAPI-PET/CT. Eur J Nucl Med Mol Imaging 2021;48(12):3918–24.

31. Zhou X, Wang S, Zhu H, et al. Imaging superiority of [68 Ga]-FAPI-04 over [18 F]-FDG PET/CT in alveolar soft part sarcoma (ASPS). Eur J Nucl Med Mol Imaging 2021;48(11):3741–2.

32. Gu B, Liu X, Wang S, et al. Head-to-head evaluation of [18 F]FDG and [68 Ga]Ga-DOTA-FAPI-04 PET/CT in recurrent soft tissue sarcoma. Eur J Nucl Med Mol Imaging 2022;49(8):2889–901.

33. Kessler L, Ferdinandus J, Hirmas N, et al. 68 Ga-FAPI as a diagnostic tool in sarcoma: data from the 68 Ga-FAPI PET prospective observational trial. J Nucl Med 2022;63(1):89–95.

34. Yoo HJ, Hong SH, Kang Y, et al. MR imaging of myxofibrosarcoma and undifferentiated sarcoma with emphasis on tail sign; diagnostic and prognostic value. Eur Radiol 2014;24(8):1749–57.

35. Wang D, Zhang Q, Eisenberg BL, et al. Significant reduction of late toxicities in patients with extremity sarcoma treated with image-guided radiation therapy to a reduced target volume: results of radiation therapy oncology group RTOG-0630 trial. J Clin Oncol 2015;33(20):2231–8.

36. Blitzer GC, Yadav P, Morris ZS. The role of MRI-guided radiotherapy for soft tissue sarcomas. J Clin Med 2022;11(4):1042.

37. Koerber SA, Staudinger F, Kratochwil C, et al. The role of 68 Ga-FAPI PET/CT for patients with malignancies of the lower gastrointestinal tract: first clinical experience. J Nucl Med 2020;61(9):1331–6.

38. Polack M, Hagenaars SC, Couwenberg A, et al. Characteristics of tumour stroma in regional lymph node metastases in colorectal cancer patients: a theoretical framework for future diagnostic imaging with FAPI PET/CT. Clin Transl Oncol 2022;24(9): 1776–84.

39. Elboga U, Sahin E, Kus T, et al. Comparison of 68 Ga-FAPI PET/CT and 18 FDG PET/CT modalities in gastrointestinal system malignancies with peritoneal involvement. Mol Imaging Biol 2022. https://doi.org/10.1007/s11307-022-01729-x.

40. Kömek H, Can C, Kaplan I, et al. Comparison of [68 Ga]Ga-DOTA-FAPI-04 PET/CT and [18 F]FDG PET/CT in colorectal cancer. Eur J Nucl Med Mol Imaging 2022;49(11):3898–909.

41. Jiang D, Chen X, You Z, et al. Comparison of [68 Ga] Ga-FAPI-04 and [18 F]-FDG for the detection of primary and metastatic lesions in patients with gastric cancer: a bicentric retrospective study. Eur J Nucl Med Mol Imaging 2022;49(2):732–42.

42. Kuten J, Levine C, Shamni O, et al. Head-to-head comparison of [68 Ga]Ga-FAPI-04 and [18 F]-FDG PET/CT in evaluating the extent of disease in gastric adenocarcinoma. Eur J Nucl Med Mol Imaging 2022;49(2):743–50.

43. Liu H, Hu Z, Yang X, et al. Comparison of [68 Ga]Ga-DOTA-FAPI-04 and [18 F]FDG uptake in esophageal cancer. Front Oncol 2022;12:875081.

44. Qin C, Shao F, Gai Y, et al. 68 Ga-DOTA-FAPI-04 PET/MR in the evaluation of gastric carcinomas: comparison with 18 F-FDG PET/CT. J Nucl Med 2022;63(1):81–8.

45. Ristau J, Giesel FL, Haefner MF, et al. Impact of primary staging with fibroblast activation protein specific enzyme inhibitor (FAPI)-PET/CT on radio-oncologic treatment planning of patients with esophageal cancer. Mol Imaging Biol 2020;22(6): 1495–500.

46. Zhang S, Wang W, Xu T, et al. Comparison of diagnostic efficacy of [68 Ga]Ga-FAPI-04 and [18 F] FDG PET/CT for staging and restaging of gastric cancer. Front Oncol 2022;12:925100.

47. Zhao L, Chen S, Chen S, et al. 68 Ga-fibroblast activation protein inhibitor PET/CT on gross tumour volume

delineation for radiotherapy planning of oesophageal cancer. Radiother Oncol 2021;158:55–61.

48. Hentschel M, Appold S, Schreiber A, et al. Serial FDG-PET on patients with head and neck cancer: implications for radiation therapy. Int J Radiat Biol 2009;85(9):796–804.

49. Promteangtrong C, Siripongsatian D, Jantarato A, et al. Head-to-head comparison of 68 Ga-FAPI-46 and 18 F-FDG PET/CT for evaluation of head and neck squamous cell carcinoma: a single-center exploratory study. J Nucl Med 2022;63(8): 1155–61.

50. Chen S, Chen Z, Zou G, et al. Accurate preoperative staging with [68 Ga]Ga-FAPI PET/CT for patients with oral squamous cell carcinoma: a comparison to 2-[18 F]FDG PET/CT. Eur Radiol 2022. https://doi.org/10.1007/s00330-022-08686-7.

51. Linz C, Brands RC, Kertels O, et al. Targeting fibroblast activation protein in newly diagnosed squamous cell carcinoma of the oral cavity - initial experience and comparison to [18 F]FDG PET/CT and MRI. Eur J Nucl Med Mol Imaging 2021; 48(12):3951–60.

52. Gu B, Xu X, Zhang J, et al. The added value of 68 Ga-FAPI PET/CT in patients with head and neck cancer of unknown primary with 18 F-FDG-negative findings. J Nucl Med 2022;63(6):875–81.

53. Serfling S, Zhi Y, Schirbel A, et al. Improved cancer detection in Waldeyer's tonsillar ring by 68 Ga-FAPI PET/CT imaging. Eur J Nucl Med Mol Imaging 2021;48(4):1178–87.

54. Qin C, Liu F, Huang J, et al. A head-to-head comparison of 68 Ga-DOTA-FAPI-04 and 18 F-FDG PET/MR in patients with nasopharyngeal carcinoma: a prospective study. Eur J Nucl Med Mol Imaging 2021; 48(10):3228–37.

55. Röhrich M, Syed M, Liew DP, et al. 68 Ga-FAPI-PET/CT improves diagnostic staging and radiotherapy planning of adenoid cystic carcinomas - imaging analysis and histological validation. Radiother Oncol 2021;160:192–201.

56. Syed M, Flechsig P, Liermann J, et al. Fibroblast activation protein inhibitor (FAPI) PET for diagnostics and advanced targeted radiotherapy in head and neck cancers. Eur J Nucl Med Mol Imaging 2020; 47(12):2836–45.

57. Wegen S, van Heek L, Linde P, et al. Head-to-Head comparison of [68 Ga]Ga-FAPI-46-PET/CT and [18 F]F-FDG-PET/CT for radiotherapy planning in head and neck cancer. Mol Imaging Biol 2022. https://doi.org/10.1007/s11307-022-01749-7.

58. Zhao L, Pang Y, Zheng H, et al. Clinical utility of [68 Ga]Ga-labeled fibroblast activation protein inhibitor (FAPI) positron emission tomography/computed tomography for primary staging and recurrence detection in nasopharyngeal carcinoma. Eur J Nucl Med Mol Imaging 2021;48(11):3606–17.

59. Li Y, Lin X, Li Y, et al. Clinical utility of F-18 labeled fibroblast activation protein inhibitor (FAPI) for primary staging in lung adenocarcinoma: a prospective study. Mol Imaging Biol 2022;24(2):309–20.

60. Röhrich M, Leitz D, Glatting FM, et al. Fibroblast activation protein-specific PET/CT imaging in fibrotic interstitial lung diseases and lung cancer: a translational exploratory study. J Nucl Med 2022;63(1): 127–33.

61. Wu J, Deng H, Zhong H, et al. Comparison of 68 Ga-FAPI and 18 F-FDG PET/CT in the evaluation of patients with newly diagnosed non-small cell lung cancer. Front Oncol 2022;12:924223.

62. Zhou X, Wang S, Xu X, et al. Higher accuracy of [68 Ga]Ga-DOTA-FAPI-04 PET/CT comparing with 2-[18 F]FDG PET/CT in clinical staging of NSCLC. Eur J Nucl Med Mol Imaging 2022;49(8):2983–93.

63. Kauhanen SP, Komar G, Seppänen MP, et al. A prospective diagnostic accuracy study of 18F-fluorodeoxyglucose positron emission tomography/computed tomography, multidetector row computed tomography, and magnetic resonance imaging in primary diagnosis and staging of pancreatic cancer. Ann Surg 2009;250(6):957–63.

64. Strobel O, Büchler MW. Pancreatic cancer: FDG-PET is not useful in early pancreatic cancer diagnosis. Nat Rev Gastroenterol Hepatol 2013;10(4): 203–5.

65. Liermann J, Syed M, Ben-Josef E, et al. Impact of FAPI-PET/CT on target volume definition in radiation therapy of locally recurrent pancreatic cancer. Cancers 2021;13(4):796.

66. Rijkers AP, Valkema R, Duivenvoorden HJ, et al. Usefulness of F-18-fluorodeoxyglucose positron emission tomography to confirm suspected pancreatic cancer: a meta-analysis. Eur J Surg Oncol 2014; 40(7):794–804.

67. Pang Y, Zhao L, Shang Q, et al. Positron emission tomography and computed tomography with [68 Ga]Ga-fibroblast activation protein inhibitors improves tumor detection and staging in patients with pancreatic cancer. Eur J Nucl Med Mol Imaging 2022;49(4): 1322–37.

68. Röhrich M, Naumann P, Giesel FL, et al. Impact of 68 Ga-FAPI PET/CT imaging on the therapeutic management of primary and recurrent pancreatic ductal adenocarcinomas. J Nucl Med 2021;62(6): 779–86.

69. Shou Y, Xue Q, Yuan J, et al. 68 Ga-FAPI-04 PET/MR is helpful in differential diagnosis of pancreatitis from pancreatic malignancy compared to 18 F-FDG PET/CT: a case report. Eur J Hybrid Imaging 2021;5(1):12.

70. Zhang Z, Jia G, Pan G, et al. Comparison of the diagnostic efficacy of 68 Ga-FAPI-04 PET/MR and 18 F-FDG PET/CT in patients with pancreatic cancer. Eur J Nucl Med Mol Imaging 2022;49(8):2877–88.

71. Zhang X, Song W, Qin C, et al. Non-malignant findings of focal 68 Ga-FAPI-04 uptake in pancreas. Eur J Nucl Med Mol Imaging 2021;48(8):2635–41.

72. Chen H, Zhao L, Ruan D, et al. Usefulness of [68 Ga] Ga-DOTA-FAPI-04 PET/CT in patients presenting with inconclusive [18 F]FDG PET/CT findings. Eur J Nucl Med Mol Imaging 2021;48(1):73–86.

73. Serfling SE, Hartrampf PE, Zhi Y, et al. Interobserver agreement rates on fibroblast activation protein inhibitor-directed molecular imaging and therapy. Clin Nucl Med 2022;47(6):512–6.

74. Zheng S, Lin R, Chen S, et al. Characterization of the benign lesions with increased 68 Ga-FAPI-04 uptake in PET/CT. Ann Nucl Med 2021;35(12):1312–20.

75. Kessler L, Ferdinandus J, Hirmas N, et al. Pitfalls and common findings in 68 Ga-FAPI PET: a pictorial analysis. J Nucl Med 2022;63(6):890–6.

76. Schaub L, Harrabi SB, Debus J. Particle therapy in the future of precision therapy. Br J Radiol 2020; 93(1114):20200183.

77. Hicks RJ, Roselt PJ, Kallur KG, et al. FAPI PET/CT: will it end the hegemony of 18 F-FDG in oncology? J Nucl Med 2021;62(3):296–302.

Imaging Fibrosis

Anna Sviridenko, MD*, Gianpaolo di Santo, MD, Irene Virgolini, MD

KEYWORDS

- ^{68}Ga-FAPI-46 PET/CT • Fibrosis • IgG4-related disease
- Persisting pulmonary lesions after COVID-19 • FAPI–Triggered antifibrosis therapies

KEY POINTS

- How to distinguish inflammatory from fibrotic activity in vivo.
- PET for fibroblast-activation protein (FAP) permits the discrimination of inflammatory from established fibrosis in fibroinflammatory pathologic condition such as IgG4-related disease, liver fibrosis, pulmonary fibrosis, kidney fibrosis, and myocardial and retroperitoneal fibrosis. How might this burden clinical practice or future developments?
- How the FAP inhibitor-PET could provide benefit to the post-COVID-19 patients with prolonged structural lung abnormalities.

INTRODUCTION

Tissue injury in nonmalignant human disease can develop from either disproportionate inflammation or exaggerated fibrotic responses. The molecular and cellular fundamental of these apparently coexisting and rather evolutionary processes, their impact on disease prognosis and the treatment concept deviates. Endogenous and exogenous damaging factors activate many cytokines, which participate in the inflammation and play a larger role in fibrogenesis.[1] As a result, the synchronous assessment and quantification of these processes in vivo is extremely desirable. To date, there is no valuable tool to assess fibrotic disease activity in humans in a noninvasive way because there is no possibility to disassemble inflammatory from fibrotic disease activity. Although noninvasive molecular techniques such as ^{18}F-fluorodeoxyglucose (^{18}F-FDG) PET offer insights into the degree of inflammatory activity, the assessment of the molecular dynamics of fibrosis remains challenging. ^{68}Ga-fibroblast activation protein inhibitor (FAPI) PET may improve noninvasive clinical diagnostic performance in patients with both fibroinflammatory pathologic condition and long-term CT-abnormalities after severe COVID-19.

DISCUSSION/EMERGING TRENDS

IgG4-Related Disease

Immune-mediated diseases, despite being inflammatory in nature, are associated with substantial activation of tissue resident fibroblasts resulting in fibrosis and organ damage. IgG4-related disease (IgG4-RD) is characterized by autoimmune inflammation associated with tumefactive tissue fibrosis that has a predilection for the pancreas and biliary tree, salivary glands, kidneys, aorta, and other organs.[2,3] The typical manifestations of IgG4-related disease are autoimmune pancreatitis, sclerosing cholangitis, sclerosing sialadenitis, Mikulicz disease, which can present with a combination of lacrimal, parotid, and submandibular gland enlargement, and idiopathic fibrosclerosis.

Recent data suggest that anti-inflammatory drugs can reduce the mass of lesions but, in some cases, the anti-inflammatory approach to treating IgG4-RD has only a limited effect on the established fibrotic component.[4,5] Unfortunately, standard-of-care diagnostic tools are neither able to distinguish between proliferative and fibrotic subtypes nor able to quantify inflammatory and fibrotic activity in the respective lesions.[6] Serum levels of fibrosis-related biomarkers as a growth differentiation factor 15, C-C motif

Department of Nuclear Medicine, Medical University of Innsbruck, Innsbruck, Austria
* Corresponding author.
E-mail address: anna.sviridenko@tirol-kliniken.at

PET Clin 18 (2023) 381–388
https://doi.org/10.1016/j.cpet.2023.02.004
1556-8598/23/© 2023 Elsevier Inc. All rights reserved.

chemokine ligand 2, hyaluronic acid, amino-terminal propeptide of type III procollagen, and tissue inhibitor of metalloproteinases 1 in IgG4-RD can only monitor the overall fibrotic disease activity irrespective of its localization.[7,8]

The recent cross-sectional clinical study by Christian Schmidkonz and colleagues[9] included 27 patients with inflammatory, fibrotic, and overlapping manifestations of IgG4-related disease. In that study ^{18}F-FDG, ^{68}Ga-FAPI-46 PET/CT, MR imaging and histopathological assessment were simultaneously performed with noninvasive evaluation of disease activity in IgG4-RD currently being primarily based on ^{18}F-FDG PET/CT. In a longitudinal approach, ^{18}F-FDG and ^{68}Ga-FAPI PET/CT data were evaluated before and after immunosuppression. The authors found that, using a combination of ^{68}Ga-FAPI and ^{18}F-FDG PET/CT, noninvasive functional tracking of IgG4-related disease evolution from inflammatory toward an established fibrotic outcome becomes feasible; these data emphasize the evolutionary pathogenic continuity from inflammation to mature fibrosis.

Histopathological assessment demonstrated that FDG-positive lesions had dense lymphoplasmacytic infiltration of IgG4 + cells, while FAPI-positive lesions showed abundant activated fibroblasts expressing fibroblast-activation protein (FAP)-α according to results from RNA-sequencing of activated fibroblasts. FDG-negative fibrotic IgG4 manifestations that had increased FAPI tracer uptake demonstrated constant or even further progression the mass of fibrotic lesions. The authors concluded that despite negative FDG findings, FAPI may indicate ongoing fibrotic activity in IgG4-RD lesions and emphasize that in the absence of ongoing inflammation, anti-inflammatory medications should be replaced by antifibrotic treatment.

Demonstration of increased FAPI uptake indicating activated fibroblasts may indicate specific treatments, such as tyrosine kinase inhibitors, pirfenidone (PFD), or inhibitors of the transcription factor PU.1.[10–12]

Pulmonary Fibrosis

Pulmonary fibrosis is the terminal phase of many interstitial lung diseases (ILDs), representing damage to normal lung structure, leading to lung function impairment, degradation of the quality of life, and may lead to death.[13,14] Idiopathic pulmonary fibrosis (IPF) is a progressive fibrotic ILD, with a median survival time of 2 to 5 years.[15,16] Its cause is unclear but related to activated fibroblasts and accumulation of extracellular matrix. Other ILDs

are identified by association with other diseases. These include rheumatoid arthritis,[17] and systemic sclerosis (SSc),[18] silica-associated lung disease,[19] immune checkpoint inhibitor therapy-related pneumonitis,[20] radiation-induced lung injury[21] but also some remain unclassifiable ILD.[22] Progression has been observed in a proportion of patients. Lung cancer is a frequent complication of ILD and crucially contributes the poor prognosis of these patients.[23]

Currently, clinicians utilize a combination of imaging, pulmonary function testing, and biopsy/histology to detect, monitor, and manage ILD.[24] The standard imaging technique for the assessment of ILD is high-resolution CT.[25] However, computed tomography (CT) is unable to assess disease activity in ILDs. Besides CT, ^{18}F-FDG PET/CT is used for the imaging of ILDs, based on increased glucose metabolism in sites of active inflammatory change that may lead to fibrosis. There is evidence that it may provide incremental diagnostic information to CT with respect to risk stratification or evaluation of antifibrotic therapies.[26]

However, both CT and ^{18}F-FDG PET have inherent limitations for the evaluation of ILDs because CT can show only established morphologic changes of the lung, which occur relatively late and does not provide adequate information regarding ongoing disease activity.[27] However, ^{18}F-FDG PET/CT depicts inflammatory reactions that may lead to fibrosis but not whether the fibrotic process is active.[27]

Therefore, there is an urgent clinical need for a sensitive noninvasive tool to diagnose early disease activity, monitor therapeutic response, and advance our understanding of the course of this debilitating group of diseases.

FAP is a serine protease selectively expressed on activated stromal fibroblasts during tissue remodeling and is associated with pulmonary fibrosis.[28] The recent study conducted by M. Röhrich and colleagues[29] analyzed 15 patients with different ILD subtypes with ^{68}Ga-FAPI PET/CT and confirmed FAP expression in ILD lesions by FAP immunohistochemistry. The authors concluded that FAPI PET/CT is a promising imaging modality for ILDs due its ability to detect abnormality earlier than CT, presumably reflecting the process that subsequently leads to the fibrosis apparent morphologically on CT.

Another recent study has evaluated the potential of FAPI tracer in detecting of IPF in a murine model. Pulmonary fibrosis was induced by intratracheal administration of bleomycin (1 U/kg) while intratracheal saline was administered to control mice.[30] CT was unable to assess disease activity in a murine model of IPF. Conversely, FAPI PET demonstrated that increased FAPI uptake qualitatively correlated with increased FAP expression and the degree of lung fibrosis by histopathological characterization. Finally, because activated fibroblasts are the initiators of active as opposed to established or "burnt-out" tissue fibrosis, FAPI PET could more sensitively detect profibrotic disease earlier than other techniques allowing more timely interventions and potentially better treatment outcomes.

Liver Fibrosis

Liver fibrosis is the consequence of chronic liver injury of any etiology.[31–33] End-stage liver fibrosis (ie, cirrhosis) is the leading cause of liver disease-related deaths globally and the most important risk factor for developing liver cancer. Current methods of staging liver fibrosis have notable limitations. Laboratory markers are unreliable[34] and liver biopsy (the current gold standard) carries morbidity and mortality risks and is prone to undersampling and variability in sampling and interpretation.[35–37] MR elastography is the best validated noninvasive tool for the histologic fibrosis stage.[38] However, MR elastography has lower sensitivity for the detection of early stages of fibrosis, can be nondiagnostic because of liver iron-overload or operator error, and cannot differentiate fibrosis from concurrent liver inflammation because both processes increase liver stiffness.[39,40] Hence, there remains a clear unmet need for a noninvasive, quantitative, and accurate tool for evaluating the activity of liver fibrosis.

^{18}F-FDG PET currently plays only a limited role in the evaluation of liver fibrosis, mainly due to altered liver glucose metabolism in the setting of chronic liver disease.[41] Reduced activity in the liver relative to the spleen, especially is associated with splenomegaly and nodularity of the hepatic surface on correlative CT can indicate advanced cirrhosis with portal hypertension but are late findings. ^{68}Ga-FAPI PET can offer several key potential advantages for the evaluation of liver fibrosis. These include the ability to detect early fibrotic changes due to the minimal uptake in normal human liver, which would be advantageous over elastography.

Indeed, in the recent study conducted by Ali Pirasteh and colleagues, the authors investigated the utility of PET in staging liver fibrosis by correlating liver uptake of ^{68}Ga-FAPI with histology in a human-sized swine model. Five pigs underwent baseline ^{68}Ga-FAPI PET/MR imaging and liver biopsy, followed by liver parenchymal embolization, 8 weeks of oral alcohol intake, with the study endpoints being correlation of ^{68}Ga-FAPI PET/MR imaging with necropsy findings.[42] The strong correlation observed between liver ^{68}Ga-FAPI uptake and the histologic stage of liver fibrosis suggests that ^{68}Ga-FAPI PET may play an impactful role in noninvasive staging of liver fibrosis, pending validation in patients.

RETROPERITONEAL FIBROSIS

One recent case report revealed a potential role for ^{68}Ga-FAPI-04 in idiopathic retroperitoneal fibrosis. In agreement with ^{18}F-FDG PET, the FAPI tracer showed the intense and homogeneous avidity of retroperitoneal mass. After treatment, follow-up CT showed significant decrease in size of the retroperitoneal mass suggesting an active but reversible process.[43]

Kidney Fibrosis

Renal fibrosis leads to a progressive reduction in kidney function ultimately resulting in kidney failure. Noninvasive imaging examinations, such as B-ultrasound, indirectly reflect renal fibrosis through renal anatomical changes, making it difficult to accurately determine the degree of renal fibrosis early in the disease process. Due to the potential influence of contrast agents on renal function, enhanced CT is also unsuitable for evaluating renal fibrosis. Accordingly, the detection of kidney fibrosis is generally based on histological validation by the way of renal biopsy, which is highly demanding for the patient, suffers from risks complications, and is time-consuming. Earlier attempts to noninvasively detect kidney fibrosis have been done with MR imaging but this technique has not yet entered routine clinical use.[44] The feasibility of PET imaging in kidney fibrosis detection has been evaluated, and the ^{18}F-FDG PET tracer was able to identify kidney cyst infections. It also showed potential in diagnosing acute rejection after kidney transplantation.[45]

In the recent retrospective study by Patrick Cone and colleagues,[46] the diagnostic value of 3 different radiotracers for the noninvasive prediction of kidney fibrosis was analyzed by correlating glomerular filtration rate with the intrarenal parenchymal radiotracer retention. In 81 patients receiving any of the following molecular imaging probes: ^{68}Ga-FAPI, the Gallium-68 labeled prostate-specific membrane antigen (^{68}Ga-PSMA) or ^{68}Ga-DOTATOC, kidney function was correlated with the maximum and mean standard uptake value of the renal parenchyma and background activity measured in lung parenchyma, myocardium, gluteal muscle, and the abdominal aorta. Patients were collected according to their grade of chronic kidney disease. They found a significant negative correlation between renal parenchymal ^{68}Ga-FAPI uptake and grade of chronic kidney disease, which was not the case for either ^{68}Ga-DOTATOC or ^{68}Ga-PSMA. This correlation suggests a specific binding of FAPI rather than a potential unspecific retention in the renal parenchyma, underlining the potential value of ^{68}Ga-FAPI for the noninvasive quantitative evaluation of kidney fibrosis. It should be noted that there was no histopathological confirmation of nephrosclerosis in this study.

Another retrospective study by Yue Zhou and colleagues[47] analyzed 13 patients who had undergone ^{68}Ga-FAPI PET/CT examination based on compassionate use criteria and subsequently had renal biopsy. High retention of radiotracer was found in almost all (12 of 13) patients with the degree of FAPI uptake of most patients corresponding to the pathology of kidney tissue. The results of this preliminary study indicate that radiolabeled FAPI can be used to image active renal fibrosis. The authors declared the quality of ^{68}Ga-FAPI PET/CT scans in patients with moderate-to-severe renal fibrosis may be superior to other examination methods but additional clinical trials are needed for further evaluation. Whether end-stage renal disease or earlier renal scarring from infection or vascular injury would remain positive on FAPI PET/CT is currently unknown.

Myocardial Fibrosis

Myocardial fibrosis (MF) occurs in response to a variety of triggers and in systemic diseases. SSc is a prototypical fibrosing disorder with a high case-related mortality. Repetitive impairment of the myocardial microcirculation due to increased vascular reactivity is thought to trigger diffuse MF in this disease.[48] Histologically, MF is characterized by the accumulation of fibroblasts and myofibroblasts. The latter express alpha-smooth-muscle actin and secrete abundant collagen. Moreover, fibroblast activation prompts the upregulation of FAP. The collagen disrupts the myocardial tissue structure with consequent alterations of the conduction system occur, and cardiac contractility is impaired. The direct, noninvasive monitoring of the current molecular activity of fibrotic remodeling in the heart has not previously been feasible.

In a recent study by Christoph Treutlein and colleagues,[49] 14 patients with SSc underwent ^{68}Ga-FAPI PET/CT, cardiac MR imaging, and clinical/serologic investigations to assist the assessment of the presence of MF.

This provided first in-human evidence that ^{68}Ga-FAPI uptake can visualize fibroblast activation in SSc-related MF and may be a diagnostic option to monitor cardiac fibroblast activity in vivo. As proof-of-principle, they showed that ^{68}Ga-FAPI tracer uptake corresponds histologically to myocardial regions with the accumulation of FAP + myofibroblasts. Moreover, the authors observed that changes of ^{68}Ga-FAPI-04 uptake between baseline and follow-up paralleled the changes of clinical parameters.

Another study by Penguin Qiao and colleagues[50] aimed to evaluate the feasibility of ^{68}Ga-FAPI for monitoring reparative fibrosis and reactive fibrosis after myocardial infarction (MI). Cardiac remodeling includes hypertrophy of the left ventricle and cardiac fibrosis involving the infarct zone and possibly extending into peri-infarction myocardium that remains viable.[51] MF is characterized by excessive deposition of extracellular matrix proteins in the myocardium, which distorts myocardial structure, promotes arrhythmia and may lead to cardiac insufficiency with heart failure.[52,53] Cardiac fibrosis can be divided into reparative fibrosis and reactive fibrosis. Reparative fibrosis (where collagen deposition replaces damaged myocardium) and reactive fibrosis (where typically diffuse collagen deposition occurs without myocardial damage) are experienced successively after MI. Reparative fibrosis is stimulated by injury and cardiomyocyte necrosis and is an essential reparative response as a consequence of MI, resulting in a fibrous scar in the infarcted area, which causes further geometric, biomechanical, and biochemical changes in the ventricular wall in the undamaged area, causing reactive fibrosis, which is the diffuse depositions of collagen throughout the myocardium remote from the infarct zone. This may be stimulated by prolonged periods of stress or by exposure to profibrotic mediators. Activated fibroblasts can predict cardiac remodeling after MI. Therefore, noninvasive monitoring of activated fibroblasts is of great significance for the study of MF and cardiac remodeling after MI. FAP has been demonstrated as a marker for fibroblast activation and plays a potential role in cardiac wound healing and cardiac remodeling after MI.[54]

In the study of Penguin Qiao, MI models were prepared by ligation of the left anterior descending coronary artery and validated by electrocardiogram and ^{18}F-FDG PET/CT one day after MI and hematoxylin and eosin staining. The infarcted area with decreased or defective myocardial metabolic activity in ^{18}F-FDG PET/CT correspondingly showed high ^{68}Ga-FAPI-04 uptake in the MI rats. The myocardial tracer uptake was

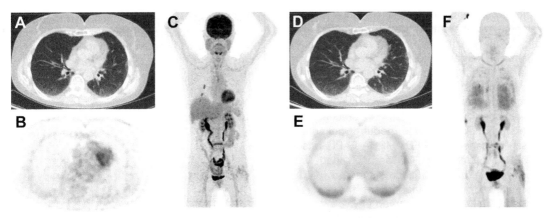

Fig. 1. FDG-FAPI-PETCT. Comparison of 18F-FDG PET/CT (*A–C*) and 68Ga-FAPI-46 PET/CT (*D–F*): the corresponding transaxial low-dose CT scans (*A* and *D*) and PET emission scans (*B* and *E*), together with the coronal MIPs (*C* and *F*). Showing no relevant accumulation of FDG but an accumulation of FAPI-46, 19 weeks after discharge from hospital, in residual peripheral ground-glass opacities and subtle reticular changes shown in the corresponding low dose CT scans. In addition, a serial rib fractures rights and inflammatory changes in left hip were detected on both scans.

significantly different between MI and sham-operated rats from day 1 to 28 after MI and reached peak value 6 days after MI. ^{68}Ga-FAPI uptake was not observed in the distal uninjured myocardium throughout the observation period. The authors concluded that the ^{68}Ga-FAPI PET could noninvasively monitor the activated fibroblasts in the early-stage postacute MI and that it may be helpful for evaluating the degree of reparative fibrosis, whereas the evolution of reactive fibrosis monitoring still needs further study. Therefore, FAPI PET is beneficial to anti-inflammatory and antifibrotic treatments after MI for the modulation of reactive fibrosis in patients with an ongoing deterioration of cardiac function in the postinfarct setting and has potential value in evaluating treatment response. Moreover, it may be useful to identify subjects with progressive fibrotic remodeling who may benefit from interventions targeting the fibroblasts.[55]

Persisting Pulmonary Lesions after COVID-19

A severe acute respiratory syndrome can be associated with the coronavirus-2 (SARS-CoV-2) pandemic, which has already infected more than 650 million people worldwide. Even though in most patients surviving COVID-19 pneumonia, initial pulmonary CT abnormalities recede over time, in some individuals, particularly after a severe episode of COVID-19, the pulmonary injury seems to persist,[56–58] and complications may become an extensive health burden.

Whether those prolonged structural lung abnormalities in patients with COVID-19 are mainly triggered by underlying inflammatory or fibrotic repair processes has not yet been answered. Within

incidental acute SARS-CoV-2, ^{18}F-FDG PET/CT has already been proven to be able to discriminate between morpho-metabolic patterns reflecting the evolutionary phases of inflammatory processes.[59] However, the role of ^{18}F-FDG PET/CT within the diagnostic pathway of long-term pulmonary changes after SARS-CoV-2 infection remains unclear. A recent study explored the potential diagnostic benefit of PET/CT in order to establish the underlying inflammatory or fibrotic repair processes in prolonged structural lung abnormalities in patients with COVID-19.[60]

This study included dual-tracer imaging with FDG and FAPI PET/CT in a small cohort of post-COVID-19 patients in comparison to a control group and demonstrated the low ^{18}F-FDG-avidity in areas of residual CT abnormality but a clear positivity on ^{68}Ga-FAPI PET/CT (**Fig. 1**). They concluded that this likely reflected ongoing fibrotic repair, and that ^{68}Ga-FAPI PET/CT may improve noninvasive clinical diagnostic performance in patients with long-term CT-abnormalities after severe COVID-19.

USING FIBROBLAST ACTIVATION PROTEIN INHIBITOR TO SELECT AND MONITOR ANTIFIBROTIC THERAPIES

It has been reported that FAP inhibitor PT100 manifests antifibrotic properties in pulmonary fibrosis induced by bleomycin in mice.[61] A further antifibrotic agent, PFD, has become an approved treatment of IPF in humans following a phase III trial that demonstrated benefits with respect to lung function but often comes along with gastrointestinal adverse events, which may be brought on by the oral administration. This limitation may be overcome by alternative drug formulations. For example, the use of nanoparticles as drug delivery carriers for targeting lesions, releasing drugs, improving pharmacokinetics, biocompatibility, and bioavailability has recently been described.[62] The mesoporous polydopamine (MPDA) is one of the most popular nanoparticles.[63] In a recent innovative study using a murine model of pulmonary fibrosis, a nanodrug, PFD@MPDA-FAPI, based on MPDA, loaded with PFD as a payload, was linked with FAPI as an antifibrosis therapy.[64] The accumulation of the nanodrug at the sites of fibrosis in the lung was observed in vivo by near-infrared imaging. This study found that the antifibrotic properties of PFD@MPDA-FAPI were better than those of pure PFD and PFD@MPDA without PFD loading in case of translation to humans.

Finally, the authors showed that the easily produced and biocompatible nanodrug PFD@MPDA-FAPI developed in the study is promising for further antifibrotic therapy and suggested that MPDA-FAPI loaded with an anticancer drug may provide an opportunity for combination with photothermal therapy.

SUMMARY

Overall, current diagnostic methods detecting morphological and functional features of organ fibrosis are often nonspecific. In addition, changes tend to only appear at later stages of the disease, resulting in delayed diagnosis, repeated diagnostic testing, and unnecessary or ineffective treatments. Alternatively, biopsies can characterize disease activity but are invasive and carry inherent risks of morbidity and mortality.

In this context, FAPI PET/CT represents the feasible tool for assessing ongoing fibrotic activity in human disease in cases with residual morphological abnormality but without evidence of ongoing inflammation. Clinical scenarios include important diseases such as IgG4-related pathologic condition and SSc. Its role in the management of ILDs requires further evaluation but this approach may provide the appropriate selection of specific antifibrotic agents rather than broad-spectrum anti-inflammatory treatments as glucocorticoids.

CLINICS CARE POINTS

- PET for FAP permits the discrimination of inflammatory from fibrotic activity in fibroinflammatory pathology.

- Benefit of appropriate selection of treatment strategies toward antifibrotic agents rather than broad-spectrum anti-inflammatory treatments.
- Additionally, target FAPI nanodrug is promising for further clinical translations in antifibrosis therapy.

DISCLOSURE

The authors have nothing to disclose.

REFERENCES

1. Zhang WJ, Chen SJ, Zhou SC, et al. Inflammasomes and fibrosis. Front Immunol 2021;12:643149.
2. Stone JH, Zen Y, Deshpande V. IgG4-Related disease. N Engl J Med 2012;366:539–51.
3. Umehara H, Okazaki K, Masaki Y, et al. A novel clinical entity, IgG4-related disease (IgG4RD): general concept and details. Mod Rheumatol 2012;22:1–14.
4. Della-Torre E, Feeney E, Deshpande V, et al. B-Cell depletion attenuates serological biomarkers of fibrosis and myofibroblast activation in IgG4-related disease. Ann Rheum Dis 2015;74:2236–43.
5. Della-Torre E, Rigamonti E, Perugino C, et al. B lymphocytes directly contribute to tissue fibrosis in patients with IgG4-related disease. J Allergy Clin Immunol 2020;145:968–81.
6. Carruthers MN, Khosroshahi A, Augustin T, et al. The diagnostic utility of serum IgG4 concentrations in IgG4-related disease. Ann Rheum Dis 2015;74:14–8.
7. Tang J, Cai S, Ye C, et al. Biomarkers in IgG4-related disease: a systematic review. Semin Arthritis Rheum 2020;50(2):354–9.
8. Kawashiri S-Y, Origuchi T, Umeda M, et al. Association of serum levels of fibrosis-related biomarkers with disease activity in patients with IgG4-related disease. Arthritis Res Ther 2018;20:277.
9. Schmidkonz C, Rauber S, Atzinger A, et al. Disentangling inflammatory from fibrotic disease activity by fibroblast activation protein imaging. Ann Rheum Dis 2020;79(11):1485–91.
10. Distler O, Highland KB, Gahlemann M, et al. Nintedanib for systemic sclerosis-associated interstitial lung disease. N Engl J Med 2019;380:2518–28.
11. King TE, Bradford WZ, Castro-Bernardini S, et al. A phase 3 trial of pirfenidone in patients with idiopathic pulmonary fibrosis. N Engl J Med 2014;370:2083–92.
12. Wohlfahrt T, Rauber S, Uebe S, et al. Pu.1 controls fibroblast polarization and tissue fibrosis. Nature 2019;566:344–9.

13. Rockey DC, Bell PD, Hill JA. Fibrosis–a common pathway to organ injury and failure. N Engl J Med 2015;372(12):1138–49.

14. Lai Y, Wei X, Ye T, et al. Interrelation between fibroblasts and T cells in fibrosing interstitial lung diseases. Front Immunol 2021;12:747335.

15. Fernández Pérez ER, Daniels CE, Schroeder DR, et al. Incidence, prevalence, and clinical course of idiopathic pulmonary fibrosis: a population-based study. Chest 2010;137(1):129–37.

16. Ley B, Collard HR, King TE Jr. Clinical course and prediction of survival in idiopathic pulmonary fibrosis. Am J Respir Crit Care Med 2011;183(4):431–40.

17. Zamora-Legoff JA, Krause ML, Crowson CS, et al. Progressive decline of lung function in rheumatoid arthritis-associated interstitial lung disease. Arthritis Rheumatol 2017;69(3):542–9.

18. Hoffmann-Vold AM, Allanore Y, Alves M, et al. Progressive interstitial lung disease in patients with systemic sclerosis-associated interstitial lung disease in the EUSTAR database. Ann Rheum Dis 2021;80(2):219–27.

19. Barnes H, Goh NSL, Leong TL, et al. Silica-associated lung disease: an old-world exposure in modern industries. Respirology 2019;24(12):1165–75.

20. Kalisz KR, Ramaiya NH, Laukamp KR, et al. Immune checkpoint inhibitor therapy-related pneumonitis: patterns and management. Radiographics 2019;39(7):1923–37.

21. Hanania AN, Mainwaring W, Ghebre YT, et al. Radiation-induced lung injury: assessment and management. Chest 2019;156(1):150–62.

22. Guler SA, Ellison K, Algamdi M, et al. Heterogeneity in unclassifiable interstitial lung disease. A systematic review and meta-analysis. Ann Am Thorac Soc 2018;15(7):854–63.

23. Kreuter M, Ehlers-Tenenbaum S, Palmowski K, et al. Impact of comorbidities on mortality in patients with idiopathic pulmonary fibrosis. PLoS One 2016;11(3):e0151425.

24. Raghu G, Remy-Jardin M, Myers JL, et al. Diagnosis of idiopathic pulmonary fibrosis. An official ATS/ERS/JRS/ALAT clinical practice guideline. Am J Respir Crit Care Med 2018;198(5):e44–68.

25. Hansell DM, Goldin JG, King TE Jr, et al. CT staging and monitoring of fibrotic interstitial lung diseases in clinical practice and treatment trials: a position paper from the Fleischner Society. Lancet Respir Med 2015;3(6):483–96.

26. Win T, Screaton NJ, Porter JC, et al. Pulmonary ^{18}F-FDG uptake helps refine current risk stratification in idiopathic pulmonary fibrosis (IPF). Eur J Nucl Med Mol Imaging 2018;45(5):806–15.

27. Win T, Thomas BA, Lambrou T, et al. Areas of normal pulmonary parenchyma on HRCT exhibit increased FDG PET signal in IPF patients. Eur J Nucl Med Mol Imaging 2014;41(2):337–42.

28. Acharya PS, Zukas A, Chandan V, et al. Fibroblast activation protein: a serine protease expressed at the remodeling interface in idiopathic pulmonary fibrosis. Hum Pathol 2006;37(3):352–60.

29. Röhrich M, Leitz D, Glatting FM, et al. Fibroblast activation protein-specific PET/CT imaging in fibrotic interstitial lung diseases and lung cancer: a translational exploratory study. J Nucl Med 2022;63(1):127–33.

30. Rosenkrans ZT, Massey CF, Bernau K, et al. [68Ga]Ga-FAPI-46 PET for non-invasive detection of pulmonary fibrosis disease activity. Eur J Nucl Med Mol Imaging 2022;49(11):3705–16.

31. GBD 2017 Cirrhosis Collaborators. The global, regional, and national burden of cirrhosis by cause in 195 countries and territories, 1990-2017: a systematic analysis for the Global Burden of Disease Study 2017. Lancet Gastroenterol Hepatol 2020;5:245–66.

32. Ge PS, Runyon BA. Treatment of patients with cirrhosis. N Engl J Med 2016;375:767–77.

33. Alberti A, Noventa F, Benvegnu L, et al. Prevalence of liver diseasein a population of asymptomatic persons with hepatitis C virus infection. Ann Intern Med 2002;137:961–4.

34. Harris R, Harman DJ, Card TR, et al. Prevalence of clinically significant liver disease within the general population, as defined by non-invasive markers of liver fibrosis: a systematic review. Lancet Gastroenterol Hepatol 2017;2:288–97.

35. Goldin RD, Goldin JG, Burt AD, et al. Intra-observer variation in the histopathological assessment of chronic viral hepatitis. J Hepatol 1996;25:649–54.

36. Maharaj B, Maharaj RJ, Leary WP, et al. Sampling variability and its influence on the diagnostic yield of percutaneous needle biopsy of the liver. Lancet 1986;1:523–5.

37. Regev A, Berho M, Jeffers LJ, et al. Sampling error and intraobserver variation in liver biopsy in patients with chronic HCV infection. Am J Gastroenterol 2002;97:2614–8.

38. Singh S, Venkatesh SK, Wang Z, et al. Diagnostic performance of magnetic resonance elastography in staging liver fibrosis: a systematic review and meta-analysis of individual participant data. Clin Gastroenterol Hepatol 2015;13:440–51.e6.

39. Yin M, Glaser KJ, Talwalkar JA, et al. Hepatic MR elastography: clinical performance in a series of 1377 consecutive examinations. Radiology 2016;278:114–24.

40. Shi Y, Qi YF, Lan GY, et al. Three-dimensional MR elastography depicts liver inflammation, fibrosis, and portal hypertension in chronic hepatitis B or C. Radiology 2021;301:154–62.

41. Verloh N, Einspieler I, Utpatel K, et al. In vivo confirmation of altered hepatic glucose metabolism in patients with liver fibrosis/cirrhosis by 18F-FDG PET/CT. EJNMMI Res 2018;8:98.

42. Pirasteh A, Periyasamy S, Meudt JJ, et al. Staging liver fibrosis by fibroblast activation protein inhibitor PET in a human-sized swine model. J Nucl Med 2022;63(12):1956–61.

43. Pan Q, Luo Y, Zhang W. Idiopathic retroperitoneal fibrosis with intense uptake of 68Ga-fibroblast activation protein inhibitor and 18F-FDG. Clin Nucl Med 2021;46(2):175–6.

44. Sun Q, Baues M, Klinkhammer BM, et al. Elastin imaging enables noninvasive staging and treatment monitoring of kidney fibrosis. Sci Transl Med 2019; 11:eaat4865.

45. Hanssen O, Lovinfosse P, Weekers L, et al. (18)F-FDG positron emission tomography in non-oncological renal pathology: current indications and perspectives. Nephrol Ther 2019;15:430–8.

46. Conen P, Pennetta F, Dendl K, et al. [^{68}Ga]Ga-FAPI uptake correlates with the state of chronic kidney disease. Eur J Nucl Med Mol Imaging 2022;49(10): 3365–72.

47. Zhou Y, Yang X, Liu H, et al. Value of [^{68}Ga]Ga-FAPI-04 imaging in the diagnosis of renal fibrosis. Eur J Nucl Med Mol Imaging 2021;48(11):3493–501. Treutlein C, Distler JHW, Tascilar K, et al.

48. Meune C, Vignaux O, Kahan A, et al. Heart involvement in systemic sclerosis: evolving concept and diagnostic methodologies. Arch Cardiovasc Dis 2010;103(1):46–52.

49. Treutlein C, Distler JHW, Tascilar K, et al. Assessment of myocardial fibrosis in patients with systemic sclerosis using [^{68}Ga]Ga-FAPI-04-PET-CT. Eur J Nucl Med Mol Imaging 2022. https://doi.org/10.1007/s00259-022-06081-4.

50. Qiao P, Wang Y, Zhu K, et al. Noninvasive monitoring of reparative fibrosis after myocardial infarction in rats using ^{68}Ga-FAPI-04 PET/CT. Mol Pharm 2022; 19(11):4171–8.

51. Leanca SA, Crisu D, Petris AO, et al. Left ventricular remodeling after myocardial infarction: from physiopathology to treatment. Life 2022;12(8):1111.

52. Li L, Zhao Q, Kong W. Extracellular matrix remodeling and cardiac fibrosis. Matrix Biol 2018;68-69: 490–506.

53. Cowling RT, Kupsky D, Kahn AM, et al. Mechanisms of cardiac collagen deposition in experimental models and human disease. Transl Res 2019;209: 138–55.

54. Venugopal H, Hanna A, Humeres C, et al. Properties and functions of fibroblasts and myofibroblasts in myocardial infarction. Cells 2022;11(9):1386.

55. Tillmanns J, Hoffmann D, Habbaba Y, et al. Fibroblast activation protein alpha expression identifies activated fibroblasts after myocardial infarction. J Mol Cell Cardiol 2015;87:194–203.

56. Ng CK, Chan JW, Kwan TL, et al. Six month radiological and physiological outcomes in severe acute respiratory syndrome (SARS) survivors. Thorax 2004; 59:889–91.

57. Mo X, Jian W, Su Z, et al. Abnormal pulmonary function in COVID-19 patients at time of hospital discharge. Eur Respir J 2020;55(6):2001217.

58. Pogatchnik BP, Swenson KE, Sharifi H, et al. Radiology-pathology correlation in recovered COVID-19, demonstrating organizing pneumonia. Am J Respir Crit Care Med 2020;202(4):598–9.

59. Ajuria-Illarramendi O, Martinez-Lorca A, Del Prado Orduña-Diez M. [18F] FDG-PET/CT in different COVID-19 phases. ID Cases 2020;21:e00869.

60. Sviridenko A, Boehm A, di Santo G, et al. Enhancing clinical diagnosis for patients with persistent pulmonary abnormalities after COVID-19 infection: the potential benefit of 68 Ga-FAPI PET/CT. Clin Nucl Med 2022;47(12):1026–9.

61. Egger C, Cannet C, Gérard C, et al. Effects of the fibroblast activation protein inhibitor, PT100, in a murine model of pulmonary fibrosis. Eur J Pharmacol 2017;809:64–72.

62. George A, Shah PA, Shrivastav PS. Natural biodegradable polymers based nano-formulations for drug delivery: a review. Int J Pharm 2019;561: 244–64.

63. Lin K, Gan Y, Zhu P, et al. Hollow mesoporous polydopamine nanospheres: synthesis, biocompatibility and drug delivery. Nanotechnology 2021;32(28). https://doi.org/10.1088/1361-6528/abf4a9.

64. Fang Q, Liu S, Cui J, et al. Mesoporous polydopamine loaded pirfenidone target to fibroblast activation protein for pulmonary fibrosis therapy. Front Bioeng Biotechnol 2022;10:920766.

Cardiac Applications of Fibroblast Activation Protein Imaging

Johanna Diekmann, MD*, Frank M. Bengel, MD

KEYWORDS

- Fibroblast activation protein • PET • Acute myocardial infarction
- Cardiac magnetic resonance tomography • Molecular imaging • Heart failure

KEY POINTS

- The use of fibroblast activation protein (FAP)-targeted PET imaging is emerging beyond tumor imaging.
- In cardiac diseases imaging fibrosis using FAP-tracers gives important new insights into pathogenesis and treatment response.
- Molecular FAP-imaging in patients with acute myocardial infarction is predictive of later cardiac function and could be used for guiding antifibrotic therapies in the future.
- Altered myocardial FAP-uptake in various cardiac diseases has been shown in preliminary studies.

OVERVIEW

Beyond tumor imaging, several promising applications of molecular fibroblast activation protein (FAP) imaging are emerging. Especially in cardiac diseases, FAP imaging is gaining attention, as indicated by the growing number of articles and case reports.[1] Myocardial fibrosis plays a key role in the complex process of cardiac remodeling and can lead to adverse clinical outcomes such as left ventricular dysfunction, propensity to arrhythmias, and reduction of perfusion. Ultimately, if fibrosis becomes irreversible, patients can develop heart failure. Fibroblast activation can be induced by various factors including ischemic, mechanical, or metabolic injuries.[2] Excitingly, molecular imaging of activated fibroblasts now expands the established methods for imaging of cardiac fibrosis, magnetic resonance tomography (T1/T2 mapping, late gadolinium enhancement [LGE]) and echocardiography (strain analysis), by providing a new selective biomarker. **Table 1** gives an overview of published articles and case reports on cardiac FAP imaging. Most relevant literature is summarized below.

Acute Myocardial Infarction

Revascularization therapy early after acute myocardial infarction (AMI) aims to restore blood flow to the damaged region and is the most important acute intervention in improving survival in the short-term. However, long-term outcome after AMI is dependent on factors beyond reperfusion alone. Acute injury of the myocardial tissue triggers an immediate inflammatory response leading to the activation of quiescent fibroblasts. The activated (myo)fibroblasts mediate this inflammatory cascade via secretion of growth factors, chemokines, and cytokines and migrate to injured tissue to deposit cross-linked collagen fibers as part of the reparative process.[3–5] However, excessive profibrotic response and involvement of remote myocardium support adverse cardiac remodeling.

Writing/Original draft preparation: J. Diekmann: Review, editing and supervision: F.M. Bengel: All authors have read and agreed to the published version of the article.

Department of Nuclear Medicine, Hannover Medical School, Carl-Neuberg-Street. 1, Hannover 30625, Germany

* Corresponding author.

E-mail address: diekmann.johanna@mh-hannover.de

PET Clin 18 (2023) 389–396
https://doi.org/10.1016/j.cpet.2023.03.004

Table 1
Overview of existing literature

Condition	FAP Tracer	FAPI-PET Key Findings
Acute myocardial infarction		
Varasteh Z et al.[10] 2019: Molecular Imaging of Fibroblast Activity After Myocardial Infarction Using a ^{68}Ga-Labeled Fibroblast Activation Protein Inhibitor, FAPI-04	^{68}Ga-FAPI-04	Preclinical study (AMI mice): tracer uptake in the injured myocardium peaked on day 6 after coronary ligation. Autoradiography and H&E staining of cross-sections showed tracer accumulation mainly at the border zone of the infarcted myocardium
Langer L et al.[11] 2021: Molecular imaging of fibroblast activation protein after myocardial infarction using the novel radiotracer ^{68}Ga-MHLL1	^{68}Ga-MHLL1	Preclinical study (AMI mice): 7 days after coronary artery ligation significant tracer uptake in the infarct area, signal persisted to 21 days. Autoradiography and histology confirmed regional uptake in the infarct and border zone regions. Immunostaining delineated persistent FAP expression at 7 days and 21 days
Diekmann J et al.[13] 2021: Molecular Imaging Identifies Fibroblast Activation Beyond the Infarct Region After Acute Myocardial Infarction	^{68}Ga-FAPI-46	Activation of fibroblasts markedly exceeds the infarct region in patients after AMI. High interindividual variability. No exact regional matching with CMR parameters of fibrosis (LGE, wall thickness)
Kessler L et al.[14] 2021: Visualization of Fibroblast Activation After Myocardial Infarction Using ^{68}Ga-FAPI PET	^{68}Ga-FAPI-04	Increased myocardial tracer uptake corresponded to the supply area of the culprit coronary vessel as well as to biomarker levels of myocardial injury
Notohamiprodjo S et al.[15] 2022: Imaging of cardiac fibroblast activation in a patient after acute myocardial infarction using ^{68}Ga-FAPI-04	^{68}Ga-FAPI-04	Case report: Dynamic PET/CMR for 60 min. No uptake found in normal myocardium and in mature scar. Focal intense tracer uptake with continuous washout in the infarct territory of coronary occlusion correlating with T1 and ECV mapping. Uptake extended beyond the actual infarcted area
Diekmann J et al.[16] 2022: Cardiac Fibroblast Activation in Patients Early After Acute Myocardial Infarction: Integration with MR Tissue Characterization and Subsequent Functional Outcome	^{68}Ga-FAPI-46	Myocardial area of FAP upregulation significantly larger than the SPECT perfusion defect size and infarct area by LGE. No exact regional matching between FAP signal and T1/T2 relaxation from CMR. Significant inverse correlation between FAP volume and left ventricular ejection fraction at follow up
Heart failure		
Song W et al.[20] 2023: ^{68}Ga-FAPI PET visualize heart failure: from mechanism to clinic	^{68}Ga-FAPI	Translational study: rats: ^{68}Ga-FAPI uptake and ventricular wall motion decreased over time as cardiac fibrosis and degree of myocardial injury gradually increased. Human studies: ^{68}Ga-FAPI PET imaging identified varying degrees of ^{68}Ga-FAPI uptake in the myocardium, no precise match with ^{13}N-NH3 myocardial perfusion

Cardiovascular risk factors

Reference	Tracer	Findings
Heckmann MB et al. [17] 2020: Relationship Between Cardiac Fibroblast Activation Protein Activity by Positron Emission Tomography and Cardiovascular Disease	^{68}Ga-FAPI	Oncologic patients. High myocardial FAP-signal intensities correlate with cardiovascular risk factors and metabolic disease
Siebermair J et al. [27] 2021: Cardiac fibroblast activation detected by Ga-68 FAPI PET imaging as a potential novel biomarker of cardiac injury/ remodeling	^{68}Ga-FAPI-04	Oncologic patients. Association of CAD, age, and LVEF with cardiac FAP uptake
Lin et al. [28]2022: Diffuse uptake of ^{68}Ga-FAPI in the left heart in a patient with hypertensive heart disease by PET/CT	^{68}Ga-FAPI	Case report: Significant diffuse heterogeneity uptake of ^{68}Ga-FAPI was observed in the myocardium of left ventricle and left atrium. No uptake in the right atrial and ventricular myocardium

Cardiac sarcoidosis

Reference	Tracer	Findings
Siebermair J et al. [18] 2022: Cardiac fibroblast activation detected by ^{68}Gallium-FAPI-46 positron emission tomography-magnetic resonance imaging as a sign of chronic activity in cardiac sarcoidosis	^{68}Ga-FAPI-46	Case report: Six months after diagnosis FDG–PET revealed no tracer uptake. MR imaging findings were stable showing persistent LGE. FAPI PET-MR imaging demonstrated pronounced tracer uptake indicating intense fibroblast activation in the basal septum/ posterior wall. These areas matched the regions of LGE/FDG uptake from 6 months before

Cardiac amyloidosis

Reference	Tracer	Findings
Guo W et al. [19] 2022: ^{68}Ga FAPI PET/MR imaging in Cardiac Amyloidosis	^{68}Ga-FAPI	Case report: Diffuse and inhomogeneous ^{68}Ga-FAPI uptake in the thickened left ventricle myocardium and tongue. Tongue biopsy results showed positive Congo red staining consistent with amyloid involvement

Cardio-oncology

Reference	Tracer	Findings
Totzeck M et al. [22] 2020: Cardiac fibroblast activation detected by positron emission tomography/computed tomography as a possible sign of cardiotoxicity	^{68}Ga-FAPI	Case report: intense FAP expression in the area of the primary tumor, multiple liver metastases, and peritoneal nodules indicating peritoneal carcinomatosis. Incisive tracer accumulation of the left ventricular myocardium was detectable
Finke D et al. [23] 2021: Early Detection of Checkpoint Inhibitor-Associated Myocarditis Using ^{68}Ga-FAPI PET/CT	^{68}Ga-FAPI	Patients with myocarditis undergoing checkpoint inhibitor therapy showed cardiac enrichment of 68Ga-FAPI, which was less distinct or absent in patients receiving checkpoint inhibitors without any signs of immunological adverse effects or cardiac impairment

(continued on next page)

Table 1
(continued)

Condition	FAP Tracer	FAPI-PET Key Findings
Others		
Treutlein C et al.[21] 2022: Assessment of myocardial fibrosis in patients with systemic sclerosis using ^{68}Ga-FAPI-04-PET-CT	^{68}Ga-FAPI-04	Increased tracer uptake in SSc-related MF with higher uptake in SSc patients with arrhythmias, elevated serum-NT-pro-BNP, and increased LGE in CMR. Histologically, myocardial biopsies from CMR imaging-positive and ^{68}Ga-FAPI-04-positive regions confirmed the accumulation of FAP + fibroblasts surrounded by collagen deposits
Wang L et al.[29] 2022: ^{68}Ga-FAPI right heart uptake in a patient with idiopathic pulmonary arterial hypertension	^{68}Ga-FAPI	Significant tracer uptake in the myocardium of the right heart including RV free wall and right atrium. RV insertion point presented with focal uptake. No uptake of ^{68}Ga-FAPI in the left ventricular myocardium
Shi et al.[30] 2022: Cardiac fibroblast activation in dilated cardiomyopathy detected by positron emission tomography	^{68}Ga-FAPI-04	Case report: Heterogeneous myocardial ^{68}Ga-FAPI-04 uptake pattern, significant cardiac uptake, the most prominent uptake was detected at LV inferior wall
Xing et al.[31] 2022: Comparison of ^{68}Ga-FAPI imaging and cardiac magnetic resonance in detection of myocardial fibrosis in a patient with chronic thromboembolic pulmonary hypertension	^{68}Ga-FAPI-04	Case report: Intense but inhomogenous uptake in the myocardium of the free wall of RV and milder uptake in the insert point of RV. No discernible uptake in the left ventricular myocardium
Chen et al.[32] 2022: Imaging of cardiac fibroblast activation in patients with chronic thromboembolic pulmonary hypertension	^{68}Ga-FAPI-04	Tracer uptake mainly localized in the RV free wall. Enhanced fibroblast activation reflects the thickening of the RV wall and decreased RV contractile function

Abbreviations: AMI, acute myocardial infarction; CAD, coronary artery disease; CMR, cardiac magnet resonance tomography; FAPI, fibroblast activation protein inhibitor; FDG, fluordesoxyglucose; Ga, Gallium; LGE, late gadolinium enhancement; LV, left ventricle; LVEF, left ventricular ejection fraction; RV, right ventricle; SPECT, single photon emission computed tomography.

Activated (myo)fibroblasts express the homodimeric membrane bound serine protease FAP, which regulates remodeling by stimulating fibrosis and deposition of extracellular matrix.[6–8] With the new FAP-directed PET radiotracers, imaging of fibroblast activation has become possible.

Consequently, FAP-targeted imaging enables substantial new insights into pathogenesis of ventricular remodeling. In 2015, Tillmanns and colleagues demonstrated that FAP is highly expressed in the first week after myocardial infarction when the stable scar is being built.[9] Recently, experimental studies supported the feasibility of ^{68}Ga-FAPI PET to identify fibroblast activation in animal models of AMI. Varasteh and colleagues examined AMI and sham-operated rats with ^{68}Ga-FAPI-04 PET and found a peak uptake 6 days after coronary ligation. Autoradiography and hematoxylin and eosin staining revealed highest tracer accumulation in the infarct border zone.[10] Langer and colleagues studied the biodistribution of ^{68}Ga-MHLL1 (which also targets FAP) in healthy mice and after coronary ligation.[11] Seven days after coronary artery ligation, ^{68}Ga-MHLL1 uptake was elevated in the infarct compared with remote myocardium and that this signal persisted on repeat imaging up to 21 days after AMI. Again, FAP expression was predominately found in the infarct border zone. These first results highlight that targeting FAP allows for new diagnostic and therapeutic possibilities.[12]

Some clinical reports already exist on FAP-imaging in patients with AMI. After initial proof that activated fibroblasts in the myocardium can be detected with ^{68}Ga-FAPI-PET,[10,13–15] in a multimodal imaging study, 35 patients with AMI underwent ^{68}Ga-FAPI-46 PET within 11 days of revascularization for in-depth analysis of global and regional myocardial FAP distribution in comparison with single photon emission computed tomography (SPECT) at rest using ^{99m}Tc-tetrofosmin, cardiac resonance tomography (CMR) and echocardiography results.[16] Determined myocardial FAP volume and area showed a high interindividual variance but despite correlating with SPECT-derived perfusion defect size and LGE volume, substantially exceeded the infarct area by involving substantial parts of the border zone as well as remote myocardium (Fig. 1). These findings prove that fibroblast activation and remodeling processes occur outside the infarcted myocardium and suggest that FAP upregulation plays a role not only in replacement fibrosis in the primary injured region but also in reactive fibrosis that may compromise noninfarcted myocardium. In a segmental analysis, FAP signal did not completely match regional tissue characteristics from CMR (T1/T2 relaxation times and LGE) and FAP-positive segments demonstrated impaired contractility as determined by wall thickening. A significant fraction of FAP-positive segments did not show LGE or prolongation of T1 and T2 relaxation times, which suggests that results of ^{68}Ga-FAPI PET are not interchangeable with CMR tissue characteristics. Potentially, ^{68}Ga-FAPI PET represents a new biomarker by adding further biologically distinct information. Finally, it was demonstrated that the myocardial FAP-volume significantly and inversely correlated with left ventricular ejection fraction at follow-up (see Fig. 1). This result suggests that the amount of activated fibroblasts in the infarcted and noninfarcted myocardium directly affects subsequent (adverse) remodeling. Prospective studies will reveal prognostic power of cardiac FAPI-PET in patients with AMI.

Cardiovascular Comorbidities, Heart Failure, Systemic Diseases, and Cardio-Oncology

Value of FAP imaging in other cardiac diseases is currently under investigation. However, specific myocardial tracer uptake has been described for a spectrum of cardiac diseases. An evaluation of cardiac FAP signal in oncologic patients revealed altered myocardial FAP uptake depending on the presence of cardiovascular comorbidities including arterial hypertension, diabetes mellitus, and obesity.[17] Case reports on cardiac sarcoidosis[18] and amyloidosis showed intense FAP uptake in affected myocardial areas. First studies described varying degrees of myocardial FAP uptake in patients with heart failure[20] and in systemic sclerosis.[21] A potential use in cardio-oncology has been demonstrated with FAPI-PET showing increased myocardial tracer uptake in a patient with chemotherapy-induced cardiotoxicity[22] and in checkpoint-inhibitor associated myocarditis.[23] All listed findings represent initial reports that demonstrate general feasibility of using FAP-tracers for imaging activated fibroblasts in the myocardium.

FIBROBLAST ACTIVATION PROTEIN PET IMAGING VERSUS ESTABLISHED FIBROSIS-IMAGING TOOLS

In patients with AMI, CMR not only detects the presence and severity of remodeling but also offers an array of novel approaches for differentiation of infarcted, viably injured, and noninfarcted myocardium.[24] Next to widely used cardiac function measures (left ventricular ejection fraction [LVEF]), CMR has the capacity to characterize tissue composition. T1-mapping may detect diffuse fibrosis while T2-imaging mainly identifies edema

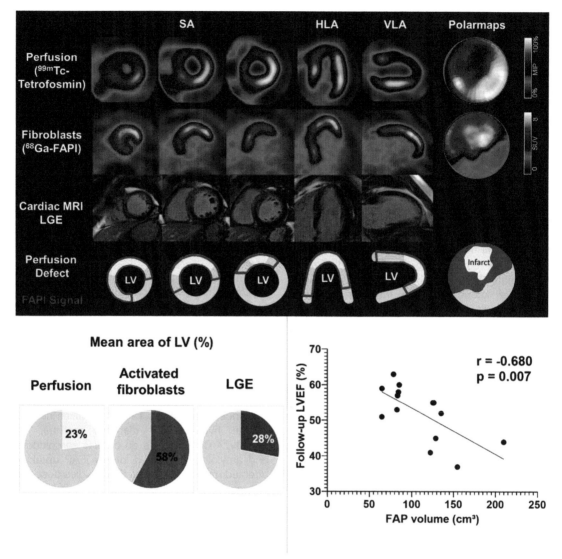

Fig. 1. Representative case with acute anterior wall myocardial infarction: Myocardial perfusion images using ^{99m}Tc-tetrofosmin at rest (*first row*), ^{68}Ga-FAPI-46 PET (*second row*), LGE from cardiac magnetic resonance (*third row*), and schematic drawings of the left ventricle (*fourth row*). Area of fibroblast activation exceeds infarct area and LGE signal, most common type of myocardial FAP-distribution. Bottom left: Mean areas of perfusion defect, FAPI-signal and LGE of 35 studied patients. Bottom right: Global myocardial FAP volume early after acute myocardial infarction inversely correlates with LVEF at follow-up in the chronic stage. (*Adapted from* Diekmann J, Koenig T, Thackeray JT, et al. Cardiac Fibroblast Activation in Patients Early After Acute Myocardial Infarction: Integration with MR Tissue Characterization and Subsequent Functional Outcome. J Nucl Med. 2022;63(9):1415-1423.)

occurring, for example, in inflammation. LGE from contrast agent imaging is used as marker for scar detection and assessing myocardial viability. Echocardiography also enables the assessment of left ventricular (LV)-geometry and LVEF quantification and is easily accessible. Strain imaging gives global and regional information on myocardial contractility as indirect markers of fibrosis. Of note, these established imaging methods provide important diagnostic and prognostic information but do not enable visualization of active fibrogenesis. A first study has described relevant discrepancies between regional FAP tracer accumulation and presence of indirect fibrosis markers from CMR in patients with AMI.[16] Consequently, FAPI-PET imaging serves as distinct biomarker extending the diagnostic toolbox for image-based assessment of cardiac fibrosis. Prospective studies will have to confirm these initial findings. Characterizing myocardial FAP distribution and exploring its role in imaging fibrosis for other cardiac diseases will be the subject of future research.

Antifibrotic Therapies—Current and Future Strategies

Development of new antifibrotic therapies is a current research focus in cardiovascular science.[24] Despite optimized acute revascularization, AMI remains a major cause of chronic heart failure. After AMI stimulation of quiescent (myo)fibroblasts induces progressive replacement fibrosis. As described above, inflammation and other triggers (eg, mechanical, metabolic) stimulate fibroblast activation. On the one hand, fibrosis is needed for sufficient scar formation; on the other hand, excessive fibrosis may impair myocardial oxygen supply and contribute to adverse remodeling.[24] After acute treatment including revascularization, platelet inhibition, and thrombolysis, wound healing in the subacute and chronic phase is currently pharmacologically regulated using angiotensin-converting enzyme inhibitors, beta-blockers, mineralocorticoid receptor antagonists, and statins. In the future, new therapies could essentially change subacute and chronic therapeutic management. Recently, Rurik and colleagues demonstrated successful use of FAP-targeted chimeric antigen receptor T-cell technologies restoring cardiac function in animals.[25,26] Here lays a great potential in FAPI-PET imaging as a distinct biomarker enabling new insights into pathogenesis and potential therapy or disease progression monitoring. Speculatively, FAP imaging could be used for patient selection for antifibrotic therapies in the future.

CLINICS CARE POINTS

- Myocardial fibrosis plays a key role in the complex process of cardiac remodeling in different diseases and can lead to adverse clinical outcomes.

- With new PET-radiotracers targeting fibroblast activation protein (FAP) molecular imaging of cardiac remodeling processes becomes feasible.

- In the future, FAP-targeted PET imaging might be useful to select patients for specific antifibrotic treatments.

FUNDING

Supported by the Deutsche Forschungsgemeinschaft (DFG, Clinical Research Unit KFO 311, FMB and Clinician Scientist Program PRACTIS, JD), the Leducq Foundation (Transatlantic Network „Immunofib", FMB, JD), and "REBIRTH – Research Center for Translational Regenerative Medicine" (State of Lower Saxony; FMB)

DISCLOSURE

The authors have no relationships relevant to the contents of this paper to disclose.

REFERENCES

1. Barton AK, Tzolos E, Bing R, et al. Emerging molecular imaging targets and tools for myocardial fibrosis detection. Eur Heart J Cardiovasc Imaging 2023;24: 261–75.
2. Gonzalez A, Schelbert EB, Diez J, et al. Myocardial interstitial fibrosis in heart failure: biological and translational perspectives. J Am Coll Cardiol 2018; 71:1696–706.
3. Virag JI, Murry CE. Myofibroblast and endothelial cell proliferation during murine myocardial infarct repair. Am J Pathol 2003;163:2433–40.
4. Sun Y, Weber KT. Angiotensin converting enzyme and myofibroblasts during tissue repair in the rat heart. J Mol Cell Cardiol 1996;28:851–8.
5. Turner NA, Das A, Warburton P, et al. Interleukin-1alpha stimulates proinflammatory cytokine expression in human cardiac myofibroblasts. Am J Physiol Heart Circ Physiol 2009;297:H1117–27.
6. Niedermeyer J, Kriz M, Hilberg F, et al. Targeted disruption of mouse fibroblast activation protein. Mol Cell Biol 2000;20:1089–94.
7. Rettig WJ, Garin-Chesa P, Healey JH, et al. Regulation and heteromeric structure of the fibroblast activation protein in normal and transformed cells of mesenchymal and neuroectodermal origin. Cancer Res 1993;53:3327–35.
8. Park JE, Lenter MC, Zimmermann RN, et al. Fibroblast activation protein, a dual specificity serine protease expressed in reactive human tumor stromal fibroblasts. J Biol Chem 1999;274:36505–12.
9. Tillmanns J, Hoffmann D, Habbaba Y, et al. Fibroblast activation protein alpha expression identifies activated fibroblasts after myocardial infarction. J Mol Cell Cardiol 2015;87:194–203.
10. Varasteh Z, Mohanta S, Robu S, et al. Molecular imaging of fibroblast activity after myocardial infarction using a (68)Ga-labeled fibroblast activation protein inhibitor, FAPI-04. J Nucl Med 2019;60:1743–9.
11. Langer LBN, Hess A, Korkmaz Z, et al. Molecular imaging of fibroblast activation protein after

myocardial infarction using the novel radiotracer [(68)Ga]MHLL1. Theranostics 2021;11:7755–66.

12. Travers JG, Kamal FA, Robbins J, et al. Cardiac fibrosis: the fibroblast awakens. Circ Res 2016; 118:1021–40.

13. Diekmann J, Koenig T, Zwadlo C, et al. Molecular imaging identifies fibroblast activation beyond the infarct region after acute myocardial infarction. J Am Coll Cardiol 2021;77:1835–7.

14. Kessler L, Kupusovic J, Ferdinandus J, et al. Visualization of fibroblast activation after myocardial infarction using 68Ga-FAPI PET. Clin Nucl Med 2021;46:807–13.

15. Notohamiprodjo S, Nekolla SG, Robu S, et al. Imaging of cardiac fibroblast activation in a patient after acute myocardial infarction using (68)Ga-FAPI-04. J Nucl Cardiol 2022;29:2254–61.

16. Diekmann J, Koenig T, Thackeray JT, et al. Cardiac fibroblast activation in patients early after acute myocardial infarction: integration with MR tissue characterization and subsequent functional outcome. J Nucl Med 2022;63:1415–23.

17. Heckmann MB, Reinhardt F, Finke D, et al. Relationship between cardiac fibroblast activation protein activity by positron emission tomography and cardiovascular disease. Circ Cardiovasc Imaging 2020;13:e010628.

18. Siebermair J, Kessler L, Kupusovic J, et al. Cardiac fibroblast activation detected by (68)Gallium-FAPI-46 positron emission tomography-magnetic resonance imaging as a sign of chronic activity in cardiac sarcoidosis. Eur Heart J Case Rep 2022;6: ytac005.

19. Guo W, Chen H. 68)Ga FAPI PET/MRI in cardiac amyloidosis. Radiology 2022;303:51.

20. Song W, Zhang X, He S, et al. 68)Ga-FAPI PET visualize heart failure: from mechanism to clinic. Eur J Nucl Med Mol Imaging 2023;50:475–85.

21. Treutlein C, Distler JHW, Tascilar K, et al. Assessment of myocardial fibrosis in patients with systemic sclerosis using [(68)Ga]Ga-FAPI-04-PET-CT. Eur J Nucl Med Mol Imaging 2022.

22. Totzeck M, Siebermair J, Rassaf T, et al. Cardiac fibroblast activation detected by positron emission tomography/computed tomography as a possible sign of cardiotoxicity. Eur Heart J 2020;41:1060.

23. Finke D, Heckmann MB, Herpel E, et al. Early detection of checkpoint inhibitor-associated myocarditis using (68)Ga-FAPI PET/CT. Front Cardiovasc Med 2021;8:614997.

24. Frantz S, Hundertmark MJ, Schulz-Menger J, et al. Left ventricular remodelling post-myocardial infarction: pathophysiology, imaging, and novel therapies. Eur Heart J 2022;43:2549–61.

25. Aghajanian H, Rurik JG, Epstein JA. CAR-based therapies: opportunities for immuno-medicine beyond cancer. Nat Metab 2022;4:163–9.

26. Rurik JG, Tombacz I, Yadegari A, et al. CAR T cells produced in vivo to treat cardiac injury. Science 2022;375:91–6.

27. Siebermair J, Kohler MI, Kupusovic J, et al. Cardiac fibroblast activation detected by Ga-68 FAPI PET imaging as a potential novel biomarker of cardiac injury/remodeling. J Nucl Cardiol 2021;28:812–21.

28. Lin K, Chen X, Xue Q, et al. Diffuse uptake of [(68)Ga]Ga-FAPI in the left heart in a patient with hypertensive heart disease by PET/CT. J Nucl Cardiol 2022;29:3596–8.

29. Wang L, Zhang Z, Zhao Z, et al. (68)Ga-FAPI right heart uptake in a patient with idiopathic pulmonary arterial hypertension. J Nucl Cardiol 2022;29: 1475–7.

30. Shi X, Lin X, Huo L, Li X. Cardiac fibroblast activation in dilated cardiomyopathy detected by positron emission tomography. J Nucl Cardiol 2022;29: 881–4.

31. Xing HQ, Gong JN, Chen BX, et al. Comparison of (68)Ga-FAPI imaging and cardiac magnetic resonance in detection of myocardial fibrosis in a patient with chronic thromboembolic pulmonary hypertension. J Nucl Cardiol 2022;29:2728–30.

32. Chen BX, Xing HQ, Gong JN, et al. Imaging of cardiac fibroblast activation in patients with chronic thromboembolic pulmonary hypertension. Eur J Nucl Med Mol Imaging 2022;49:1211–22.

Fibroblast Activation Protein Inhibitor Theranostics
Preclinical Considerations

Kazuko Kaneda-Nakashima, PhD[a,b,*], Yoshifumi Shirakami, PhD[a,b],
Yuichiro Kadonaga, PhD[b,c], Tadashi Watabe, MD PhD[a,c]

KEYWORDS

- FAP inhibitors • Tumor-bearing model • Antitumor effect • Targeted radiotherapy • Theranostics
- Actinium-225 • Lutetium-177 • Astatine-211

KEY POINTS

- Fibroblast activation protein (FAP) is overexpressed on the surface of cancer-associated fibroblasts.
- FAP thus represents a novel target for molecular imaging of several tumors.
- FAP inhibitors (FAPI) are potential theranostic molecular probes for various cancers.
- A tumor model expressing FAP is available to verify or confirm the usefulness of FAPI experimentally and provides a means to compare radiopharmaceuticals before clinical translation for both diagnostic and therapeutic applications.

INTRODUCTION

Fibroblast activation protein (FAP) was first reported in 1986 by Rettig and colleagues[1] as a membrane antigen expressed by reactive stromal fibroblasts of epithelial cancers, soft tissue sarcomas, granulation tissue of wound healing, and certain fetal mesenchymal fibroblasts. However, FAP is not expressed in normal fibroblasts, normal or malignant epithelial cells, or in the stroma of benign epithelial tumors. Recent studies have reported that FAP is related to health and pathology.[2] Although FAP is present in malignant tissues and is currently a molecular target for cancer treatment, the role of FAP in cancer tissues is still incompletely understood as its impact on disease prognosis has been inconsistent in the literature.[3] Nevertheless, most data support the concept that high expression of FAP generally promotes cancer progression and reduces responsiveness to chemotherapy, radiotherapy, and immunotherapy, and, consequently, has adverse prognostic implications.

FAP is a cell membrane-bound serine peptidase overexpressed on the surface of cancer-associated fibroblasts (CAFs). FAP is consequently, a novel pan-tumor target for molecular imaging in oncology. In particular, FAP inhibitors (FAPI) have been developed as potential theranostic molecular probes for various cancers. The number of published papers on FAPI for radiopharmaceuticals has significantly increased since their first description in 2018 (**Fig. 1**).

Fibroblast activation protein alpha (FAPα) is expressed in more than 90% of cancers and has consequently attracted attention as a therapeutic target for cancer. In addition to radiopharmaceuticals, various cancer treatments have been

[a] Division of Radiation Science, Institute for Radiation Sciences, Osaka University, 2-4 Yamadaoka, Suita, Osaka 565-0871, Japan; [b] MS-CORE, Forefront Research Center, Graduate School of Science, Osaka University, 1-1 Machikaneyama, Toyonaka, Osaka 560-0043, Japan; [c] Department of Nuclear Medicine and Tracer Kinetics, Graduate School of Medicine, Osaka University, 2-2 Yamadaoka, Suita, Osaka 565-0871, Japan
* Corresponding author.
E-mail address: kkaneda@irs.osaka-u.ac.jp

PET Clin 18 (2023) 397–408
https://doi.org/10.1016/j.cpet.2023.02.005
1556-8598/23/© 2023 Elsevier Inc. All rights reserved.

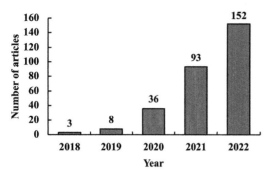

Fig. 1. Number of articles for FAPI from 2018 to 2022. These numbers were retrieved using the database Pubmed.gov (https://pubmed.ncbi.nlm.nih.gov).

developed to target FAP. These include vaccines, monoclonal antibodies, small-molecule inhibitors, nanoparticles, and peptides targeting the peptidase activity of FAP.[4]

Recent reviews have summarized clinical studies of various FAP-targeting radiopharmaceuticals,[5–7] and recent advances in this field are detailed elsewhere in this edition of *PET Clinics* (Editorial staff can insert citation for Chapter 1 by Babich). The current review focuses on experimental studies on FAPI agents involving preclinical models.[8–14] Specifically, tumor models expressing FAP have been used to verify or confirm the usefulness of FAPI experimentally. As FAP is generally not expressed in cancer cell lines suitable for xenografting, cultured cells were stimulated to express FAP using transfection techniques. The primary exception is sarcoma, in which several subtypes directly express FAP on the malignant cells. In human tumors, FAP is highly expressed in CAFs in the stroma as they progress, but it is unclear whether this is sufficiently recapitulated in the murine stroma that develops in the xenograft setting to allow robust testing of FAPI agents. A patient-derived xenograft (PDX) model may be more appropriate for creating a preclinical model in which both epithelial and human stromal elements, including CAFs, are directly implanted. Using PDX models, it is theoretically possible to perform preclinical experiments to check the efficacy of the FAP-targeting compounds that mimic the conditions in patients.

Diagnostic FAPI compounds labeled with gallium-68 (^{68}Ga) and fluorine-18 (^{18}F) are not described in detail in this article, as they have already been reported in detail in other reviews. The physiological accumulation of FAPI is minimal in normal organs, except for the uterus.[14] Lutetium-177 (^{177}Lu) is mainly used for the therapeutic purpose of FAPI labeling in preclinical and clinical situations because of its widespread use

in other approved forms of radionuclide therapy, including the treatment of metastatic neuroendocrine tumors and prostate cancer. Notwithstanding that its half-life is relatively long compared with the biological residence time of most FAPI radiopharmaceuticals described thus far, it has the clinical advantages of being a low-energy beta emitter providing a significant crossfire effect and a convenient gamma emission allowing post-treatment imaging. However, the production of ^{177}Lu requires a nuclear reactor, and the supply of nuclear reactors is limited and unstable. Thus, it is necessary to consider the use of different nuclides (eg, ^{212}Pb or ^{47}Sc). In recent years, nuclear medicine treatment using alpha rays and ^{225}Ac[8,9] and ^{211}At has been investigated.[15] Half-lives of ^{47}Sc is 3.35 days,[16] and ^{212}Pb is 10.64 h.[17,18] These nuclides can be produced in nuclear reactors, generators, or high-energy cyclotrons.

In this review, we introduce the current situation and prospects for the preclinical development and evaluation of FAPI, focusing on its therapeutic purpose.

PRECLINICAL EVALUATION OF FIBROBLAST ACTIVATION PROTEIN INHIBITOR IN ANIMAL MODELS

As shown in **Table 1**, subcutaneous implantation models (s.c.) have been mainly used for the preclinical evaluation of FAPI in several previous reports. This model is often used because changes in tumor size are easy to measure; however, they differ largely from the actual clinical pathology of cancer in terms of cancer stroma formation. An in vitro experimental system using cultured cells is also effective for compound screening because nonspecific uptake can be reduced as low as possible by using cells that artificially express the target protein of FAP.[12,13] However, they are different from the in vivo situation in which FAP expression is observed in CAFs in the stroma, and not in the cancer cell itself. Therefore, the PDX model is considered more appropriate for connecting animal experiments and clinical applications. By transplanting a patient sample into mice, it is possible to mimic the behavior of a patient's cancer lesion.[12,14]

Nevertheless, it is still difficult to reproduce the exact cancer tissues/cells of patients with cancer, even in PDX models. There are large differences in the growth rate of tumors, microenvironment formation within cancer tissues, and blood components, and these factors might affect the differences in therapeutic responses between patients and preclinical models. One of the reasons

Table 1
Summary of therapeutic animal studies of fibroblast activation protein inhibitor

Radiopharmaceutical	Mice (Strain)	Tumor Cell	Tumor Type	Ref.
FAPI-04 (^{225}Ac)	Balb/c-nu/nu	PANC1 (s.c.)	Pancreatic cancer	Watabe et al,[8] 2020
FAPI-46 (^{225}Ac)	Balb/c-nu/nu	PANC1 (s.c.)	Pancreatic cancer	Liu et al,[9] 2022
FAPI-46 (^{177}Lu)	Balb/c-nu/nu	PANC1 (s.c.)	Pancreatic cancer	
FAPI-04 (I-131)	Balb/c-nu/nu	U87 MG (s.c.)	Glioma	Ma et al,[10] 2021
EB-FAPI-B1 (^{177}Lu)	Balb/c-nu/nu	U87 MG (s.c.)	Glioma	Wen et al,[11] 2022
FAP-2286 (^{177}Lu-)	Balb/c-nu/nu	HEK-FAP (s.c.)	Kidney	Zboralski et al,[12] 2022
FAP-2286 (^{177}Lu)	SCID beige mice	HEK-FAP (s.c.)	Kidney	
FAP-2286 (^{177}Lu)	NMRI nu/nu	PDX	Sarcoma	
FAPI-04 (^{177}Lu)	Balb/c-nu/nu	A549-FAP (s.c.)	Lung cancer	Li et al,[13] 2022
Lu-ND-bisFAPI (^{177}Lu)	Balb/c-nu/nu	A549-FAP (s.c.)	Lung cancer	
TEFAPI-06 (^{177}Lu)	NOD/SCID	PDX	Pancreatic cancer	Xu et al,[14] 2022
TEFAPI-06 (^{177}Lu)	NOD/SCID	PDX	Pancreatic cancer	
FAPI-04 (^{177}Lu)	NOD/SCID	PDX	Pancreatic cancer	

Abbreviations: FAP, fibroblast activation protein; FAPI, fibroblast activation protein inhibitor; PANC, pancreatic cancer cell; PDX, patient-derived xenograft.

for this is that the cell lines were originally established as cells that grow in vitro. In other words, cells can increase without depending on the microenvironment of the body. In traditional two-dimensional (2D) cultures, cells adhere to an artificial solid phase, such as plastic or glass, and only touch the other cells at their outer edges. In addition, unlike living tissues, the cellular environment is uniform because there are no gradients of oxygen, nutrients, or excretion. Cultures using extracellular matrix (ECM)-coated dishes and co-cultures in which two or more types of cells are cultured together provide a more in vivo-like state; however, cells on a flat surface become three-dimensional (3D) and this interferes with structure formation. In other words, cells grown in a flat layer on a plastic surface do not reflect the in vivo micro-environment. Meanwhile, the 2D culture of tumor cell lines has certainly yielded a tremendous amount of knowledge regarding cancer mechanisms. However, it is largely different from the in vivo situation in the cancer lesions of patients whose cancer cells are growing natively in a heterogeneous population, which is insufficient for the evaluation of anticancer drugs.

Animal models allow us to observe how human tumors behave within an individual. Mice implanted with tumor cells or manipulated for gene expression to generate tumors, similar to those of humans, are mainly used. At first glance, such models appear to mimic human disease. However, even with this expensive animal model, which is widely used for screening, clinical translation of anticancer drugs can fail.[19–21] In addition, for some cancers, such as those of the brain, kidney, and skin, no qualified animal models currently exist.[22] Establishing an appropriate animal model for the evaluation of FAPI requires tremendous effort and trials which are still underway.

For these reasons, many cell lines have low expression of FAP. Because FAP is generally not expressed in cancer cell lines suitable for xenografting, cultured cells were engineered to express FAP through transfection techniques. The primary exception is sarcoma, in which several subtypes directly express FAP on the malignant cells themselves. In human tumors, FAP is highly expressed in CAFs in the stroma as they progress, but it is unclear whether this is sufficiently recapitulated in the murine stroma that develops in the xenograft setting to allow robust testing of FAPI agents.

DEVELOPMENT OF FIBROBLAST ACTIVATION PROTEIN INHIBITOR CHEMICALS

FAPα is widely expressed on CAF surfaces in various cancers. In this article, we review preclinical studies of FAPIs (**Table 2**)[23–31] labeled with therapeutic radionuclides for targeted radionuclide therapy (TRT), as shown in **Table 1** and **Fig. 2**. One of the earliest reports on radionuclide-labeled FAPI was radioiodine-labeled MIP-1232, a benzamido-glycine-boronoproline derivative synthesized and evaluated by Marquis and Meletta.[23,24] Radioactive iodines (^{123}I, ^{125}I, and ^{131}I) were labeled using an electrophilic aromatic substitution reaction from the trialkyl stannyl precursor (radiochemical yield: 10% to 12%), and HPLC purification yielded the product (radiochemical purity: >90%). They showed

Table 2
Preclinical studies on radiolabeled fibroblast activation protein inhibitors for theranostics

Radiolabeled Therapeutics	Tumor Cells and Murine Xenografts	Biodistribution in Mice % ID/h in Tumor	Treatment of Mice with Tumor Xenograft	Ref.
MIP-1232 (^{125}I)	SK-Mel-187 IC50:0.6 nM(h.FAP)	Significantly accumulated in FAP (+) legions	No data	Meletta et al,[23] 2025 & Marquis et al,[24] 2009
FAPI-04 (^{68}Ga) FAPI-04 (^{177}Lu) FAPI-04 (^{90}Y)	HT-1080(FAP+)	[^{68}Ga] FAPI-04: 4.9 ± 0.82% ID/g (1 h) 5.4 ± 1.51% ID/g (4 h) 3.0 ± 0.23% ID/g (24 h)	No data	Lindner et al,[25] 2018
FAPI-04 (^{225}Ac)	PANC-1	0.251 ± 0.010% ID/g (3 h) 0.097% ± 0.008% ID/g (24 h)	Significantly reduced tumor volume	Watabe et al,[8] 2020
FAPI-46 (^{225}Ac) FAPI-46 (^{177}Lu)	PANC-1	0.3% ID/g (3 h) 0.3% ID/g (3 h)	Significantly reduced tumor volume	Liu et al,[9] 2022
FAPI 3 (^{211}At) FAPI 4 (^{211}At)	HEK293-FAP (+) A549-FAP (+)	Significantly bound to FAP (+) cells in vitro.	No data	Aso et al,[15] 2022
FAPI-04 (^{131}I)	U87 MG	6.16 ± 1.21% ID/g @0.5 h	66% reduction of tumor volume at 15 d after iv injection of 0.55 MBq	Ma et al,[10] 2021
FAPI-04 (^{211}At)	U87 MG	4.04 ± 2.68% ID/g @0.5 h	76% reduction of tumor volume at 15 d after iv injection of 0.55 MBq	Ma et al,[26] 2022
EB-FAPI-B1 (^{177}Lu)	U87 MG IC50 = 16.5 nM	U87 MG-bearing mice: 12.42 ± 1.54% ID/g@96 h	Fold change: [^{177}Lu] EB-FAPI-B1 = 5 times Control = 15 times	Wen et al,[11] 2022
TEFAPI-06 (^{177}Lu) TEFAPI-07 (^{177}Lu)	HT-1080 (FAP+) Kd: (06)10.16 ± 2.56 nM (07) 7.81 ± 2.28 nM	Pancreatic cancer PDX model: (06)7.33 ± 2.28% ID/g@96 h (07)7.57 ± 2.68% ID/g@96 h	Both agents (1.85 and 3.7 MBq) showed remarkable growth inhibition of PDX tumors.	Xu et al,[14] 2022
FAPI-C16 (^{177}Lu)	HT-1080(FAP+)	11.22 ± 1.18% ID/g@24 h 6.50 ± 1.19% ID/g@72 h	Median survival days (29.6MBq): [^{177}Lu] FAPI-C16 = 28 d [^{177}Lu] FAPI-04 = 10 d	Zhang et al,[27] 2022
Onco FAP (^{177}Lu)	SK-RC-52. hFAP HT-1080(FAP+) Kd:0.68 nM	SK-RC-52. hFAP xenografted mice: >30% ID/g (10 min to 3 h)	No data	Millul et al,[28] 2021

Agent	Model	Biodistribution	Findings	Reference
FAP-2286 ([177Lu]FAP-2286 (68Ga))	HEK-FAP Sarcoma PDX Kd:0.2 to 1.4 nM (h.FAP)	21.1% ID/g (3 h) 16.4% ID/g (24 h)	Significant reduction of tumor volume was observed with 30 and 60 MBq of [177Lu] FAP-2286	Zboralski et al,[12] 2022
[177Lu]-DOTAGA.(SA.FAPI)2	No data	No data	First in Human	Ballal et al,[29] 2021
[68Ga]/[177Lu]-DOTA-2P(FAPI)2	HCC PDX HT-1080-FAP	8.28 ± 2.43% ID/g at 4 h 2.85 ± 1.32% ID/g at 48 h 19.71 ± 2.87% ID/g at 48 h	DOTA-2P(FAPI)2 has increased tumor uptake and retention compared with FAPI-46, allowing improved theranostics	Zhao et al,[30] 2022
[68Ga]FAPI-RGD	PANC02	6.16 ± 0.46% ID/g at 0.5 h 5.79 ± 0.22% ID/g at 4 h	Tumor SUV: 6 to 8 in six patients	Zang et al,[31] 2020

Abbreviations: % ID, % of injection dose; FAP, fibroblast activation protein; FAPI, fibroblast activation protein inhibitor; h, hours; PDX, patient-derived xenograft.

A

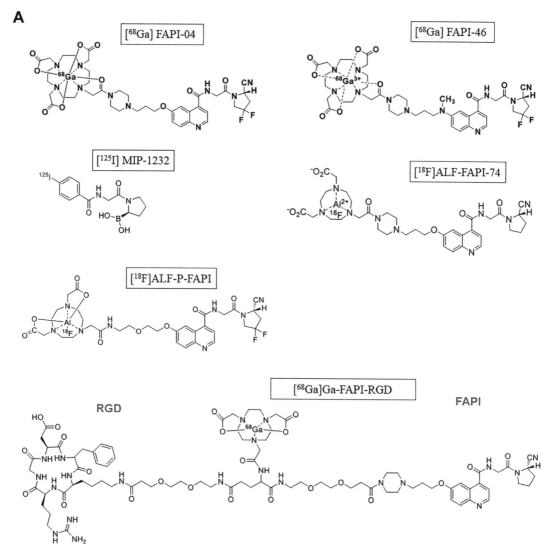

Fig. 2. Radiolabeled FAPI compounds for radio-theranostics. (*A*) Diagnostic compounds suitable for PET. (*B,C*) Therapeutic compounds suitable for radionuclide therapy.

that [125I] MIP-1232 binds to FAPα-positive melanoma cell (SK-Mel-187) xenograft sections in experiments in vitro and that the binding site is consistent with FAPα immunostaining, suggesting that the radiolabeled FAPI may be useful for tumor treatment and imaging.

Lindner and colleagues[25] synthesized a series of quinoline-based FAPIs incorporating a 1,4,7,10-tetraazacyclododecane-1,4,7,10-tetraacetic acid (DOTA) chelate and found that [68Ga] FAPI-04 was the most suitable PET imaging agent of that initial series due to a combination of high uptake and longer tumor retention than other agents, rendering therapeutic applications more practical. Consequently, they further synthesized FAPI-04

labeled with 177Lu, a promising β-ray emitter for TRT, and confirmed its tumor accumulation by biodistribution studies in tumor-implanted mice. They stated that the 4,4-difluoroproline structure is important for inhibiting enzyme activity, and that the heterocyclic segment is required for intratumor retention of the radionuclide.

We also used the FAPI-04 to expand α-ray therapy research.[8] [225Ac] FAPI-04 injected intravenously at 34 kBq into pancreatic cancer cell (PANC-1)-transplanted mice showed marked tumor growth suppression for approximately 1 month after administration, despite relatively low tumor accumulation based on preclinical Cu-64 PET imaging (**Fig. 3**). [225Ac] FAPI-04 targets

B

Fig. 2. (*continued*)

C

[^{177}Lu] DOTA-2P-(FAPI)$_2$

DOTA

PEG3

PEG3

FAPI binding motif

FAPI binding motif

Fig. 2. (*continued*)

cancer stromal cells and does not directly target tumor cells, and the short range of α-rays makes it unlikely to the α-rays reach cancer cells sufficiently. The short range of the α-rays suggests that they may indirectly injure tumor tissues by injuring cancer stromal cells. However, the details of these therapeutic mechanisms have not yet been elucidated.

Comparative experiments were performed with [^{225}Ac] FAPI-46 and [^{177}Lu] FAPI-46 to compare

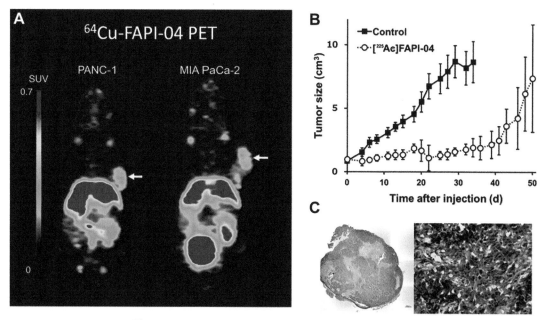

Fig. 3. (*A*) PET imaging of ^{64}Cu-FAPI-04 (2.5 h post-injection) in PANC-1 and MIA PaCa-2 xenograft models. (*B*) Treatment effect in PANC-1 xenograft mice after the injection of ^{225}Ac-FAPI-04. (*C*) Immunohistochemical staining of the PANC-1 and tumor xenograft using an FAPα antibody (left: low magnification, right: high magnification). *Arrows* indicate tumors. (Data from Watabe and colleagues[7] according to open access policy).

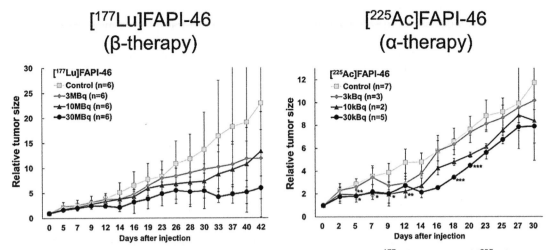

Fig. 4. Relative tumor size changes in PANC-1 xenograft mice treated with [^{177}Lu] FAPI-46 and [^{225}Ac] FAPI-46. (*$P < 0.05$ between 10 kBq and control group; **$P < 0.05$ between 30 kBq and control group; and ***$P < 0.05$ between 3 kBq and 30 kBq group.) (Data from Liu and colleagues[8] according to open access policy).

the effects of α- and β-radioligand therapies in the same animal models.[9] Both dose-dependent suppression of tumor growth. However, [^{177}Lu] FAPI-46 tended toward more sustained effects (**Fig. 4**). In contrast, [^{225}Ac] FAPI-46 showed relatively rapid tumor growth suppression followed by faster regrowth.

FAPI-46 is a compound in which a methylamino group replaced the ether oxygen in the linker moiety of FAPI-04. [^{68}Ga]-or [^{177}Lu]-labeled FAPI-46 showed a higher tumor accumulation rate, and their retention was improved over [^{68}Ga]-or [^{177}Lu]-labeled FAPI-04.[32] However, the tumor growth-inhibitory effect of [^{177}Lu] FAPI-46 did not improve significantly. The prolongation of tumor retention by introducing methylamino groups may still be inadequate given the half-life of ^{177}Lu (6.6 d).

Aso and colleagues[15] selected ^{211}At as the α-ray nuclide, replacing the DOTA chelate structure of FAPI-02 with a boronophenyl group, and synthesized [^{211}At] FAPI 4 by the borono-astatin exchange reaction method in the presence of potassium iodide as a catalyst. [^{211}At] FAPI 4 was specifically taken up by FAPα/HEK293 and FAPα/A549 cells in cell-binding experiments in vitro.

Ma and colleagues[10,26] synthesized [^{131}I] FAPI-04 and [^{211}At] FAPI-04 using trialkyltin transgenic precursors. In mice transplanted with the human

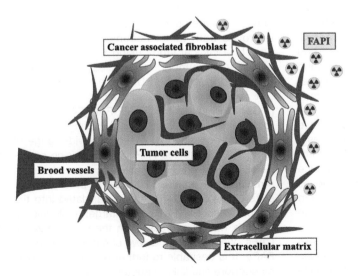

Fig. 5. Schematic representation of the relationship between CAFs, blood vessels, and intracellular matrix in tumor tissue. FAP inhibitor reaches CAFs but might not be enough to attack inside cancer cells.

glioma cell line (U87 MG), the tumor accumulation rates of [^{131}I] FAPI-04 and [^{211}At] FAPI-04 at 30 min were 6.16 ± 1.21% ID/g and 4.04 ± 2.68% ID/g, respectively. The tumor shrinkage rates of [^{131}I] FAPI-04 (5 MBq) and [^{211}At] FAPI-04 (0.55 MBq) in the same mouse model were 66% and 76%, respectively, 15 d after the administration of [^{131}I] FAPI-04 (5 MBq) and [^{211}At] FAPI-04 (0.55 MBq). The total urinary and fecal excretion rates of [^{131}I] FAPI-04 at 6 h after administration were as high as 75.8%, and the urinary radioactivity was highly polar.

These preclinical results indicate that quinoline-based FAPIs labeled with α- or β-emitting radionuclides inhibit tumor growth. The quinoline-based FAPI tumor accumulation rate and tumor retention are adequate for PET diagnostics, but further improvement is desirable for therapeutic use. Therefore, FAPI derivatives incorporating Evans blue, 4-p-iodophenylbutyric acid, or fatty acids were synthesized to enhance blood retention.[11,14,27] Tumor accumulation and retention by these [^{177}Lu]-conjugated derivatives in tumor-implanted mice were greatly improved compared with those of FAPI-04, which also showed marked tumor growth inhibition.

Currently, the most advanced compounds in the developmental stage are [^{177}Lu] OncoFAP and [^{177}Lu] FAP-2286. [^{177}Lu] OncoFAP is a quinoline-based FAPI derivative with ultra-high affinity (Kd = 0.68 nM) for FAP and showed the highest tumor accumulation rate of greater than 30% ID/g in SK-RC-52h, FAP transplantation mice in a biodistribution study (10 min to 3 h after administration).[28] [^{177}Lu] FAP-2286 is a novel FAPI with a cyclic peptide (Cys-Pro-Pro-Ser-Gln-Phe-Cys) as the pharmacophore, which has the second highest tumor uptake after [^{177}Lu] OncoFAP. Administration of this compound (30 or 60 MBq) to HEK-FAP and sarcoma PDX mice showed marked tumor growth inhibitory effects in both animal models. Both compounds were screened and discovered for their high affinity for FAP, resulting in high tumor accumulation and retention. Further translational research on both the compounds is required.

Several unique complex structures have recently been developed. Ballal and colleagues[29] designed and synthesized a dimeric FAPI compound, [^{177}Lu] Lu-DOTAGA.(SA.FAPi)$_2$ to enhance tumor accumulation. The tumor-absorbed doses in patients treated with the compound averaged 6.70 Gy/GBq, which was 5.16 times higher than that of the equivalent monomer.

Zhao and colleagues discovered another FAPI dimer, DOTA-2P(FAPI)$_2$, and performed diagnostic and therapeutic experiments in FAP-positive hepatocellular carcinoma PDX mice and HT-1080-FAP cell-transplanted mice using ^{68}Ga and ^{177}Lu-conjugates [26]. [^{68}Ga] and [^{177}Lu] Lu-DOTA-2P(FAPI)$_2$ were stable in PBS for 4 h. Tumor retention of [^{68}Ga] Ga-DOTA-2P(FAPI)$_2$ in HT-1080 transplanted mice were superior to that of [^{68}Ga] Ga-FAPI-46. Similarly, the tumor accumulation rate and retention of [^{177}Lu] Lu-DOTA-2P(FAPI)$_2$ administered to HT-1080 transplanted mice were superior to that of [^{177}Lu] Lu-FAPI-46 (19.71 ± 2.87% ID/g vs 2.69 ± 1.25% ID/g at 48 h) to FAP positive tumors. These data showed that ^{68}Ga- and ^{177}Lu-labeled DOTA-2P(FAPI)$_2$ are excellent diagnostic and therapeutic agents, respectively. When [^{177}Lu] Lu-DOTA-2P(FAPI)$_2$ or [^{68}Ga] Ga-DOTA-2P(FAPI)$_2$ was administered to FAP-positive hepatocellular carcinoma PDX mice at 29.6 MBq, [^{177}Lu] Lu-DOTA-2P(FAPI)$_2$ showed a stronger inhibitory effect on tumor growth. In conclusion, dimerization of FAPI enhances tumor accumulation and prolongs retention.

Zang and colleagues[31] discovered a dual-targeting PET tracer, [^{68}Ga] Ga-FAPI-RGD (Arg-Gly-Asp motif), which targets both FAP and αVβ3 and conducted preclinical and clinical studies. This compound is a complex of the quinoline-type compound FAPI-02 skeleton and RGD. The cancer cell uptake rate of [^{68}Ga] Ga-FAPI-RGD was approximately twice that of [^{68}Ga] Ga-RGDfK (a single-targeting PET tracer). Tumor accumulation in mice transplanted with mouse pancreatic cancer cells (PANC02) was 6.16 ± 0.46 %ID/g (0.5 h), 5.95 ± 0.43 %ID/g (1 h), 5.78 ± 0.28 %ID/g (2h), and 5.79 ± 0.22 %ID/g (4 h) for [^{68}Ga] Ga-FAPI-RGD. In contrast, the accumulation of [^{68}Ga] Ga-RGDfK and [^{68}Ga] Ga-FAPI-02 in the same mice was 3.51 ± 0.47 %ID/g (1 h) and 0.97 ± 0.09 %ID/g (1 h), respectively. These results showed that dual targeting improved both tumor accumulation and retention. In a clinical study using the compound in 6 patients, tumors were clearly delineated (SUV 6 to 9), and the SUV increased over time.

It is well demonstrated that [^{68}Ga] FAPI-04, [^{68}Ga] FAPI-46, and [^{18}F]-AlF-FAPI-74 are useful for PET imaging in a clinical setting, because FAPα is frequently expressed in a wide range of tumors. Radiolabeled FAPIs are promising candidates for use in TRT. However, several issues remain to be resolved before the preclinical results of the FAPI TAT can be translated into the clinical practice. FAPα, the target molecule of FAPI, is mainly expressed on the membranes of CAFs, whereas only a few carcinomas express FAPα. It is desirable to further optimize the pharmacophore and linker structures, and improve the affinity of the ligand for FAPα. The combination of α- and β -radionuclides should be investigated in the future.

COMPOUND STRUCTURE AND BIOLOGICAL AFFINITY

Through investigations by many researchers, the structure required for FAP binding has been clarified. The feasibility of labeling, post-labeling stability, and anticancer efficacy must be achieved while maintaining the essential structure. The major FAPI compounds reported to have high selectivity are shown in **Fig. 2**. In addition to high selectivity, long retention time and stability are necessary for successful treatment. As described in the previous section, one of the disadvantages of the FAPI is its short retention time. To be a more effective drug, it is necessary to consider a matching of the half-time of the labeling radionuclide coupled with the biological half-life of the FAPI compound, while maintaining chemical stability. In other words, FAPI compounds labeled with short-lived therapeutic nuclides are considered likely to be more effective in addition to achieving longer retention.

DISCUSSION IN THE FUTURE

Diagnostic PET reports by various international research groups have clearly shown that FAP is an excellent molecular target for cancer.[33] However, several experimental and clinical issues must be addressed to increase its therapeutic effect. CAFs are the main components of cancer lesions and represent the scaffold of the tumor microenvironment. Therefore, if only CAFs are damaged without affecting the cancer cells, they will re-proliferate and generate new CAFs; thus, the therapeutic effect will be insufficient (**Fig. 5**). This problem might be solved by establishing novel compounds and repeating the compound administration. It is because by gradually damaging the scaffold of cancer, even if CAFs are radioresistant, it might be possible to prevent regrowth and achieve better therapeutic effects. A combination of anticancer drugs may also be effective. By destroying CAFs with FAPI and facilitating drug delivery to cancer cells, it may be possible to make anticancer drugs function effectively at lower concentrations. Reducing the amount of the drug used would reduce the incidence of side effects, leading to a higher therapeutic effect at the same concentration. The unremitting efforts of researchers who develop therapeutic FAPI might lead to considerable treatment success in clinical situations. We hope this will be an effective treatment option to improve the prognosis of patients.

SUMMARY

Because FAPI agents show high accumulation in cancer lesions with minimal expression in normal organs, they represent excellent molecular probes for PET imaging. However, owing to their short retention times and predominant targeting of stromal cells rather than cancer cells, they are difficult to use as therapeutic probes. Various researchers, including our group, have designed compounds that target FAP as radioligand therapeutics. However, there are still many challenges in the preclinical evaluation of therapeutic FAPI to realize clinical translation with sufficient therapeutic effects in patients. We strongly believe that FAPI can be used as a pan-tumor therapeutic for next-generation radioligand therapy.

CONFLICT OF INTEREST

The authors have declared no conflicts of interest.

DISCLOSURE

No potential conflict of interest relevant to this article was reported.

REFERENCES

1. Rettig WJ, Chesa PG, Beresford HR, et al. Differential expression of cell surface antigens and glial fibrillary acidic protein in human astrocytoma subsets. Cancer Res 1986;46(12 Part 1):6406.
2. Fitzgerald AA, Weiner LM. The role of fibroblast activation protein in health and malignancy. Cancer Metastasis Rev 2020;39(3):783.
3. Sahai E, Astsaturov I, Cukierman E, et al. A framework for advancing our understanding of cancer-associated fibroblasts. Nat Rev Cancer 2020;20:174–86.
4. Xin L, Gao J, Zheng Z, et al. Fibroblast activation protein-α as a target in the bench-to-bedside diagnosis and treatment of tumors: a narrative review. Front Oncol 2021;11:648187.
5. Sharma P, Singh SS, Gayana S. Fibroblast activation protein inhibitor PET/CT: a promising molecular imaging tool. Clin Nucl Med 2021;46(3):e141–50.
6. Altmann A, Haberkorn U, Siveke J. The latest developments in imaging of fibroblast activation protein. J Nucl Med 2021;62(2):160–7.
7. Li M, Younis MH, Zhang Y, et al. Clinical summary of fibroblast activation protein inhibitor-based radiopharmaceuticals: cancer and beyond. Eur J Nucl Med Mol Imaging 2022;49(8):2844–68.
8. Watabe T, Liu Y, Kaneda-Nakashima K, et al. Theranostics targeting fibroblast activation protein in the tumor stroma: ^{64}Cu- and ^{225}Ac-labeled FAPI-04 in

pancreatic cancer xenograft mouse models. J Nucl Med 2020;61(4):563–9.

9. Liu Y, Watabe T, Kaneda-Nakashima K, et al. Fibroblast activation protein targeted therapy using [^{177}Lu]FAPI-46 compared with [^{225}Ac]FAPI-46 in a pancreatic cancer model. Eur J Nucl Med Mol Imaging 2022;49(3):871–80.

10. Ma H, Li F, Shen G, et al. Synthesis and preliminary evaluation of ^{131}I-labeled FAPI tracers for cancer theranostics. Mol Pharm 2021;18(11):4179–87.

11. Wen X, Xu P, Shi M, et al. Evans blue-modified radiolabeled fibroblast activation protein inhibitor as long-acting cancer therapeutics. Theranostics 2022; 12(1):422–33.

12. Zboralski D, Hoehne A, Bredenbeck A, et al. Preclinical evaluation of FAP-2286 for fibroblast activation protein targeted radionuclide imaging and therapy. Eur J Nucl Med Mol Imaging 2022;49(11):3651–67.

13. Li H, Ye S, Li L, et al. ^{18}F- or ^{177}Lu-labeled bivalent ligand of fibroblast activation protein with high tumor uptake and retention. Eur J Nucl Med Mol Imaging 2022;49(8):2705–15.

14. Xu M, Zhang P, Ding J, et al. Albumin binder–conjugated fibroblast activation protein inhibitor radiopharmaceuticals for cancer therapy. J Nucl Med 2022;63(6):952–8.

15. Aso A, Kaneda-Nakashima K, Nabetani H, et al. Substrate study for dihydroxyboryl astatine substitution reaction with fibroblast activation protein inhibitor (FAPI). Chem Lett 2022;51:1091–4.

16. Sadler AWE, Hogan L, Fraser B, et al. Cutting edge rare earth radiometals: prospects for cancer theranostics. EJNMMI Radiopharm Chem 2022;7(1):21.

17. Kokov KV, Egorova BV, German MN, et al. ^{212}Pb: production approaches and targeted therapy applications. Pharmaceutics 2022;14(1):189.

18. Hutchinson L, Kirk R. High drug attrition rates—where are we going wrong? Nat Rev Clin Oncol 2011;8(4):189–90.

19. Aggarwal B, Danda D, Gupta S, et al. Models for prevention and treatment of cancer: problems vs promises. Biochem Pharmacol 2009;78(9):1083–94.

20. Hait WN. Anticancer drug development: the grand challenges. Nat Rev Drug Discov 2010;9(4):253–4.

21. van der Worp HB, Howells DW, Sena ES, et al. Can animal models of disease reliably inform human studies? PLoS Med 2010;7(3):e1000245.

22. Steele VE, Lubet RA. The use of animal models for cancer chemoprevention drug development. Semin Oncol 2010;37(4):327–38.

23. Meletta R, Herde AM, Chiotellis A, et al. Evaluation of the radiolabeled boronic acid-based FAP inhibitor MIP-1232 for atherosclerotic plaque imaging. Molecules 2015;20:2081–99.

24. Marquis J, Wang J, Maresca K, et al. Targeting tumor microenvironment with radiolabeled inhibitors of seprase. Cancer Res 2009;69(9 Supplement): 4467.

25. Lindner T, Loktev A, Altmann A, et al. Development of quinoline-based theranostic ligands for the targeting of fibroblast activation protein. J Nucl Med 2018; 59:1415–22.

26. Ma H, Li F, Shen G, et al. *In vitro* and *in vivo* evaluation of ^{211}At-labeled fibroblast activation protein inhibitor for glioma treatment. Bioorg Med Chem 2022;55:116600.

27. Zhang P, Xu M, Ding J, et al. Fatty acid-conjugated radiopharmaceuticals for fibroblast activation protein-targeted radiotherapy. Eur J Nucl Med 2022;49:1985–96.

28. Millul J, Bassi G, Mock J, et al. An ultra-high-affinity small organic ligand of fibroblast activation protein for tumor-targeting applications. Proc Natl Acad Sci USA 2021;118. e2101852118.

29. Ballal S, Yadav MP, Moon ES, et al. First-In-Human results on the biodistribution, pharmacokinetics, and dosimetry of [^{177}Lu] Lu-DOTA.SA.FAPi and [^{177}Lu] Lu-DOTAGA.(SA.FAPi)$_2$. Pharmaceuticals 2021;14:1212.

30. Zhao L, Chen J, Pang Y, et al. Development of fibroblast activation protein inhibitor-based dimeric radiotracers with improved tumor retention and antitumor efficacy. Mol Pharmaceutics 2022;19: 3640–51.

31. Zang J, Wen X, Lin R, et al. Synthesis, preclinical evaluation and radiation dosimetry of a dual targeting PET tracer [^{68}Ga] Ga-FAPI-RGD. Theranostics 2022;12:7180–90.

32. Loktev A, Lindner T, Burger EM, et al. Development of fibroblast activation protein-targeted radiotracers with improved tumor retention. J Nucl Med 2019; 60:1421–9.

33. Kratochwil C, Flechsig P, Lindner T, et al. ^{68}Ga-FAPI PET/CT: tracer uptake in 28 different kinds of cancer. J Nucl Med 2019;60(6):801–5.

Fibroblast Activation Protein Inhibitor Theranostics
Preclinical Combination Treatment

Katharina Lückerath, PhD[a,*], Marija Trajkovic-Arsic, PhD[b,c], Christine E. Mona, PhD[d]

KEYWORDS

- Fibroblast activation protein • Radioligand • Theranostics • Combination therapy
- Tumor microenvironment

KEY POINTS

- Fibroblast activation protein (FAP)-radioligands hold promise for detection and therapy of diverse cancer entities but are unlikely to be curative.
- Combination therapies are one approach to improve outcomes after FAP therapy.
- The interaction between radioligands and the tumor tissue—that is, tumor cells, cancer-associated fibroblasts, immune cells, and other components of the tumor microenvironment—need to be understood in detail before rationale and more effective combination regimens can be developed.

INTRODUCTION

Fibroblast activation protein (FAP) is expressed on myofibroblastic cancer-associated fibroblasts (myCAF; CAF) in the tumor microenvironment (TME), and on tumor cells in some mesenchymal cancers, such as sarcoma, glioblastoma, mesothelioma, and uterine cancer.[1,2] Radioligands binding to FAP have recently come into focus for imaging and therapy as almost all cancers have a stromal component, and diagnostic imaging with FAP-radioligands may outperform ^{18}F-FDG imaging.[3–6] Data on the clinical efficacy of FAP-targeted radioligands are still scarce; current data indicate that FAP-radioligands might hold promise for cancer treatment but are very unlikely to be curative.[7–10] As for other radioligand therapies (RLT), such as prostate-specific membrane antigene (PSMA)- or somatostatin receptor (SSTR)-targeted RLT,[11,12] inherent and acquired resistance to FAP-RLT will likely pose a significant challenge resulting in early or late treatment failure. Thus, improved RLT approaches are urgently needed.

Success of RLT depends on multiple factors, including optimization of radiotherapeutic strategy, overcoming tumor cell-intrinsic resistance mechanisms, and modulating the TME. For example, the choice of radioisotope and suboptimal pharmacokinetics of the ligand may result in insufficient tumor radiation dose delivery. Tumor

[a] Department of Nuclear Medicine, University of Duisburg-Essen and German Cancer Consortium (DKTK)-University Hospital Essen, Hufelandstrasse 55, 45147 Essen, Germany; [b] Division of Solid Tumor Translational Oncology, DKTK and German Cancer Research Center (DKFZ) Partner Side Essen, Hufelandstrasse 15, 45147, Germany; [c] Bridge Institute of Experimental Tumor Therapy, West German Cancer Center, University Hospital Essen, Hufelandstrasse 55, 45147 Essen, Germany; [d] Ahmanson Translational Theranostic Division, Department of Molecular and Medical Pharmacology, University of California Los Angeles, 650 Charles E Young Drive S, Los Angeles, CA 90095, USA
* Corresponding author.
E-mail address: katharina.lueckerath@uk-essen.de

PET Clin 18 (2023) 409–418
https://doi.org/10.1016/j.cpet.2023.02.006
1556-8598/23/© 2023 Elsevier Inc. All rights reserved.

cell-intrinsic resistance may be driven by the regulation of target availability, DNA damage repair capacity, stress response signaling, mutations, proliferation, and redox balance, among others. In the TME, CAF, immune cells, extracellular matrix composition (ECM), fibrosis, hypoxia, and vascularization might contribute to RLT resistance.

FIBROBLAST ACTIVATION PROTEIN RADIOLIGAND THERAPY

Based on the expression of FAP on CAF and on some tumor cells, FAP-radioligands can act through different mechanisms. Radioligands bound to FAP$^+$ CAF deliver ionizing radiation directly to CAF and may irradiate tumor cells in the vicinity via crossfire-effects; vice versa, binding to FAP$^+$ tumor cells irradiates tumor cells directly and targets close-by CAF by cross-fire effects. In addition, radioligands can induce bystander effects, and cross-fire radiation can target other components of the TME, such as immune cells. The relative contribution of these mechanisms to FAP-RLT efficacy has not been investigated yet. Responsiveness may differ with the cell type(s) expressing FAP, tumor architecture, FAP-radioligand characteristics, and tumor (radio)biology. However, general assumptions that hold true for other RLT also hold true for FAP-RLT. These are that radioligands can induce DNA damage in directly or indirectly targeted cells, and that target expression levels, which can vary between and within lesions, and radiation type impact overall tumor radiation dose and the distribution and severity (eg, clustered double-strand DNA breaks [DSB]) of radioligand-induced DNA damage.[13–15] The likelihood of cell death, which is needed for curing cancer, relates to the amount and type of DNA damage and the ability of the cell to survive this insult through DNA-damage repair (DDR) and replication stress response (RSR) pathways.

The following sections will discuss the potential to improve (FAP–)RLT through rational combination therapies that leverage the effects of (direct and indirect) irradiation of tumor cells and CAF. These considerations are not exclusive to FAP-radioligands. The data presented in this review reflect experiences with other radioligands as no data are available specifically supporting these concepts for FAP-radioligands. Furthermore, (individual) tumor biology is diverse and may determine the optimal RLT combination for a patient. This may be especially relevant for FAP-RLT due to the broad expression of FAP across cancer entities and anatomical locations.

LEVERAGING RESPONSES TO DNA DAMAGE

Radioligands induce cell stress responses in tumor cells that allow the tumor cells to survive RLT-induced cytotoxicity. Thus, targeting these compensatory responses is an attractive option for combination therapies.

The cytotoxicity of radioligands is due to the induction of DNA damage, mainly single-strand and double-strand breaks, as indicated by accumulation of phospho-H2A.X and 53BP1 foci in tumors after RLT exposure.[13,16,17] In response to radiation, the kinases Ataxia Telangiectasia Mutated (ATM) and Ataxia Telangiectasia and Rad3-Related Protein (ATR) primarily recognize DNA double-strand breaks and coordinate the signaling cascades that mediate DDR through either homologous recombination (HR) or nonhomologous end-joining (NHEJ). Single-strand DNA breaks are repaired by the base-excision repair (BER) pathway.[18] Cell viability is also influenced by its response to replication stress (RSR). Cell death is initiated when the extent of DNA damage exceeds the repair capacity of the cell. Consistently, RLT activated signaling through ATM and ATR, induced cell cycle arrest, increased TP53 signaling (unless mutated), and decreased DNA-nucleotide pools in mouse models of prostate cancer[19] and neuroendocrine tumors.[20]

Increased DDR/RSR activity can protect tumors from RLT-induced cytotoxicity; at the same time, it is a tumor vulnerability that can be targeted with clinical-stage inhibitors of key effectors in these pathways. This is especially relevant in patients who already have inactivating mutations in DDR/RSR proteins at either a somatic or germline level. These patients have an increased reliance on parallel DDR pathways and pharmacological inhibition of an additional effector might cause synthetic lethality (eg, poly(ADP-ribose)-polymerase [PARP] inhibitors in the HR deficiency setting).[21–23] In addition, these patients might per se present with more radiosensitive tumors because DDR/RSR mutation(s) reduce the ability to cope with RLT-induced stress.[24]

Inhibition of ATR, which primarily impacts HR, DNA-protein kinase, which is a key gene regulating NHEJ, or PARP, a key gene in BER (and alternative end-joining), in the context of RLT has successfully been applied in genetically unselected preclinical tumor models[25–27] and is being investigated in clinical trials (eg, NCT05053854 and NCT03874884). The benefit of these strategies may depend on the type of radiation damage (eg, predominantly single- vs double-strand DNA breaks), the dependence of a cell on HR (occurring primarily in actively cycling cells) versus NHEJ (active throughout the cell cycle and therefore, potentially more important for tumors with a low proliferative fraction), and on underlying mutations in DDR/RSR genes (see above). Likewise, inhibitors of the kinases CHK1 and WEE1, which act downstream of ATM and ATR, have been used as radiosensitizers, although not in the context of RLT. CHK1 and WEE1 inhibitors might sensitize tumors to RLT by overriding the G2 cell cycle checkpoint to allow cell cycle progression despite DNA damage.[28–30] Interestingly, DDR inhibitors have been shown to increase micronuclei formation in CAF, suggesting that they might radiosensitize both, tumor cells and CAF.[31]

Antimetabolites like capecitabine[32] and inhibitors of enzymes essential for nucleotide biosynthesis, such as ribonucleotide reductase or thymidylate synthase inhibitors, are combined with RLT to further reduce nucleotide pools needed for repair and synthesis of new DNA (eg, NCT04234568 and NCT0419412).

Targeting pathways regulating DDR/RSR signaling may impair initiation and execution of damage repair by restraining the tumor's ability to deal with diverse cell stresses as these pathways include important tumor drivers such as RAS/MAPK/MEK, PI3K/AKT/mTOR, heat shock protein 90, or androgen receptor pathways.[33–37]

Standard chemotherapies, such as the alkylating agent temozolomide and taxanes, and targeted therapies, such as Aurora kinase inhibitors, that inhibit cell cycle might improve RLT-efficacy by inducing additional DNA damage and thus, by promoting cell death due to a massive amount of unrepaired DNA.[38–41] Cell cycle inhibitors can also exert radiosensitizing effects by locking cells in more radiosensitive phases of the cell cycle (eg, G2/M phase).

Besides exhausting the tumor cells' capacity to repair damaged DNA, interference with DNA damage repair might promote more error-prone DNA repair and thus, accumulation of genomic aberrations, which may increase tumor immunogenicity.[42,43] Although these aberrations may be deleterious, there is also a possibility that novel mutations may provide cells with a survival advantage. The most error-prone repair mechanism is NHEJ.[44] NHEJ would be particularly important in repairing DSB that follow fork collapse induced by PARP inhibition in cells attempting to repair single-strand DNA breaks.

Taken together, co-targeting the DDR/RSR and/or adding therapies that further increase DNA damage may radiosensitize tumors and thus, be the most obvious approach for RLT-combination regimens. It is, however, not a trivial approach; genome integrity is protected on many levels and by various players, which can act in parallel and compensate for one another. Furthermore, severe side effects need to be avoided. This is important because normal cells are highly dependent on DNA-repair mechanisms. Therefore, elucidating the specific DNA repair pathways involved in resolving DNA damage after RLT in a given tumor, their activation kinetics, and interdependencies is warranted to select the most promising RLT combination and to inform on how therapies should be sequenced relative to one another.

EXPLOITING RADIOLIGAND THERAPY-INDUCED IMMUNOMODULATION

Fueled by reports (i) suggesting synergy between RLT and programmed cell death protein 1/programmed death ligand 1 (PD-1/PD-L1) and/or cytotoxic T-lymphocyte-associated protein 4 (CTLA-4) immune-checkpoint blockade (ICB) in murine tumor models and patients,[45–55] and (ii) indicating that a functional immune system is required to achieve deep and durable responses to RLT,[51,56] data on RLT-mediated immune-modulation are emerging.

RLT may induce immunogenic cell death[51] which can increase tumor infiltration by CD8[+] T cells[51,56] and antigen-presenting cells,[45] and elevate CD8[+] T cell: regulatory T cell ratios.[56] Mice with prostate cancer, melanoma, breast cancer or neuroblastoma showing complete response to RLT were immune to tumor re-challenge,[48,50,56] and co-culturing of splenocytes from immune-competent melanoma-bearing mice with tumor cells increased interferon-gamma (IFN-γ) production.[56] These findings suggest the generation of tumor-specific T-cell responses and immunological antitumor memory. Mechanistically, stimulator of interferon genes (STING)/IFN type 1 signaling might be central in orchestrating the changes in immune repertoire as RLT upregulated STING/IFN1 target gene expression in melanoma.[50,53] Although RLT-treated tumor cells induced IFN-γ production by CD8[+] T cells independent of tumor cell STING expression,[53] tumoral STING signaling seemed to be required for optimal RLT efficacy and synergy of RLT with CTLA-4 ICB.[50,53] Direct and indirect STING agonists have shown to possess potent efficacy in multiple preclinical cancer models and entered clinical trials.[57–59]

The outcome of RLT-induced immunomodulation might be shaped by several factors, including delivered tumor dose, subcellular localization of radiation (damage), sequencing of therapies, tumor entity, and stage, and the TME context. Low-dose RLT as monotherapy did not or only moderately increase T cell recruitment and functionality in melanoma mouse models,[50,60] whereas higher tumor doses facilitated profound tumor-specific T-cell responses and prolonged survival of mice with non-Hodgkin lymphoma.[56] However, combining low tumor doses with ICB was sufficient to launch durable tumor cell-specific CD8+ T cell responses with increased tumor immune infiltration of CD8+ T cells, CD8+ CD103+ effector memory T cells and $\gamma\delta$T cells, and reduced CD8+PD-1+ exhausted T cells.[50,60] Several studies report improved efficacy of RLT plus PD-1/PD-L1 ICB but preponderance of tolerogenic changes over immune effector exhaustion can render this combination not superior to either monotherapy.[50,51,61] Adding CTLA-4 blockade and/or direct or indirect STING activation to RLT might prove beneficial in these cases.[49–51,59,62] In addition, the relative timing of RLT and immunotherapy may determine therapeutic responses as concurrent RLT and PD-L1 ICB administration in mice with colon cancer outperformed a regimen in which ICB was initiated 11 days after RLT.[46] Contrarily, pre-, peri-, or post-RLT treatment with CTLA-4 ICB did not impact the outcome in a melanoma model.[50] More preclinical and clinical studies exploring the relative timing of RLT and specific immunotherapies are warranted.

Lastly, subcellular localization of radiation (damage) might be important, especially in the context of alpha-particle and Auger electron emitters with short ranges and a potentially heterogeneous distribution within a cell. For instance, radiation targeted to the radiosensitive cell membrane can impact lipid raft-dependent signaling, leading, among others, to nuclear factor kappa B activation, oxidative stress, and increased intracellular calcium levels that can influence mitochondrial ATP synthesis, and thus, to bystander effects and modulation of the TME.[63–65]

Summarizing, several, mostly preclinical studies indicate the ability of RLT to activate antitumor immune responses and to facilitate responses to immunotherapies, even in immunologically "cold" tumor entities. RLT might rely less on abscopal effects for launching successful systemic antitumor immune responses than radiotherapy.[66] Even then, by targeting multiple deposits simultaneously, a broader spectrum of potential metastatic subclones may enhance the likelihood of abscopal effects. However, important gaps in knowledge that need to be addressed to fully leverage RLT-induced immune-modulation include (i) the spatiotemporal dynamics of immune-modulation, (ii) the interdependencies between lymphoid and myeloid populations in the response to RLT, (iii) the interplay of immune-activating versus -suppressing processes in immune-, tumor- and stroma (CAF) cells, (iv) a requirement for eliciting immunogenic cell death versus sufficiency of DNA damage induction for launching antitumor immunity (v) the impact of physical properties of RLT (eg, tumor dose, retention time, linear energy transfer, range in tissue), and tumor immunophenotype,[67] degree of dissemination, and anatomical location on the immunological outcome, and (vi) the degree to which we can extend knowledge on radiotherapy to RLT. Addressing these knowledge gaps will be essential to inform clinical evaluation of RLT/immunotherapy combination regimens.

RADIATION RESPONSES OF CANCER-ASSOCIATED FIBROBLASTS AND THEIR POTENTIAL UTILIZATION IN COMBINATION THERAPY

FAP-radioligands deliver radiation directly to FAP+ CAF and may profoundly alter CAF biology. However, the impact of radioligands on CAF has not been investigated yet. Several studies analyzed the cross-talk between CAF and tumor cells under external beam radiotherapy. This has been reviewed in detail elsewhere[68–70] but the major findings will be briefly summarized here.

As in tumor cells, ionizing radiation induces DNA damage and cell cycle arrest in CAF but this usually does not result in cell death, potentially due to defective TP53/p21 signaling that limits apoptosis, and high survivin expression in CAF.[71] However, it might also not be the goal to eliminate CAF with radioligands. Although some studies found that elimination of (FAP+) CAF reduced tumor growth and increased immunogenicity,[72–74] other studies observed enhanced invasion in mouse models of pancreatic cancer when CAF were depleted and increased immunosuppression leading to poorer outcomes in pancreatic cancer patients with a lower CAF content.[75,76]

In agreement with this discrepancy, data on the functional outcome of exposing CAF to ionizing radiation are heterogeneous. Several studies reported that radiation enhanced tumor-promoting functions of CAF, including (i) upregulation of DDR in tumor cells leading to increased radioresistance and survival[77]; (ii) elevated metabolic activity of tumors, thereby (further) rising glutamine and glucose consumption[78]; and (iii) induction of a senescence-associated secretory phenotype in CAF that promotes secretion and/or expression of cytokines (eg, CXCL1, CXCL12, interleukin 6), growth factors (eg, transforming growth factor beta [TGF-β]), ECM factors (eg, matrix metalloproteases, integrins, collagens) and cargo-loaded exosomes that collectively can facilitate cancer cell proliferation, migration/invasion, resistance to therapies, neoangiogenesis, fibrosis, and increased immunosuppression.[79–84] Induction of senescence might depend on radiation dose as a low dose was found to transiently increase DDR, whereas a high dose triggered constitutive DDR and thereby, senescence.[85] A recent report suggests that it might be feasible to exploit senescence in CAF; a cell-penetrating peptide that disrupts the interaction of FOXO4, a protein specifically upregulated in the nucleus of senescent cells, with TP53 was shown to specifically induce apoptosis of senescent CAF and radiosensitize lung tumors in mice.[86]

In contrast, other studies either did not observe significant changes in most protumorigenic and immunosuppressive functions of CAF after radiation, or found a reversal of tumor-promoting activities[87–91]—which could be an important aspect for RLT.

In summary, the current consensus is that CAF are likely to survive radiation exposure. The functional consequences of exposure are not well defined and discrepancies between studies might be explained by the use of different radiation doses, administration schedules (single dose vs fractionation), and in vivo and in vitro experimental models, and lack of discrimination between CAF subpopulations. Responses of CAF to radioligands may differ from those to radiotherapy as the former deliver a lower dose rate, different quality of radiation, and can continuously irradiate tumors for hours to days. Techniques for spatiotemporal tracking of interactions and changes in tumor tissue, including lineage shifts and evolutionary trajectories, may allow for a systematic analysis of RLT-induced responses in CAF and thus, for identification of rationale (FAP-)RLT combinations.

CO-TARGETING THE TUMOR MICROENVIRONMENT

Although gaps in knowledge on RLT-induced alterations in CAF prevent specific exploitation of these CAF responses, it is possible and attractive to co-target CAF in cancer therapy. CAF can constitute over 90% of the stroma, are the central mediators of the desmoplastic reaction in tumors and communicate with tumor and immune cells. CAF can thus impact tumor differentiation state, progression and invasiveness, immune cell infiltration, and function, oxygenation, and drug delivery, among other biological effects.[92,93]

As described above, depletion of CAF from the TME has been explored but with mixed results. Modulating CAF function might be more promising. The outcome of CAF-signaling may be pro- or antitumorigenic, and immunosuppressive or -supportive, depending on the balance of tumor-promoting versus -restraining CAF subpopulations present in the TME (eg, myCAF, inflammatory CAF, and antigen-presenting CAF[92,94]). This balance might itself be a product of the interplay between tumor cells, immune cells, and CAF. When attempting to therapeutically address CAF it is, therefore, imperative to understand tumor tissue composition and interdependencies of its components, and to specifically target tumor-supportive subpopulations and functions. MyCAF often are the dominant CAF subtype in cancer and localized in the vicinity of tumor cells.[95–97] MyCAF are involved in ECM organization, collagen deposition, and contractility. Their characteristics include high expression levels of collagens, alpha-smooth muscle actin, FAP (although FAP may not be restricted to myCAF[95]), ECM-modifying factors (eg, matrix metalloproteases), genes mediating tumor survival and metastasis, and TGF-β signaling.[95,97,98] TGF-β neutralization diminished myCAF, reduced fibrosis, and opened the TME niche for the emergence of an immunosupportive CAF population termed IFN-licensed CAF. IFN-licensed CAF seem to be involved in antigen-processing and presentation. As a consequence, activated effector T cells were recruited to previously immune-excluded tumors, and response to treatment with PD-1 ICB was facilitated.[95,97,98] Toxicity associated with TGF-β/R inhibitors can be challenging for clinical application.[99] Interference of adenosine signaling using adenosine receptor inhibitors may be a promising alternative option. Adenosine is a potent immunosuppressive and tumorigenic metabolite; it regulates and is regulated by TGF-β, and is additionally produced from ATP released by dying cells, for instance by tumor cells following RLT.[100] CXCL12 (SDF-1) and interleukin 6 are further cytokines produced by CAF that signal through CXCR4 and JAK/STAT3, respectively. Interfering with CXCL12 (eg, plerixafor) or interleukin 6 (eg, siltuximab, tocilizumab) signals might reverse CAF-induced tumor growth, treatment resistance, and immunosuppression, normalize tumor vasculature, and (radiotherapy-induced) invasion.[80,101–103]

In addition, normalization of the TME has been explored pre-clinically using agents like all-*trans*-retinoic acid, Minnelide, and vitamin D receptor agonists. These treatments have been shown to reprogram CAF from an active to a quiescent state associated with loss of protumorigenic signaling, fibrotic activity, and immunosuppression, as well as normalization of vasculature and improved drug delivery.[104–107]

To summarize, the TME is very complex as it includes multiple interacting, interdependent, and variable cellular and acellular components. Knowledge of this ecosystem and how to target its effectors is only beginning to emerge. Though fibroblasts are essential and abundant in the TME, the impact of radioligands on CAF and the TME has to be systematically investigated before RLT-specific combination therapy will be feasible.

DISCUSSION AND CONCLUSION

The possibility to specifically target FAP-expressing cells using radioligands is an attractive therapeutic option because (i) almost all tumors have a stromal component and FAP$^+$ CAF in the stroma have been associated with diverse pro-tumor and immunosuppressive functions; (ii) diagnostic FAP-radioligands allow imaging-based selection of patients with FAP$^+$ tumor lesions for subsequent FAP-RLT; and (iii) therapeutic FAP-radioligands may act through multiple mechanisms, as they can directly and indirectly (crossfire, bystander) irradiate tumor cells, CAF and other TME components. First clinical data suggest that FAP-targeted radioligands may produce beneficial therapeutic effects in patients with FAP$^+$ tumor cells and/or FAP$^+$ CAF. However, efficacy of FAP-radioligands has been rather moderate so far, rendering improvement of FAP theranostics imperative. One option for improving outcomes after FAP-RLT is the combination with other therapeutics. This, however, requires a detailed understanding of the interaction of FAP-radioligands with the tumor tissue.

In a first step, this may include investigating which radiotherapeutic strategy could be optimal in a given setting, for instance, which type of radioligand and radioisotope would best be suited. Second, the impact of FAP-radioligands on CAF, tumor cells, and immune cells needs to be elucidated on a molecular and cellular level. This could be especially relevant when only FAP$^+$ CAF (and not FAP$^+$ tumor cells) are being targeted. CAF are generally radioresistant and RLT might not induce CAF death. Controversial results have been reported as to whether ionizing radiation renders CAF even more tumor-supportive, for instance through eliciting bystander effects in tumor cells, or reprograms them to tumorsuppressive phenotypes. Along those lines, different CAF subpopulations with different phenotypes and functionalities have been identified.[92,94]

Radioligands may or may not alter the balance of these tumorsupportive and tumorsuppressive subpopulations and/or induce plasticity, and might affect the subpopulations in different ways and at different times after RLT. Anatomical location and spatial organization of the tumor is likely to be important. If CAF are interspersed with tumor cells or located around tumor cell clusters, as, for example, in pancreatic cancer,[95] it might be possible to exploit crossfire-effects; this might not be feasible in tumors in which (FAP$^+$) CAF are more distant to tumor cells, especially for alpha particle therapies with limited tissue penetration. Importantly, sub-TMEs coexisting in a tumor have been identified that differ in composition and functionality and thus, introduce another level of complexity and heterogeneity.[108]

Summarizing, we are beginning to gain experience in targeting the TME with radioligands. To exploit the full potential of (TME-targeted) radioligands we will have to understand the impact a specific radioligand has on tumor tissue. It is conceivable that when attempting to enhance RLT through combination therapies similar considerations apply to tumor cell- and TME-targeted approaches. All factors in the tumor tissue act in a concerted manner, so that targeting one aspect of the tumor tissue leads to a change in most others. Optimal RLT and RLT combination approaches facilitating deep and durable responses can only successfully be developed if we adopt a more holistic view of cancer that (i) shifts the focus from tumor cells to the intricate codependencies of the tumor ecosystem and (ii) considers the specific characteristics of the theranostic agents.

DISCLOSURE

K. Lückerath is a consultant to Sofie Biosciences.

REFERENCES

1. Garin-Chesa P, Old LJ, Rettig WJ. Cell surface glycoprotein of reactive stromal fibroblasts as a potential antibody target in human epithelial cancers. Proc Natl Acad Sci U S A 1990;87(18):7235–9.
2. The human protein atlas: FAP pathology. Available at: https://www.proteinatlas.org/ENSG00000078098-FAP/pathology. Accessed September 12, 2022.
3. Kratochwil C, Flechsig P, Lindner T, et al. FAPI-PET/CT: mean intensity of tracer-uptake (SUV) in 28 different kinds of cancer. J Nucl Med 2019. https://doi.org/10.2967/jnumed.119.227967.
4. Treglia G, Muoio B, Roustaei H, et al. Head-to-Head comparison of fibroblast activation protein inhibitors (FAPI) radiotracers versus [^{18}F]-FDG in Oncology: A Systematic Review. Int J Mol Sci

2021;22(20). https://doi.org/10.3390/ijms222011192.

5. Roustaei H, Kiamanesh Z, Askari E, et al. Could fibroblast activation protein (FAP)-Specific radioligands Be considered as pan-tumor agents? Contrast Media Mol Imaging 2022;2022:3948873.

6. Sollini M, Kirienko M, Gelardi F, et al. State-of-the-art of FAPI-PET imaging: a systematic review and meta-analysis. Eur J Nucl Med Mol Imaging 2021; 48(13):4396–414.

7. Fendler WP, Pabst KM, Kessler L, et al. Safety and efficacy of 90Y-FAPI-46 radioligand therapy in patients with advanced sarcoma and other cancer entities. Clin Cancer Res 2022. https://doi.org/10.1158/1078-0432.CCR-22-1432.

8. Ferdinandus J, Costa PF, Kessler L, et al. Initial clinical experience with 90Y-FAPI-46 Radioligand Therapy for Advanced-Stage Solid Tumors: A Case Series of 9 Patients. J Nucl Med 2022;63(5): 727–34.

9. Assadi M, Rekabpour SJ, Jafari E, et al. Feasibility and therapeutic potential of 177Lu-fibroblast activation protein inhibitor-46 for patients with relapsed or refractory cancers: a preliminary study. Clin Nucl Med 2021;46(11):e523–30.

10. Baum RP, Schuchardt C, Singh A, et al. Feasibility, biodistribution, and preliminary dosimetry in peptide-targeted radionuclide therapy of diverse adenocarcinomas using 177Lu-FAP-2286: First-in-Humans Results. J Nucl Med 2022;63(3):415–23.

11. Sartor O, de Bono J, Chi KN, et al. Lutetium-177-PSMA-617 for metastatic castration-resistant prostate cancer. N Engl J Med 2021. https://doi.org/10.1056/NEJMoa2107322.

12. Strosberg J, El-Haddad G, Wolin E, et al. Phase 3 trial of 177Lu-dotatate for midgut neuroendocrine tumors. N Engl J Med 2017;376(2):125–35.

13. Current K, Meyer C, Magyar CE, et al. Investigating PSMA-targeted radioligand therapy efficacy as a function of cellular PSMA levels and intra-tumoral PSMA heterogeneity. Clin Cancer Res 2020. https://doi.org/10.1158/1078-0432.CCR-19-1485.

14. Feijtel D, Doeswijk GN, Verkaik NS, et al. Inter and intra-tumor somatostatin receptor 2 heterogeneity influences peptide receptor radionuclide therapy response. Theranostics 2021;11(2):491–505.

15. Mavragani IV, Nikitaki Z, Souli MP, et al. Complex DNA damage: a route to radiation-induced genomic instability and carcinogenesis. Cancers 2017;9(7). https://doi.org/10.3390/cancers9070091.

16. Ruigrok EAM, Tamborino G, de Blois E, et al. In vitro dose effect relationships of actinium-225- and lutetium-177-labeled PSMA-I&T. Eur J Nucl Med Mol Imaging 2022;49(11):3627–38.

17. Idrissou MB, Pichard A, Tee B, et al. Targeted radionuclide therapy using auger electron emitters: the quest for the right vector and the right radionuclide. Pharmaceutics 2021;13(7). https://doi.org/10.3390/pharmaceutics13070980.

18. Pilié PG, Tang C, Mills GB, et al. State-of-the-art strategies for targeting the DNA damage response in cancer. Nat Rev Clin Oncol 2019;16(2):81–104.

19. Stuparu AD, Capri JR, Meyer CAL, et al. Mechanisms of resistance to prostate-specific membrane antigen-targeted radioligand therapy in a mouse model of prostate cancer. J Nucl Med 2021;62(7): 989–95.

20. Purohit NK, Shah RG, Adant S, et al. Potentiation of 177Lu-octreotate peptide receptor radionuclide therapy of human neuroendocrine tumor cells by PARP inhibitor. Oncotarget 2018;9(37):24693–706.

21. Wengner AM, Siemeister G, Lücking U, et al. The novel ATR inhibitor BAY 1895344 is efficacious as monotherapy and combined with DNA damage-inducing or repair-compromising therapies in preclinical cancer models. Mol Cancer Ther 2020; 19(1):26–38.

22. Mateo J, Porta N, Bianchini D, et al. Olaparib in patients with metastatic castration-resistant prostate cancer with DNA repair gene aberrations (TOPARP-B): a multicentre, open-label, randomised, phase 2 trial. Lancet Oncol 2020; 21(1):162–74.

23. Reinhardt HC, Aslanian AS, Lees JA, et al. p53-deficient cells rely on ATM- and ATR-mediated checkpoint signaling through the p38MAPK/MK2 pathway for survival after DNA damage. Cancer Cell 2007;11(2):175–89.

24. van der Doelen MJ, Isaacsson Velho P, Slootbeek PHJ, et al. Impact of DNA damage repair defects on response to radium-223 and overall survival in metastatic castration-resistant prostate cancer. Eur J Cancer 2020;136:16–24.

25. Wickstroem K, Karlsson J, Ellingsen C, et al. Synergistic effect of a HER2 targeted thorium-227 conjugate in combination with olaparib in a BRCA2 deficient xenograft model. Pharmaceuticals 2019; 12(4). https://doi.org/10.3390/ph12040155.

26. Wickstroem K, Hagemann UB, Cruciani V, et al. Synergistic effect of a Mesothelin-Targeted 227Th Conjugate in Combination with DNA Damage Response Inhibitors in Ovarian Cancer Xenograft Models. J Nucl Med 2019;60(9):1293–300.

27. Cullinane C, Waldeck K, Kirby L, et al. Enhancing the anti-tumour activity of 177 Lu-DOTA-octreotate radionuclide therapy in somatostatin receptor-2 expressing tumour models by targeting PARP. Sci Rep 2020;10(1):10196.

28. Patel R, Barker HE, Kyula J, et al. An orally bioavailable Chk1 inhibitor, CCT244747, sensitizes bladder and head and neck cancer cell lines to radiation. Radiother Oncol 2017;122(3):470–5.

29. Zhou ZR, Yang ZZ, Wang SJ, et al. The Chk1 inhibitor MK-8776 increases the radiosensitivity of

human triple-negative breast cancer by inhibiting autophagy. Acta Pharmacol Sin 2017;38(4):513–23.

30. Cuneo KC, Morgan MA, Davis MA, et al. Wee1 kinase inhibitor AZD1775 radiosensitizes hepatocellular carcinoma regardless of TP53 mutational status through induction of replication stress. Int J Radiat Oncol Biol Phys 2016;95(2):782–90.

31. Domogauer JD, de Toledo SM, Howell RW, et al. Acquired radioresistance in cancer associated fibroblasts is concomitant with enhanced antioxidant potential and DNA repair capacity. Cell Commun Signal 2021;19(1):30.

32. Ballal S, Yadav MP, Damle NA, et al. Concomitant 177Lu-dotatate and capecitabine therapy in patients with advanced neuroendocrine tumors: a long-term-outcome, toxicity, survival, and quality-of-life study. Clin Nucl Med 2017;42(11):e457–66.

33. Cáceres-Gutiérrez RE, Alfaro-Mora Y, Andonegui MA, et al. The influence of oncogenic RAS on chemotherapy and radiotherapy resistance through DNA repair pathways. Front Cell Dev Biol 2022;10:751367.

34. Toulany M, Rodemann HP. Phosphatidylinositol 3-kinase/Akt signaling as a key mediator of tumor cell responsiveness to radiation. Semin Cancer Biol 2015;35:180–90.

35. Maier P, Hartmann L, Wenz F, et al. Cellular pathways in response to ionizing radiation and their targetability for tumor radiosensitization. Int J Mol Sci 2016;17(1). https://doi.org/10.3390/ijms17010102.

36. Polkinghorn WR, Parker JS, Lee MX, et al. Androgen receptor signaling regulates DNA repair in prostate cancers. Cancer Discov 2013;3(11):1245–53.

37. Lundsten S, Spiegelberg D, Raval NR, et al. The radiosensitizer Onalespib increases complete remission in 177Lu-DOTATATE-treated mice bearing neuroendocrine tumor xenografts. Eur J Nucl Med Mol Imaging 2020;47(4):980–90.

38. Golden EB, Formenti SC, Schiff PB. Taxanes as radiosensitizers. Anti Cancer Drugs 2014;25(5):502–11.

39. Yordanova A, Ahrens H, Feldmann G, et al. Peptide receptor radionuclide therapy combined with chemotherapy in patients with neuroendocrine tumors. Clin Nucl Med 2019;44(5):e329–35.

40. Tao Y, Zhang P, Girdler F, et al. Enhancement of radiation response in p53-deficient cancer cells by the Aurora-B kinase inhibitor AZD1152. Oncogene 2008;27(23):3244–55.

41. Yao M, Rogers L, Suchowerska N, et al. Sensitization of prostate cancer to radiation therapy: molecules and pathways to target. Radiother Oncol 2018;128(2):283–300.

42. Vendetti FP, Karukonda P, Clump DA, et al. ATR kinase inhibitor AZD6738 potentiates CD8+ T cell-dependent antitumor activity following radiation. J Clin Invest 2018;128(9):3926–40.

43. McGrail DJ, Pilié PG, Dai H, et al. Replication stress response defects are associated with response to immune checkpoint blockade in nonhypermutated cancers. Sci Transl Med 2021;13(617):eabe6201.

44. Ceccaldi R, Rondinelli B, D'Andrea AD. Repair pathway choices and consequences at the double-strand break. Trends Cell Biol 2016;26(1):52–64.

45. Wu Y, Pfeifer AK, Myschetzky R, et al. Induction of anti-tumor immune responses by peptide receptor radionuclide therapy with (177)Lu-dotatate in a murine model of a human neuroendocrine tumor. Diagnostics 2013;3(4):344–55.

46. Chen H, Zhao L, Fu K, et al. Integrin αvb3-targeted radionuclide therapy combined with immune checkpoint blockade immunotherapy synergistically enhances anti-tumor efficacy. Theranostics 2019;9(25):7948–60.

47. Choi J, Beaino W, Fecek RJ, et al. Combined VLA-4-targeted radionuclide therapy and immunotherapy in a mouse model of melanoma. J Nucl Med 2018;59(12):1843–9.

48. Czernin J, Current K, Mona CE, et al. Immune-checkpoint blockade enhances 225Ac-PSMA617 efficacy in a mouse model of prostate cancer. J Nucl Med 2020. https://doi.org/10.2967/jnumed.120.246041.

49. Vito A, Rathmann S, Mercanti N, et al. Combined radionuclide therapy and immunotherapy for treatment of triple negative breast cancer. Int J Mol Sci 2021;22(9). https://doi.org/10.3390/ijms22094843.

50. Patel RB, Hernandez R, Carlson P, et al. Low-dose targeted radionuclide therapy renders immunologically cold tumors responsive to immune checkpoint blockade. Sci Transl Med 2021;13(602). https://doi.org/10.1126/scitranslmed.abb3631.

51. Rouanet J, Benboubker V, Akil H, et al. Immune checkpoint inhibitors reverse tolerogenic mechanisms induced by melanoma targeted radionuclide therapy. Cancer Immunol Immunother 2020;69(10):2075–88.

52. Guzik P, Siwowska K, Fang HY, et al. Promising potential of [177Lu]Lu-DOTA-folate to enhance tumor response to immunotherapy-a preclinical study using a syngeneic breast cancer model. Eur J Nucl Med Mol Imaging 2021;48(4):984–94.

53. Jagodinsky JC, Jin WJ, Bates AM, et al. Temporal analysis of type 1 interferon activation in tumor cells following external beam radiotherapy or targeted radionuclide therapy. Theranostics 2021;11(13):6120–37.

54. Lin AL, Tabar V, Young RJ, et al. Synergism of checkpoint inhibitors and peptide receptor radionuclide therapy in the treatment of pituitary carcinoma. J Endocr Soc 2021;5(10):bvab133.

55. Ferdinandus J, Fendler WP, Lueckerath K, et al. Response to combined peptide receptor radionu-clide therapy and checkpoint immunotherapy with ipilimumab plus nivolumab in metastatic merkel cell carcinoma. J Nucl Med 2022;63(3):396–8.

56. Hernandez R, Walker KL, Grudzinski JJ, et al. Y-NM600 targeted radionuclide therapy induces immunologic memory in syngeneic models of T-cell Non-Hodgkin's Lymphoma. Commun Biol 2019;2:79.

57. Li J, Duran MA, Dhanota N, et al. Metastasis and immune evasion from extracellular cGAMP hydroly-sis. Cancer Discov 2021;11(5):1212–27.

58. Ruiz-Fernández de Córdoba B, Moreno H, Valencia K, et al. Tumor ENPP1 (CD203a)/Haptoglobin Axis ex-ploits myeloid-derived suppressor cells to promote post-radiotherapy local recurrence in breast cancer. Cancer Discov 2022;12(5):1356–77.

59. Amouzegar A, Chelvanambi M, Filderman JN, et al. STING agonists as cancer therapeutics. Cancers 2021;13(11). https://doi.org/10.3390/cancers13112695.

60. Clark PA, Sriramaneni RN, Bates AM, et al. Low-dose radiation potentiates the propagation of anti-tumor immunity against melanoma tumor in the brain after in situ vaccination at a tumor outside the brain. Radiat Res 2021;195(6):522–40.

61. Bolli E, D'Huyvetter M, Murgaski A, et al. Stromal-targeting radioimmunotherapy mitigates the pro-gression of therapy-resistant tumors. J Control Release 2019;314:1–11.

62. Onyedibe KI, Wang M, Sintim HO. ENPP1, an old enzyme with new functions, and small molecule inhibitors-A STING in the tale of ENPP1. Molecules 2019;24(22). https://doi.org/10.3390/molecules24224192.

63. Paillas S, Ladjohounlou R, Lozza C, et al. Localized irradiation of cell membrane by auger electrons is cytotoxic through oxidative stress-mediated non-targeted effects. Antioxid Redox Signal 2016; 25(8):467–84.

64. Pouget JP, Constanzo J. Revisiting the radiobiology of targeted alpha therapy. Front Med 2021;8: 692436.

65. Pouget JP, Santoro L, Piron B, et al. From the target cell theory to a more integrated view of radiobi-ology in Targeted radionuclide therapy: the Mont-pellier group's experience. Nucl Med Biol 2022; 104-105:53–64.

66. Dudzinski SO, Cameron BD, Wang J, et al. Combi-nation immunotherapy and radiotherapy causes an abscopal treatment response in a mouse model of castration resistant prostate cancer. J Immunother Cancer 2019;7(1):218.

67. Hegde PS, Chen DS. Top 10 challenges in cancer immunotherapy. Immunity 2020;52(1):17–35.

68. Wang Z, Tang Y, Tan Y, et al. Cancer-associated fi-broblasts in radiotherapy: challenges and new op-portunities. Cell Commun Signal 2019;17(1):47.

69. Ansems M, Span PN. The tumor microenvironment and radiotherapy response; a central role for cancer-associated fibroblasts. Clin Transl Radiat Oncol 2020;22:90–7.

70. Ragunathan K, Upfold NLE, Oksenych V. Interac-tion between fibroblasts and immune cells following DNA damage induced by ionizing radia-tion. Int J Mol Sci 2020;21(22). https://doi.org/10.3390/ijms21228635.

71. Hawsawi NM, Ghebeh H, Hendrayani SF, et al. Breast carcinoma-associated fibroblasts and their counterparts display neoplastic-specific changes. Cancer Res 2008;68(8):2717–25.

72. Feig C, Jones JO, Kraman M, et al. Targeting CXCL12 from FAP-expressing carcinoma-associ-ated fibroblasts synergizes with anti-PD-L1 immu-notherapy in pancreatic cancer. Proc Natl Acad Sci U S A 2013;110(50):20212–7.

73. Lo A, Wang LS, Scholler J, et al. Tumor-promoting desmoplasia is disrupted by depleting FAP-expressing stromal cells. Cancer Res 2015; 75(14):2800–10.

74. Lo A, Li CP, Buza EL, et al. Fibroblast activation protein augments progression and metastasis of pancreatic ductal adenocarcinoma. JCI Insight 2017;2(19). https://doi.org/10.1172/jci.insight.92232.

75. Özdemir BC, Pentcheva-Hoang T, Carstens JL, et al. Depletion of carcinoma-associated fibro-blasts and fibrosis induces immunosuppression and accelerates pancreas cancer with reduced survival. Cancer Cell 2014;25(6):719–34.

76. Rhim AD, Oberstein PE, Thomas DH, et al. Stromal elements act to restrain, rather than support, pancreatic ductal adenocarcinoma. Cancer Cell 2014;25(6):735–47.

77. Wang Y, Gan G, Wang B, et al. Cancer-associated fibroblasts promote irradiated cancer cell recovery through autophagy. EBioMedicine 2017;17:45–56.

78. Tommelein J, De Vlieghere E, Verset L, et al. Radio-therapy-activated cancer-associated fibroblasts promote tumor progression through paracrine IGF1R activation. Cancer Res 2018;78(3):659–70.

79. Zhang H, Yue J, Jiang Z, et al. CAF-secreted CXCL1 conferred radioresistance by regulating DNA damage response in a ROS-dependent manner in esophageal squamous cell carcinoma. Cell Death Dis 2017;8(5):e2790.

80. Li D, Qu C, Ning Z, et al. Radiation promotes epithelial-to-mesenchymal transition and invasion of pancreatic cancer cell by activating carcinoma-associated fibroblasts. Am J Cancer Res 2016;6(10):2192–206.

81. Boelens MC, Wu TJ, Nabet BY, et al. Exosome transfer from stromal to breast cancer cells regu-lates therapy resistance pathways. Cell 2014; 159(3):499–513.

82. Puthawala K, Hadjiangelis N, Jacoby SC, et al. Inhibition of integrin alpha(v)beta6, an activator of latent transforming growth factor-beta, prevents radiation-induced lung fibrosis. Am J Respir Crit Care Med 2008;177(1):82–90.

83. Kamochi N, Nakashima M, Aoki S, et al. Irradiated fibroblast-induced bystander effects on invasive growth of squamous cell carcinoma under cancer-stromal cell interaction. Cancer Sci 2008; 99(12):2417–27.

84. Weichselbaum RR, Ishwaran H, Yoon T, et al. An interferon-related gene signature for DNA damage resistance is a predictive marker for chemotherapy and radiation for breast cancer. Proc Natl Acad Sci U S A 2008;105(47):18490–5.

85. Rodier F, Coppé JP, Patil CK, et al. Persistent DNA damage signalling triggers senescence-associated inflammatory cytokine secretion. Nat Cell Biol. Aug 2009;11(8):973–9.

86. Meng J, Li Y, Wan C, et al. Targeting senescence-like fibroblasts radiosensitizes non-small cell lung cancer and reduces radiation-induced pulmonary fibrosis. JCI Insight 2021;6(23). https://doi.org/10.1172/jci.insight.146334.

87. Hellevik T, Pettersen I, Berg V, et al. Cancer-associated fibroblasts from human NSCLC survive ablative doses of radiation but their invasive capacity is reduced. Radiat Oncol 2012;7:59.

88. Hellevik T, Pettersen I, Berg V, et al. Changes in the secretory profile of NSCLC-associated fibroblasts after ablative radiotherapy: potential impact on angiogenesis and tumor growth. Transl Oncol 2013;6(1):66–74.

89. Grinde MT, Vik J, Camilio KA, et al. Ionizing radiation abrogates the pro-tumorigenic capacity of cancer-associated fibroblasts co-implanted in xenografts. Sci Rep 2017;25(7):46714.

90. Berzaghi R, Tornaas S, Lode K, et al. Ionizing radiation curtails immunosuppressive effects from cancer-associated fibroblasts on dendritic cells. Front Immunol 2021;12:662594.

91. Arshad A, Deutsch E, Vozenin MC. Simultaneous irradiation of fibroblasts and carcinoma cells repress the secretion of soluble factors able to stimulate carcinoma cell migration. PLoS One 2015;10(1):e0115447.

92. Biffi G, Tuveson DA. Diversity and biology of cancer-associated fibroblasts. Physiol Rev 2021; 101(1):147–76.

93. Geng X, Chen H, Zhao L, et al. Cancer-associated fibroblast (CAF) heterogeneity and targeting therapy of CAFs in pancreatic cancer. Front Cell Dev Biol 2021;9:655152.

94. Peltier A, Seban RD, Buvat I, et al. Fibroblast heterogeneity in solid tumors: from single cell analysis to whole-body imaging. Semin Cancer Biol 2022. https://doi.org/10.1016/j.semcancer.2022.04.008.

95. Dominguez CX, Müller S, Keerthivasan S, et al. Single-cell RNA sequencing reveals stromal evolution into LRRC15(+) myofibroblasts as a determinant of patient response to cancer immunotherapy. Cancer Discov 2020;10(2):232–53.

96. Buechler MB, Pradhan RN, Krishnamurty AT, et al. Cross-tissue organization of the fibroblast lineage. Nature 2021;593(7860):575–9.

97. Grauel AL, Nguyen B, Ruddy D, et al. TGFβ-blockade uncovers stromal plasticity in tumors by revealing the existence of a subset of interferon-licensed fibroblasts. Nat Commun 2020;11(1): 6315.

98. Kieffer Y, Hocine HR, Gentric G, et al. Single-cell analysis reveals fibroblast clusters linked to immunotherapy resistance in cancer. Cancer Discov 2020;10(9):1330–51.

99. de Streel G, Lucas S. Targeting immunosuppression by TGF-β1 for cancer immunotherapy. Biochem Pharmacol 2021;192:114697.

100. Kepp O, Bezu L, Yamazaki T, et al. ATP and cancer immunosurveillance. EMBO J 2021;40(13): e108130.

101. Johnson DE, O'Keefe RA, Grandis JR. Targeting the IL-6/JAK/STAT3 signalling axis in cancer. Nat Rev Clin Oncol 2018;15(4):234–48.

102. Chen Y, Zhang F, Tsai Y, et al. IL-6 signaling promotes DNA repair and prevents apoptosis in CD133+ stem-like cells of lung cancer after radiation. Radiat Oncol 2015;10:227.

103. Matsuoka Y, Nakayama H, Yoshida R, et al. IL-6 controls resistance to radiation by suppressing oxidative stress via the Nrf2-antioxidant pathway in oral squamous cell carcinoma. Br J Cancer 2016;115(10):1234–44.

104. Froeling FE, Feig C, Chelala C, et al. Retinoic acid-induced pancreatic stellate cell quiescence reduces paracrine Wnt-β-catenin signaling to slow tumor progression. Gastroenterology 2011;141(4): 1486–97.

105. Banerjee S, Modi S, McGinn O, et al. Impaired synthesis of stromal components in response to minnelide improves vascular function, drug delivery, and survival in pancreatic cancer. Clin Cancer Res 2016;22(2):415–25.

106. Dauer P, Zhao X, Gupta VK, et al. Inactivation of cancer-associated-fibroblasts disrupts oncogenic signaling in pancreatic cancer cells and promotes its regression. Cancer Res 2018;78(5):1321–33.

107. Sherman MH, Yu RT, Engle DD, et al. Vitamin D receptor-mediated stromal reprogramming suppresses pancreatitis and enhances pancreatic cancer therapy. Cell 2014;159(1):80–93.

108. Grünwald BT, Devisme A, Andrieux G, et al. Spatially confined sub-tumor microenvironments in pancreatic cancer. Cell 2021;184(22):5577–92. e18.

Fibroblast Activation Protein Inhibitor Theranostics: Early Clinical Translation

Yuriko Mori, MD[a],*, Clemens Kratochwil, MD[b], Uwe Haberkorn, MD[b],
Frederik L. Giesel, MD, MBA[a,b]

KEYWORDS

- Clinical translation • Fibroblast • FAPI • Radioligand therapy • Theranostic

KEY POINTS

- Fibroblast activation protein (FAP)-targeted radioligand therapy (RLT) is a novel oncological strategy, generally targeting tumor stroma.
- FAPI-04 and FAPI-46 are currently the most widely used compounds in the FAP-targeting theranostics.
- New innovative tracers such as FAPI-34 with the potential of SPECT-based diagnostic and therapy via Tc-99m/Re-188 as well as peptides and small molecules with ultra-high affinity to FAP have recently been introduced and are currently under validation.

OVERVIEW

Fibroblast activation protein (FAP)-targeted radioligand therapy (RLT) offers the possibility of a novel cancer therapeutic strategy, by generally targeting tumor stroma.[1] Early clinical translation of FAP-tracers occurred as early as in the 1990s using antibodies but did not progress beyond the clinical phase II trial. The essential step toward a theranostic approach, which conceptually combines diagnostic and therapeutic emitters to a specific tracer, began with the implementation of small-molecule FAP-enzyme inhibitors fibroblast activation protein inhibitor (FAPI) in 2018. Currently, FAPI-04 and FAPI-46, containing 1,4,7,10-tetraaza-cylclododecane-1,4,7,10-tetrayl tetraacetic acid (DOTA)-chelators, with the possibility of radionuclide combination with the radiometals Gallium-68 (Ga-68), Yttrium-90 (Y-90), and Lutetium-177 (Lu-177), are the compounds most widely used in the theranostic regimen. New innovations such as FAPI-34, which has the potential for single photon emission tomography (SPECT)-based diagnostic scanning and therapy using Tc-99m and Re-188, respectively, and other small molecules with ultra-high affinity to FAP are currently under the status of validation. Most proof-of-concept studies have thus far been performed in single institutions, and systematic validation is required.

EARLY THERANOSTIC APPLICATION OF FIBROBLAST ACTIVATION PROTEIN INHIBITOR LIGANDS

The first-in-human application of FAPI ligand was the diagnostic use of Ga-68-FAPI-02 in patients with metastasized breast, lung and pancreatic cancer, as presented by the Heidelberg group.[2] This showed robust accumulation of the tracer in the tumoral lesions with high image contrast. However, this compound was initially not applied in humans with therapeutic intention because preceding experiments with tumor-bearing xenografts showed a relatively short tumor retention time of Lu-177-FAPI-02, limiting practical use. The same group subsequently synthesized 15

[a] Department of Nuclear Medicine, Medical Faculty and University Hospital Duesseldorf, Heinrich-Heine-University Duesseldorf, Moorenstrasse 5, 40225, Duesseldorf, Germany; [b] Department of Nuclear Medicine, Heidelberg University Hospital, Im Neuenheimer Feld 400, 69120 Heidelberg, Germany
* Corresponding author.
E-mail address: yuriko.mori@med.uni-duesseldorf.de

PET Clin 18 (2023) 419–428
https://doi.org/10.1016/j.cpet.2023.02.007
1556-8598/23/© 2023 Elsevier Inc. All rights reserved.

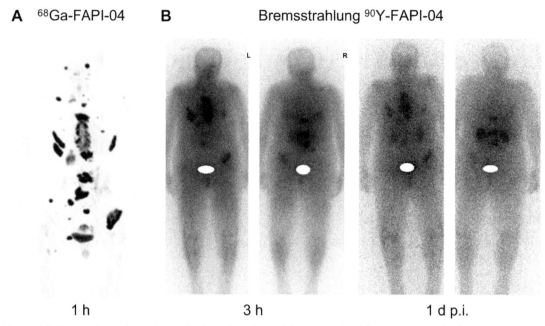

A ⁶⁸Ga-FAPI-04　　**B**　　Bremsstrahlung ⁹⁰Y-FAPI-04

1 h　　　　　　3 h　　　　　　1 d p.i.

Fig. 1. (*A*) PET maximum-intensity projection of patient with metastasized breast cancer 1 h after administration of 270 MBq of ⁶⁸Ga-FAPI-04. Intense uptake is seen in metastases. (*B*) Bremsstrahlung images showing uptake at 3 h and even 1 d after treatment with ⁹⁰Y-FAPI-04 in the same patient. This research was originally published in JNM. Loktev A et al., A Tumor-Imaging Method Targeting Cancer-Associated Fibroblasts. J Nucl Med. 2018;59(9):1423-1429. © SNMMI.

different FAPI tracers. Of those, FAPI-04 was identified as the most suitable compound for the theranostic application due to excellent stability in human serum, high specific binding affinity to FAP and higher cellular retention in vitro.[3] Based on high uptake of Ga-68-FAPI-04-PET/computed tomography (CT) (SUVmax 7 to 15.5 and 15.3 to 29.9, respectively) in two patients with metastasized breast cancer, one of these was selected to undergo a first-in-human administration of 2.9 GBq of Y-90-FAPI-04 (24 nmol/GBq). Despite a rather low administered activity, this treatment led to a significant reduction in pain medication in this patient and was well-tolerated. The bremsstrahlung images showed persistent accumulation of the therapeutic radionuclide at 3 h and 1 d after administration in the tumoral lesions (**Fig. 1**).[3]

FURTHER DEVELOPMENT OF THERANOSTIC TRACER: FAPI-46

Most subsequent reports on FAP theranostics have used FAPI-46 as the theranostic compound. As mentioned, from the 15 different FAPI tracers synthesized in the early phase of tracer development by Lindner and colleagues, FAPI-04 was initially identified as the most suitable potential theranostic tracer. As with its precursor FAPI-02, FAPI-04 showed rapid tracer internalization into

FAP-positive tumoral lesions as well as fast clearance from the blood pool. The intravenous application of the compound resulted in the rapid accumulation of the tumor with a favorable tumor-to-background ratio. Moreover, the effective tumor uptake after 24 h was considerably higher for FAPI-04 than for FAPI-02, which provides a relative advantage for therapeutic application. However, this agent's pharmacokinetics were still probably suboptimal for radionuclide therapy.

To address this issue, Loktev and colleagues[4] developed 11 further FAPI derivatives (FAPI-20 to FAPI-55), for which they evaluated the binding affinity using FAP-expressing HT-1050 cells. Of these compounds, FAPI-46 was identified as the most promising derivative as it displayed considerably longer retention in the FAP-expressing cells than the other compounds. In comparison to the lead compound FAPI-04, FAPI-46 washed out more slowly, retaining other favorable properties in regard to target binding and pharmacokinetic profile. Notably, FAPI-46 showed variable tumor retention depending on the tumor type. In the study of Loktev and colleagues, eight patients with metastasized colorectal, ovarian, oropharyngeal, and pancreatic cancer as well as a patient with carcinoma of unknown primary underwent whole-body PET/CT scans at three different time points (10 min, 1 h, and 3 h) after 216 to 242

MBq of Ga-68-FAPI-46 were administered intravenously. PET imaging revealed that the tumor activity remained relatively constant up to 3 h after injection in colorectal, ovarian, oropharyngeal and pancreatic cancer, but a continuous decrease of tumor activity was observed in breast cancer. Conversely, tumor accumulation in the patient with carcinoma of unknown primary increased from 1 to 3 h after injection. The authors consider as the possible explanation the heterogeneity of FAP distribution and expression in cancer-associated fibroblasts (CAFs), which might result in heterogenous FAP binding in tumor stroma.

RADIOLIGAND THERAPY WITH FAPI-46

Based on these results, FAPI-46 began to be more widely used in the theranostic setting. Unfortunately, currently available clinical reports are heterogeneous, occurring primarily as proof-of-concept studies in the patients with end-stage cancer.[5–11] These are described below.

Assadi and Colleagues (Radiopharmaceutical: Lu-177-FAPI-46)

Of 21 patients with advanced cancers, which were inoperable or refractory to conventional therapies, who were enrolled in this study, 18 were selected for RLT. The tumor entities included ovarian cancer, sarcoma, colon cancer, breast cancer, pancreatic cancer, prostate cancer, cervical cancer, round-cell tumor, lung cancer, anaplastic thyroid cancer, and cholangiocarcinoma[5].

Treatment included escalating doses of Lu-177-FAPI-46 (1.85 to 4.44 GBq; median injected dose 3.7 GBq) per cycle with intervals of 4 to 6 weeks between the cycles. Overall, 36 therapy cycles were administered, with the median number of 2 cycles per patient. Biodistribution and dosimetry were examined by anterior and posterior whole-body planar and limited SPECT scans. The dosimetric analysis revealed median absorbed doses of 0.026, 0.136, 0.886, and 0.02 mGy/MBq with ranges of 0.023 to 0.034, 0.001 to 0.2, 0.076 to 1.39, and 0.002 to 0.2 mGy/MBq for the whole body, liver, kidneys, and spleen, respectively. The therapy was well-tolerated except for one patient who suffered low-grade thrombocytopenia and leukopenia, and an additional case of mild anemia. Overall, the therapy resulted in 12 cases of stable disease and 6 cases of progressive disease.

Ferdinandus and Colleagues (Radiopharmaceutical: Y-90-FAPI-46)

A total of nine patients with metastatic disease from either pancreatic cancer or soft-tissue or bone sarcoma with documented high FAP expression, and who had exhausted all approved therapies based on multidisciplinary tumor board decision, were enrolled in this study.[6] High FAP expression was defined as SUVmax greater than or equal to 10 in more than half of all lesions. Patients received a median of 3.8 GBq (range 3.25 to 5.40 GBq) for the first cycle, and three patients received subsequent cycles with a median of 7.4 GBq (range 7.3 to 7.5 GBq). Overall, 13 therapy cycles were performed, with 1 to 3 cycles for each patient. Post-treatment Y-90-FAPI-46 bremsstrahlung scintigraphy showed persistent Y-90-FAPI-46 uptake in tumor lesions in 7 of 9 patients (78%). The dosimetric analysis using Y-90 PET/CT at several time-points revealed median absorbed doses of 0.52 Gy/GBq in the kidney, 0.04 Gy/GBq in bone marrow, and less than 0.26 Gy/GBq in the lung and liver. Measured tumor lesions showed up to 2.28 Gy/GBq (median, 1.28 Gy/GBq).

Grade 3 or 4 hematological toxicities were noted in four patients (44%, two patients with thrombocytopenia only, two patients with new onset of thrombocytopenia and anemia). Other adverse events reported were of kidney (G1 to G2 in three patients), liver (G1 to G4 in five patients), and pancreatobiliary system (G1 to G4 in three patients). Overall, the therapy resulted in four cases of stable disease and four cases of progressive disease.

Lindner and Colleagues (Radiopharmaceutical: Y-90-FAPI-46)

In assessing the diagnostic utility of Tc-99m FAPI-34, the authors reported post-treatment imaging of two cases who had RLT with Y-90-FAPI-46. A case each of metastasized ovarian and pancreatic cancer underwent therapy with Y-90-FAPI-46 [7](Fig 2) as a last-line treatment. The patient with metastasized ovarian cancer underwent RLT with 6 GBq of Y-90-FAPI-46. The other patient with pancreatic cancer had undergone a previous FAPI therapy and then received a further 6 GBq cycle of Y-90-FAPI-46. Tc-99m-FAPI-34 scintigraphy showed stable disease.

Kratochwil and Colleagues (Radiopharmaceutical: Sm-153-/Y-90-FAPI-46)

A patient with soft-tissue sarcoma metastasized to the lungs received three cycles with cumulative 20 GBq of Sm-153- and 8 GBq of Y-90-FAPI-46.[8] The primary tumor and the early oligo-focal metastases had previously been treated by surgery and external-beam radiotherapy. In the later metastatic stage, cyclophosphamide and pazopanib had already been applied. According to the

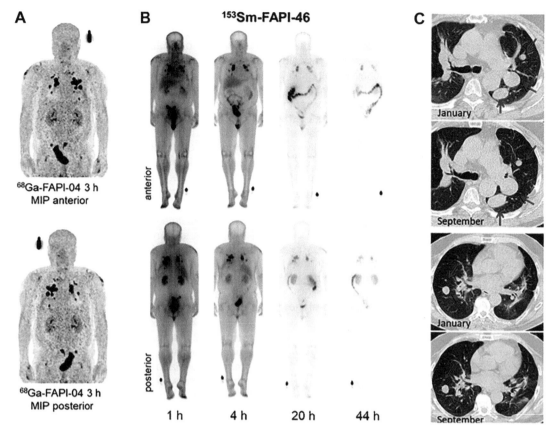

Fig. 2. (*A*) PET maximum-intensity projection of patient with lung metastasized soft-tissue sarcoma (*red arrows*) 3 h after administration of ^{68}Ga-FAPI-46. Intense uptake is seen in metastases. (*B*) ^{153}Sm emission scans during therapy demonstrate tumor targeting up to 44 h p.i. and rapid clearance from normal organs. (*C*) Axial CT images after three cycles with cumulative 20 GBq Sm-153- and 8 GBq Y-90-FAPI-46 show stable disease. This research was originally published in JNM. Lindner T et al.,Design and Development of (99m)Tc-Labeled FAPI Tracers for SPECT Imaging and (188)Re Therapy. J Nucl Med. 2020;61(10):1507-13. © SNMMI.

interdisciplinary tumor board, the patient was not suitable to receive standard chemotherapy with anthracycline. Experimental FAPI-RLT was considered as an alternative to immunotherapy.

The RLT was well-tolerated, and the patient achieved stable disease for 8 months. Subsequent immunotherapy with pembrolizumab, experimentally enhanced with oncolytic parvovirus and nab-paclitaxel, was unsuccessful with disease progression after only 3 months.

RECENT THERANOSTIC AGENT DEVELOPMENTS
Tc-99m-/Re-188-FAPI-34

The diagnostic-therapeutic pair of Tc-99m-/Re-188-FAPI-34 was developed by Lindner and colleagues,[7] to enable SPECT-based selection and monitoring of treatment with the therapeutic agent.

The background of the development of this tracer was the attempt to adjust the length of the radionuclide half-life to match the tumor retention time of the tracer. As Ga-68 labeled FAPI tracers generally show efflux, it leads to the relatively short intratumoral half-lives, resulting in a limited therapeutic effect.[7]

Fundamentally, there are two possibilities to encounter this; the one is to design a new compound with prolonged tumor residence time. The other is to adapt a radionuclide with comparable half-life in comparison with the tumor retention time.

Tc-99m-/Re-188-FAPI-34 was designed to meet the second demand; FAPI-34 can be radiolabeled with the β-emitting Re-188 with a physical half-life of 17 h, which is better suited in regard of biological half-life of the FAP tracer. Re-188 is a generator-produced radionuclide.

In their attempt, Lindner and colleagues originally synthesized six FAPI derivatives with Tc-99m labeling (Tc-99m-FAPI-19, −28, −29, −33, −34, and −43), all of which showed excellent binding properties (45% binding, 95% internalization), high affinity to FAP (half-maximal inhibitory concentration [IC50], 6.4 to 12.7 nM) and significant tumor uptake (5.4% injected dose per gram of tissue) in biodistribution studies. They then identified the lead candidate, Tc-99m-FAPI-34, which showed the lowest uptake in the liver, biliary tract, and intestine. It also showed a significant uptake in the tumor lesions in mice, which could be blocked by the injection of the unlabeled analog, confirming the target specificity of the compound.

Tc-99m-FAPI-34 was first applied for diagnostic scintigraphy and SPECT of patients with metastasized ovarian and pancreatic cancer for follow-up after therapy with Y-90 -FAPI-46 (**Fig. 3**). Tc-99m-FAPI-34 accumulated in the tumor lesions, concordant with the corresponding PET/CT imaging using Ga-68-FAPI-46, showing the practical compatibility of this compound. The efficacy of Re-188 FAPI-46 was not evaluated.

Ga-68-DOTA.SA.FAPi/Lu-177-DOTAGA.(SA.FAPi)₂

These new theranostic agents have been constructed based on the concept that dimerization may enhance the tumor retention time.

The lead structure of these FAPI tracers is UAMC1110, as described by van der Veken's group[12,13] and involves a linker unit between the chelator and FAP enzyme inhibitor, which was varied in subsequent development. The Heidelberg group used piperazine to design novel FAPI tracers.

Moon and colleagues[14] applied another modification method, using squaramide (SA). The critical subunits are the SA linker unit coupled with the DOTA/DOTA5m bifunctional chelators and an FAP inhibitor targeting moiety. The resulting SA.FAPi monomer showed a high tumor affinity, but early washout of the radiotracer, which was completely eliminated by 48 h p.i.[15] To counter this problem and prolong tumor retention, the same group further constructed the homodimer DOTAGA.(SA.FAPi)₂. In this new compound, the bifunctional chelator at the center is linked to two SA linker/target vector units. The homodimeric structure significantly increased tumor uptake and tumor retention. The background uptake was also lower at 24 h p.i. compared to the monomer. Both SA.FAPi monomer and DOTAGA.(SA.FAPi)₂ were well tolerated in patients and showed minimal toxicities.

The first application of Ga-68 PET-guided Lu-177-DOTA.SA.FAPi therapy was performed in patients with advanced-stage breast cancer.[15] Three patients were injected with 2.96 GBq (median activity) of Lu-177-DOTA.SA.FAPi as a single treatment cycle. In the Lu-177-DOTAGA.(SA.FAPi)₂ group, seven patients with various cancer entities (including thyroid cancer, breast cancer, and paraganglioma) were injected with a median activity of 1.48 GBq at the first cycle of treatment. Two cycles of treatment at a median interval of 2 months were performed in this group. The therapy was well tolerated with none of the patients showing any early adverse events. Overall, a grade 3 anemia and grade I thrombocytopenia were reported with no grade 3 or 4 toxicities noted.

Ga-68-/Lu-177-FAP-2286

Baum and colleagues[16] presented a new peptide conjugate FAP-2286, which can be used for theranostics. This compound comprises a cyclic peptide that selectively binds to FAP with low off-target activity. FAP-2286 is coupled with DOTA chelator and thus can be radiolabeled with particle emitters for theranostic purposes.

The first-in-human application of FAP-2286 was performed in 11 patients with metastasized pancreas, breast, rectal, and ovarian cancer.[16] The mean administrated activity was 5.8 GBq (range: 2.4 to 9.9 GBq) for each patient. One to three therapy cycles were performed per patient with overall 22 therapies. The whole-body effective dose was 0.07 ± 0.02 Gy/GBq (range, 0.04 to 0.1 Gy/GBq). Higher uptake and longer tumor retention was observed in bone metastases. The therapy was well tolerated with no grade 4 adverse events being observed. The major reported events were grade 3 events, which occurred in three patients with pancytopenia, leukocytopenia, and pain flare.

Post-therapy evaluation in all patients at 6 to 8 weeks after the first therapy revealed stable disease in two patients but progression in the other nine patients. This finding was in agreement with serum tumor marker levels and with correlative Ga-68-FAP-2286 PET/CT findings.

Regarding the dosimetric assessment authors give a detailed analysis of the whole-body and bone marrow absorbed doses of Lu-177-FAP-2286 (0.07 and 0.05 Gy/GBq, respectively) in comparison with other Lu-177-labeled RLT such as Lu-177-PSMA-617 (0.04 and 0.03 Gy/GBq, respectively) and Lu-177-DOTATATE (0.05 and 0.04 Gy/GBq, respectively), which show similar values. Also, the effective half-life of Lu-177-FAP-2286 in the whole body was estimated to be 35 h, which is slightly shorter than that of Lu-177-PSMA-617 (40 h) and Lu-177-DOTATATE (55 h). This compatibility gives the basis for the promising future exploration in the clinical setting.

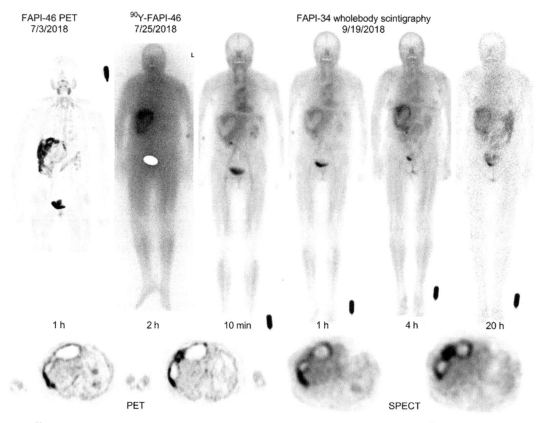

FAPI-46 PET
7/3/2018

^{90}Y-FAPI-46
7/25/2018

FAPI-34 wholebody scintigraphy
9/19/2018

1 h   2 h   10 min   1 h   4 h   20 h

PET   SPECT

Fig. 3. ^{68}Ga-FAPI-46 PET/CT imaging (bremsstrahlung) during treatment with 6 GBq of ^{90}Y-FAPI-46 and scintigraphy with ^{99m}Tc-labeled FAPI-34 (planar scintigraphy and transaxial SPECT slices) in a patient with ovarian cancer. This research was originally published in JNM. Ferdinandus J et al.,Kostbade K et al. Initial clinical experience with (90)Y-FAPI-46 radioligand therapy for advanced stage solid tumors: a case series of nine patients. J Nucl Med. 2021. 63(5) 727-734. © SNMMI.

Challenges in the Implementation of Theranostic Regimens

As FAP tracers highly selectively bind to CAFs in tumor stroma with excellent target-to-background ratio (TBR), FAP-targeted combined diagnostic and therapy (theranostic) is an attractive strategy in oncology.

The main challenges in implementation of theranostic regimens are as follows: (1) prolonging tumor retention time to achieve sufficient cumulative activity in tumor to achieve biologically effective radiation doses, (2) correct selection of the suitable radionuclide to match the physiological and biological half-life of the tracer, (3) heterogeneity, and (4) minimizing radiation toxicity.

1. Prolonging tumor retention time

To achieve high therapeutic radiation doses to target tumor lesions, high uptake followed by prolonged tumor residence time is essential. FAPI derivatives show a rapid and high rate of internalization into the target cells but have also a considerable efflux. This feature leads to a relatively short intratumoral retention and limits the area under curve of radiation delivery.

There are several strategies to optimize the tumor residence time. These are mainly achieved by the radiochemical elaboration, as described in detail by Lindner and colleagues, and summarized below. One example is the modification of the linker-inhibitor-binding agent, which may enhance binding affinity.

Of all currently known tracer options, small-molecule and peptide-based tracers are the leading groups for FAP-targeted strategy. Theoretically, there are other chemical structures that could serve as a tracer, such as antibodies. Antibodies and peptides are reported to show generally longer tumor retention but cause higher nontarget exposure. For instance, antibody-based tracers lead to higher exposure to red bone marrow and peptide-based tracers cause higher exposure to kidney.[17]

2. Correct selection of the suitable radionuclide to match the physiological and biological half-life of the tracer

For an optimal therapeutic application, the physical half-life of the radionuclide used in the tracer should be adjusted to the biologic half-life in the tumor.[17] Based on the preclinical data in cells expressing human and murine FAP and CD26, the biologic half-life of Lu-177-FAPI-04 was reported to be 3.0 h versus 1.7 h for Lu-177-FAPI-02 in the tumor. In a patient study, multifactorial effects play a pivotal role in the real tumor retention; These may include levels of tissue perfusion, the proportion of desmoplasia with the tumor mass, and biological factors such as hypoxia or pH. For example, the whole-body PET/CT scans performed 10 min, 1 h, and 3 h after intravenous administration of Ga-68-FAPI-46 in patients with metastasized mucoepidermoid, oropharynx, ovarian, and colorectal carcinoma showed constant remaining tumor activity up to 3 h after injection in colorectal, ovarian, oropharyngeal, and pancreatic carcinoma. The first clinical application of 2.9 GBq of Y-90-FAPI-04 showed accumulation of the tracer at 3 h and even at 1 d after injection in this patient, as shown in the bremsstrahlung image (see **Fig. 1**). Emission scans after the application of 8 GBq Sm-153-FAPI-46 showed tumor targeting up to 44 h p.i.[8]

Given that the tumor retention time remains relatively short, consideration of similarly short-lived isotopes such as α-emitter Bi-213 or the β-emitters Re-188 and Y-90 are rather more suitable to deliver a higher radiation dose to the tumor than longer-lived therapeutic radionuclides such as Lu-177 or Ac-225. The prior success of targeted RLT such as DOTATOC- or PSMA-ligand therapy for neuroendocrine tumors and prostate cancer with the same radionuclides reflects the long biological half-life of these agents.[18]

Further dosimetric analysis with a larger number of patients is pivotal to elucidate in vivo characterization of biological half-lives of each tracer in real-world, and necessarily, rather inhomogeneous therapeutic situations.

3. Heterogeneity

Newly synthesized FAP tracers undergo in vitro analysis using cell culture and in vivo using tumor-bearing xenografts under standardized condition. In many of these the cell lines have been transfected to overexpress FAP and do not faithfully recapitulate the human tumor microenvironment wherein FAP expression is in the benign stromal elements and not the malignant cell line. These artificial models perhaps better represent the situation for sarcoma wherein FAP is expressed in the malignant clone. Nevertheless, preclinical models allow rigorous control of experimental conditions and limit the impact of tumor heterogeneity. In the therapeutic situation in humans, heterogeneity in patient demographics, such as age, sex, immunological status, and prior therapies may interact, with variable FAP expression across different tumor types and heterogeneity within tumor stroma at different sites may play an essential role in determining the success of FAP targeted radiotherapy.

Despite these multifactorial conditions, and confounding factors, standardized and well-designed preclinical studies in vitro and in vivo are important to inform the design of human therapeutic trials, which require elaborately performed dosimetric studies in a larger number of patients with relevant patient outcomes being recorded.

4. Minimizing the radiation toxicity

For the currently available major FAP-targeting theranostic agents, the major dose-limiting organ is the kidney. Other organs at risk include the colon, liver, gall bladder, and bone marrow. To achieve the safe and tolerable limit to each organ, the maximum cumulative activity should be carefully evaluated and calculated after each therapy to determine the safety of proceeding to further treatment cycles. Bodei and colleagues[19] followed patients with neuroendocrine tumors after RLT and revealed that long-term kidney toxicities are minimal. However, individual conditions always play a role in the therapeutic situations, for example, a constipation with limited intestinal motility or a history of hepatobiliary or renal tract obstruction should be carefully evaluated and taken into consideration.

The implementation of dose fractionation protocols with the application of low administered activities over multiple therapy cycles is also an option to give organs at risk time for recovery. Such concepts, together with the question of optimal time interval between each therapy cycle, warrant future exploration.

4. Other conditions

Most studies on FAP-targeted theranostics that have been published up to now have been proof-of-concept studies from single institutions with inconsistent eligibility criteria, diverse disease types and variable treatment protocols, or have occurred as case reports.

The number of patients included in these studies is very small, and the patient cohorts are heterogeneous. This results mainly from the fact that patients generally received FAP-targeted radionuclide therapy on compassionate grounds after exhaustion of multiple cancer therapies. These factors, particularly the bias in selection of patients with a particularly poor prognosis, and likely to negatively impact the efficacy and safety reported FAP-targeted RLT compared to that which might be achieved in less physiologically-compromised and heavily pretreated patients.

There is currently no standard regimen for FAP-targeted RLT with respect to the number of therapeutic cycles, optimal administered activity, and interval between cycles. The authors believe that serial acquisition at various time-points after treatment are required to allow precise dosimetric evaluation and is pivotal for optimizing our understanding of observed therapeutic effects and refining treatment protocols to achieve a high therapeutic index.

Pathophysiological Consideration

Radionuclide therapy targeting FAP aims selectively the tumor-associated fibroblasts (CAFs) in the stroma of multiple epithelial tumors. As stroma formation only occurs from around a tumor size of 1 to 2 mm,[20] the therapeutic effects of radioligand binding to the CAFs in adjacent cancer cells is likely to be via cross-fire effect, which has potential implications for the treatment of micrometastases lacking significant stroma and for the path-length of the therapeutic radionuclide. Moreover, direct effects on other stromal elements must be considered given the essential contribution of CAFs in sustaining and enhancing immunological activity within the tumor microenvironment and regulating neovascularization.

In the therapeutic application of FAP ligands, the contributions of CAFs in the immune evasion and chemo-resistance are important factors that might influence the outcome, as CAFs are known to be the essential drivers for invasiveness and metastasis.

In a cell-culture model of pancreatic ductal adenocarcinoma, depletion of the FAP-expressing CAFs induced T-cell accumulation in cancer cells and synergistically enhanced anti-tumor effects within programmed cell death ligand 1 (PD-L1) immunotherapy.[21] Hence, future exploration of the potentially synergistic combination of immunotherapy with FAP-targeting radionuclide therapy is warranted, as are combinations with nonradioactive cancer therapeutics.

ROLE OF RADIOCHEMISTRY

Radiochemistry plays a fundamental role in the development of theranostic agents.

In the development of small-molecule FAPI tracers, the reduction of molecular weight with better tissue penetration contributed essentially to the better pharmacokinetics in comparison to the antibodies of the former generation.[17]

The highly selective and potent precursor molecule as the basic compound of the subsequent FAPI derivatives, was developed by the group of van der Veken. This compound is based on (4-quinoinolyl)glycinyl-2-cyanopyrrolidine scaffold. The Heidelberg group has chosen the quinoline positions 6 and 7 to attach the chelator moiety. The best results were obtained with a 1,3-propylen spacer between an N-piperazine and an ether oxygen or a methylamino group bound to the quinoline.[17]

The initial radiometal-based ligand, Ga-68-FAPI-02, showed a rapid washout from tumor tissues and thus was not felt suitable for therapeutic applications despite high target affinity.[17] Through the difluoro substitution at the cyanopyrrolidine moiety, a reduction of the IC50 value occurred, and the features of derivatives were much more suitable due to longer tumor retention. FAPI-46 was developed with a feature of extended tumor retention while maintaining the diagnostic benefit of a fast clearance from blood and most other organs. This was achieved by a methylated nitrogen, which replaced the bridging oxygen at the 6-quinoline position.[4]

For the design of FAPI-34, which provided the benefit of using SPECT/CT scanner for diagnostic scanning as well as leveraging the wide availability of Mo-99/Tc-99m-generators, Lindner and colleagues designed various precursors with bisimidazole chelators. The derivative with the most favorable features was FAPI-34, in which the high lipophilicity of the Tc-99m-tricarbonyl core was compensated through two carboxyglutamate residues attached to the chelating moiety.[7]

Several strategies for prolonging the retention of tracer molecules by adding albumin-binder moieties have been recently reported (these are detailed elsewhere in this edition of PET Clinics). In this strategy, series of albumin binder (truncated Evans blue) radiopharmaceuticals based on FAPI-02 or FAPI-04-based albumin binder (4-[p-iodophenyl] butyric acid moiety, truncated Evans blue moiety, lauric acid [C12], and palmitic acid [C16]) were developed. Prolonged tumor retention as well as an increased accumulation of these tracers until 96 h post-injection were reported.[22,23]

Multimerization is another strategy to enhance tumor uptake and retention. Recently developed FAPI dimer DOTA-2P(FAPI)$_2$ as described above.

FUTURE PERSPECTIVES

Currently, published data on FAP-targeted thera-nostics primarily rely on proof-of-concept studies, performed in single institutions. Patients who received RLT with FAP ligands were all end-stage cancer patients who had exhausted available therapy options. This has led to a heterogeneity in results that limit any general statements regarding the efficacy and safety of this approach.

Nevertheless, the first reports on the practical application of FAP-targeted therapy are promising. To summarize, the first-in-human RLT with FAP ligand was performed by the Heidelberg group with 2.9 GBq of Y-90-FAPI-04 in a patient with end-stage breast cancer, which led to a significant reduction in pain medication in this patient. In the further development of FAPI tracers Loktev and colleagues introduced a new derivative FAPI-46 with longer tumor retention and favorable pharmacokinetics. Several reports on FAPI-46 are published. For example, Assadi and colleagues applied Lu-177-FAPI-46 in 18 patients with an average of 3.7 GBq. Kratochwil and colleagues applied 20 GBq of Sm-153- and 8 GBq of Y-90-FAPI-46, fractioned in three cycles in a patient with metastasized soft-tissue sarcoma.

In all the reported cases, the therapy appears to have been well tolerated, and a few patients achieved stable disease. Although objective responses were lacking with current agents and many continued to progress, it must be emphasized that the patients enrolled in the reported studies had cancers that are notoriously resistant to many types of cancer treatment and had already been heavily pretreated. Expectations of efficacy in such end-stage patients must be tempered, particularly as eligibility criteria for most clinical trials of cancer therapeutics would likely exclude many such patients.

Several new options are presented. FAPI-34, developed by Lindner and colleagues, is a new FAPI-derivative that can be labeled with Tc-99m and Re-188 for theranostic use. Ballal and colleagues presented a patient study with new theranostic compound DOTAGA.(SA.FAPi)$_2$ which shows longer tumor retention due to the homodimerization. Baum and colleagues reported the clinical application of a new peptide compound Ga-68-/Lu-177-FAP-2286. Clinical validation in larger patient cohorts are eagerly awaited.

Besides addressing technical issues that will be primarily led in the field of radiochemistry, the further elucidation of pathophysiological mechanisms underlying FAP- and stroma-targeting is warranted in future research. This includes the possibility of using immune system to enhance the therapeutic effect, in a manner of concurrent or sequential radionuclide and immune therapy. Those concepts require a well-designed preclinical work together with the elaborate clinical assessment in a selected, larger cohort of patients.

AUTHOR CONTRIBUTION

Writing/original draft preparation: Y. Mori. Review and editing: C. Kratochwil. Supervision: U. Haberkorn and F. L. Giesel. All authors have read and agreed to the published version of the manuscript.

CONFLICTS OF INTEREST

F. L. Giesel, U. Haberkorn, and C. Kratochwil have filed a patent application for quinoline-based FAP-targeting agents for imaging and therapy in nuclear medicine. F. L. Giesel, U. Haberkorn, and C. Kratochwil also have shares of a consultancy group for iTheranostics. F. L. Giesel is also advisor at ABX, Telix, SOFIE Biosciences and Alpha-Fusion.

CLINICS CARE POINTS

- For an optimal therapeutic application, the physical half-life of the radionuclide used in the tracer should be adjusted to the biologic half-life in the tumor.

- In a patient study, multifactorial effects such as the levels of tissue perfusion, the proportion of desmoplasia with the tumor mass, hypoxia or pH- may play a pivotal role in the real tumor retention.

- The implementation of dose fractionation protocols over multiple therapy cycles is an option to give organs at risk time for recovery and warrant future exploration.

REFERENCES

1. Mori Y, Dendl K, Cardinale J, et al. Fapi PET: fibroblast activation protein inhibitor use in oncologic and nononcologic disease. Radiology 2023. https://doi.org/10.1148/radiol.220749. Online ahead of print.
2. Loktev A, Lindner T, Mier W, et al. A tumor-imaging method targeting cancer-associated fibroblasts. J Nucl Med 2018;59(9):1423–9.
3. Lindner T, Loktev A, Altmann A, et al. Development of quinoline-based theranostic ligands for the targeting of fibroblast activation protein. J Nucl Med 2018; 59(9):1415–22.

4. Loktev A, Lindner T, Burger EM, et al. Development of fibroblast activation protein-targeted radiotracers with improved tumor retention. J Nucl Med 2019; 60(10):1421–9.

5. Assadi M, Rekabpour SJ, Jafari E, et al. Feasibility and therapeutic potential of 177Lu-fibroblast activation protein inhibitor-46 for patients with relapsed or refractory cancers: a preliminary study. Clin Nucl Med 2021;46(11):e523–30.

6. Ferdinandus J, Fragoso Costa P, Kessler L, et al. Initial clinical experience with (90)Y-FAPI-46 radioligand therapy for advanced stage solid tumors: a case series of nine patients. J Nucl Med 2021. https://doi.org/10.2967/jnumed.121.262468.

7. Lindner T, Altmann A, Kramer S, et al. Design and development of (99m)Tc-labeled FAPI tracers for SPECT imaging and (188)Re therapy. J Nucl Med 2020;61(10):1507–13.

8. Kratochwil C, Giesel FL, Rathke H, et al. [(153)Sm] Samarium-labeled FAPI-46 radioligand therapy in a patient with lung metastases of a sarcoma. Eur J Nucl Med Mol Imaging 2021;48(9):3011–3.

9. Rathke H, Fuxius S, Giesel FL, et al. Two tumors, one target: preliminary experience with 90Y-FAPI therapy in a patient with metastasized breast and colorectal cancer. Clin Nucl Med 2021;46(10):842–4.

10. Jokar N, Velikyan I, Ahmadzadehfar H, et al. Theranostic approach in breast cancer: a treasured tailor for future oncology. Clin Nucl Med 2021;46(8): e410–20.

11. Ballal S, Yadav MP, Kramer V, et al. A theranostic approach of [(68)Ga]Ga-DOTA.SA.FAPi PET/CT-guided [(177)Lu]Lu-DOTA.SA.FAPi radionuclide therapy in an end-stage breast cancer patient: new frontier in targeted radionuclide therapy. Eur J Nucl Med Mol Imaging 2021;48(3):942–4.

12. Jansen K, De Winter H, Heirbaut L, et al. Selective inhibitors of fibroblast activation protein (FAP) with a xanthine scaffold. MedChemComm 2014;5: 1700–7.

13. Jansen K, Heirbaut L, Verkerk R, et al. Extended structure-activity relationship and pharmaco-kinetic investigation of (4-quinolinoyl)glycyl-2-cyanopyrrolidine inhibitors of fibroblast activation protein (FAP). J Med Chem 2014;57:3053–74.

14. Moon ES, Ballal S, Yadav MP, et al. Fibroblast Activation Protein (FAP) targeting homodimeric FAP inhibitor radiotheranostics: a step to improve tumor uptake and retention time. AJNMMI 2021;11(6): 476–91.

15. Ballal S, Yadav MP, Moon ES, et al. First-in-human results on the biodistribution, pharmacokinetics, and dosimetry of [177Lu]Lu-DOTA.SA.FAPi and [177Lu]Lu-DOTAGA.(SA.FAPi)2. Pharmaceuticals 2021;14(12):1212.

16. Baum RP, Schuchardt C, Singh A, et al. Feasibility, biodistribution and preliminary dosimetry in peptide-targeted radionuclide therapy (PTRT) of diverse adenocarcinomas using (177)Lu-FAP-2286: first-in-human results. J Nucl Med 2021. https://doi.org/10.2967/jnumed.120.259192.

17. Lindner T, Giesel FL, Kratochwil C, et al. Radioligands targeting fibroblast activation protein (FAP). Cancers 2021;13(22):5744.

18. Zhao L, Chen J, Pang Y, et al. Fibroblast activation protein-based theranostics in cancer research: a state-of-the-art review. Theranostics 2022;12(4): 1557–69.

19. Bodei L, Cremonesi M, Ferrari M, et al. Long-term evaluation of renal toxicity after peptide receptor radionuclide therapy with 90Y-DOTATOC and 177Lu-DOTATATE: the role ofassociated risk factors. Eur. J. Nucl. Med. Mol. Imaging 2008;35:1847–56.

20. Davidson B, Goldberg I, Kopolovic J. Inflammatory response in cervical intraepithelial neoplasia and squamous cell carcinoma of the uterine cervix. Pathol Res Pract 1997;193:491–5.

21. Feig C, Jones JO, Kraman M, et al. Targeting CXCL12 from FAP-expressing carcinoma-associated fibroblasts synergizes with anti-PD-L1 immunotherapy in pancreatic cancer. Proc Natl Acad Sci U S A 2013;110(50):20212–7.

22. Wen X, Xu P, Shi M, et al. Evans blue-modified radiolabeled fibroblast activation protein inhibitor as long-acting cancer therapeutics. Theranostics 2022; 12(1):422–33.

23. Xu M, Zhang P, Ding J, et al. Albumin binder-conjugated fibroblast activation protein inhibitor radiopharmaceuticals for cancer therapy. J Nucl Med 2021. https://doi.org/10.2967/jnumed.121.262533.

Current State of Clinical Trials and Regulatory Approvals with Fibroblast Activation Protein Targeting Interventions

Sherly Mosessian, PhD[a],*, Jessica D. Jensen, MPH[b], Aaron S. Enke, BS[c]

KEYWORDS

- Fibroblast activation protein • Clinical development • Clinical trial • Theranostic • Diagnostic
- Radioligand therapy • Cancer-associated fibroblasts • Radiopharmaceuticals

KEY POINTS

- This article examines the current state of clinical studies with interventions targeting fibroblast activation protein (FAP).
- Thirty-seven studies from clinicaltrials.gov with FAP-targeting interventions were identified using imaging, radioligand therapy, non-radioligand therapy, or other interventions.
- Imaging studies comprise the largest number of studies currently registered. [^{18}F]FAPI-74 and [^{68}Ga]FAPI-46 at Phase 2 are at the most advanced stage of development, followed by [^{68}Ga]FAP-2286 in Phase 1 and investigator-initiated studies with FAPI family of compounds in Phase 0/Phase 1.
- Currently, there are four studies with three products using ^{177}Lutetium for radioligand therapy in early phases of clinical evaluation. These products are [^{177}Lu]-PNT6555 and [^{177}Lu]-FAP-2286 and [^{177}Lu]-EB-FAPI.
- Non-radioligand therapies targeting FAP are conducted by three main companies. Avacta, Molecular Partners AG, and Roche and are in early phases of evaluation.

BACKGROUND

Fibroblast activation protein (FAP) has served as an attractive target for diagnostic and therapeutic use since its initial discovery based on evidence generated by two independent groups in the late 1980s and 1990s. The first group developed a monoclonal antibody (F19) from a mouse immunized with lung fibroblasts.[1] This antibody recognized a glycoprotein found primarily on proliferating cultured fibroblasts extracted from benign and malignant tumors and the stroma of epithelial cancers, which was absent in resting fibroblasts in normal tissues.[2,3] Concurrently, the second group identified a protease present in invasive melanoma cells.[4] Gene sequencing later demonstrated that these were the same protein.[5–8] Although the degree and extent of FAP expression varies, it has consistently shown to be highly expressed in cancer-associated fibroblasts surrounding solid carcinomas and expressed in tumor cells of some cancers, such as sarcomas.[9] In a study of pan-cancer human tissue microarray analysis, investigators assessed

[a] Sofie Biosciences Inc, 21000 Atlantic Boulevard, Ste 730, Dulles, VA 20166, USA; [b] Clinical Development, Point Biopharma, 4850 West 78th Street, Indianapolis, IN 46268, USA; [c] Clinical Development, Clovis Oncology, 5500 Flatiron Parkway, Boulder, CO 80301, USA
* Corresponding author.
E-mail address: sherly.mosessian@sofie.com

PET Clin 18 (2023) 429–439
https://doi.org/10.1016/j.cpet.2023.02.010
1556-8598/23/© 2023 Elsevier Inc. All rights reserved.

FAP expression across 14 cancer types with strong FAP expression observed in association with cancers of bile duct, bladder, colon, esophagus, stomach, lung, oropharynx, ovary, and pancreas.[10] In addition to cancer, FAP expression has also been associated with nonmalignant disease including cardiovascular disease, fibrosis in various organs, IgG4 disease, joint dysfunction, and more.[11]

Following the identification of FAP as a target, several efforts have taken place targeting FAP for oncology, including development of sibrotuzumab (also known as Sibrotuzumab [BIBH] 1) by Boehringer Ingelheim Pharma, a humanized monoclonal antibody with high affinity to bind to FAP. In 2003, studies were conducted in several solid cancers, including colorectal, non-small cell lung, breast, and head and neck cancers but failed to demonstrate sufficient efficacy in Phase 2. Since then, small molecule inhibitors have been under investigation along with newer approaches of FAP targeting including CAR T-cell therapy and prodrug approaches. To date, no FAP-targeting treatment approach has been approved by regulatory entities.

In 2018, with the development of a new class of FAP-targeting radiopharmaceutical (FAP Inhibitors), new attention has been directed to FAP as a target of radioligands for imaging and therapy, along with non-radioligand therapy (non-RLT) interventions. In this article, the authors highlight the latest efforts and clinical development progress made to date in FAP targeting.

Approach

Data for analysis of the current state of clinical trials using FAP-targeted interventions were obtained through a search of the clinicaltrials.gov website, a US government web-based resource maintained by the National Library of Medicine. Search criteria included "FAP" and "Fibroblast Activation Protein," in addition to the recruitment statuses "completed, "active, not recruiting," "recruiting," "enrolling by invitation," and "not yet recruiting." These criteria resulted in 37 studies as shown in **Fig. 1**. Further analysis of the results demonstrated 21 studies in diagnostic investigations using PET, four studies in radioligand therapy (RLT), eight studies in non-RLT, and four other studies of interventions with biologics and genetic approaches. The data from this approach are further analyzed and discussed below.

CURRENT TRIALS
Radioligands Under Investigation

Analysis of the clinicaltrials.gov data shows that radioligands for imaging and/or therapy belong to the following sets of products: (1) Fibroblast Activation Protein Inhibitor (FAPI) family of compounds, (2) FAP-2286, and (3) PNT6555. Industry-sponsored studies in support of clinical development for these products are listed in **Table 1**. A brief description of these products, along with recent clinical development efforts, is highlighted below.

FAPI Family of Compounds

Many well-documented FAPI compounds and derivatives have emerged in recent years, with the first publication in 2018 from Professor Uwe Haberkorn's laboratory at Heidelberg University. This development has followed a series of improvements focusing on achieving high tumor uptake, high tumor retention, high signal-to-background, and low activity in normal organs.

In initial studies, FAPI-02 showed superior performance with higher cellular uptake and retention over time. Subsequent work focused on prolonging the tumor retention time, resulting in the development of 12 new FAPI compounds.[12] [^{68}Ga]FAPI-04 was a marked improvement over [^{68}Ga]FAPI-02 with significantly increased tumor retention. Utility of FAPI-04 was further demonstrated in a groundbreaking study where 80 patients with 28 different types of cancer were successfully imaged with [^{68}Ga]FAPI-04, showing high image contrast and good tumor delineation.[13] To build on these promising results with [^{68}Ga]FAPI-04, researchers sought to further enhance tumor retention while maintaining high image contrast. Fifteen more FAPI compounds were developed and tested, with [^{68}Ga]FAPI-46 displaying better tumor uptake and higher tumor-to-organ ratios than FAPI-04, making [^{68}Ga]FAPI-46 the lead product for theranostic use. When labeled with gallium-68 (^{68}Ga), FAPI-46 is used for PET imaging[14]; when labeled with alpha- or beta-emitting isotopes, the product can be used for RLT. In a recent publication, [^{90}Y]-FAPI-46-RLT was shown to be safe and led to RECIST partial response in one case and stable disease in about one-third of patients with previously progressive sarcomas, pancreatic ductal adenocarcinomas, and other cancers.[15]

A second focus in the development of FAPI products for diagnostic use has been to expand from radiolabeling with [^{68}Ga] to labeling with fluorine-18 [^{18}F] to overcome limitations posed by the short half-life of [^{68}Ga] and the small batch size of [^{68}Ga]-tracers, which impedes production using good manufacturing practice (GMP) and commercial distribution. This work resulted in the identification of [^{18}F]FAPI-74 as

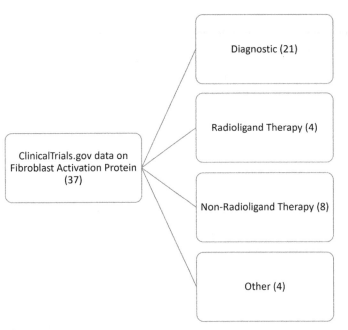

Fig. 1. ClinicalTrials.gov search results. Search results with keywords "FAP" and "Fibroblast Activation Protein" resulted in 37 studies. Further classification of the results broke down the data into 21 diagnostic studies with PET or PET/CT, four studies in radioligand therapy, eight therapeutic studies in non-radioligand therapy, followed by four studies under "Other." The other studies included three completed genetic studies and one biologic intervention study currently active.

the lead [^{18}F]-labeled product best meeting these requirements.[16]

Sofie Biosciences, Inc, has licensed the rights to use of the FAPI family of compounds in diagnostics and companion diagnostics. SOFIE's current clinical plan includes the development of the two lead ^{68}Ga- and ^{18}F-labeled compounds [^{68}Ga] FAPI-46 and [^{18}F]FAPI-74. [^{68}Ga]FAPI-46 is under clinical investigation in the US in a Phase 2 multicenter study of patients with pancreatic ductal

Table 1
Industry-sponsored trials with FAP radioligands for imaging and therapy

Sponsor	Study Title	Study Type	Intervention	Trial Phase
SOFIE	Study of [^{18}F]FAPI-74 PET in patients with gastrointestinal cancers	Diagnostic	[^{18}F]FAPI-74	Phase 2
SOFIE	Study of [^{68}Ga]FAPI-46 PET in patients with pancreatic ductal carcinoma	Diagnostic	[^{68}Ga]FAPI-46	Phase 2
Clovis Oncology, Inc	A study of ^{177}Lu-FAP-2286 in advanced tumors (LuMIERE)	Theranostic	[^{68}Ga]-FAP-2286 [^{177}Lu]-FAP-2286	Phase 1/Phase 2
POINT Biopharma	FAPi radioligand open-label, phase 1 study to evaluate safety, tolerability and dosimetry of [Lu-177]-PNT6555; A dose escalation study for treatment of patients with select solid tumors (FRONTIER)	Theranostic	[^{68}Ga]-PNT6555 [^{177}Lu]-PNT6555	Phase 1

Current active industry-sponsored clinical studies in support of clinical development of radioligands for imaging and therapy are highlighted in this table. The information provided includes the sponsoring entity, study title, study type, intervention used, and the clinical phase(s).

adenocarcinoma (NCT05262855). [18F]FAPI-74 received active investigational new drug application status from the Food and Drug Administration (FDA) for a Phase 2 multicenter imaging study of patients with gastrointestinal cancers, including gastric, cholangiocarcinoma, hepatocellular carcinoma, pancreatic cancer, and colorectal cancer (NCT05641896).

In addition to SOFIE-sponsored studies, the FAPI global outreach program enables the international community to engage in preclinical, chemistry, and clinical studies through investigator-initiated studies in various diseases. SOFIE supports investigators by providing precursors for these lead compounds (FAPI-46 and FAPI-74) and manufacturing and regulatory support for these efforts. These studies will allow further research development opportunities for investigators and provide supplemental clinical safety and efficacy data to support clinical development and regulatory approval pathways for both [68Ga] FAPI-46 and [18F]FAPI-74.

Fibroblast Activation Protein -2286

FAP-2286 was originally developed by 3B Pharmaceuticals GmBH (3BP; Berlin, Germany). Clovis Oncology, Inc, licensed FAP-2286 from 3BP in September 2019 and currently has rights for both diagnostic and therapeutic development in North America, Asia, and other territories. FAP-2286 was identified by an in vitro screening assay of 10^{14} unique peptides using mRNA display to select for affinity and stability to provide an array of FAP-binding candidate peptides, using cyclic peptides as binding motifs, which may have superior binding affinity and selectivity than linear peptides. The structure activity relationship was examined for each to identify peptide sequences optimized for in vivo biodistribution, with increased affinity and stability, and with sites for linker and radionuclide attachment. FAP-2286 is a compound made from of one of these optimized peptides plus a linker and 1,4,7,10-tetraazacyclododecane-1,4,7,10-tetraacetic acid (DOTA) moiety for chelation of a variety of radioactive metals for imaging and therapeutic applications.

In preclinical studies comparing FAP-2286 to FAP-targeting radionuclides, FAP-2286 was found to have superior biodistribution and retention. Zboralski and colleagues[17] compared the biodistribution and retention of radiolabeled FAP-2286 with that of FAPI-46 and evaluated the efficacy of [177Lu]-FAP-2286 in tumor-bearing mice. FAP-2286 labeled with ^{177}Lu displayed prolonged tumor retention ($\geq$72 h) compared with FAPI-46 after injection in an HEK-FAP tumor-bearing mouse model as measured by Single-Photon Emission Computerized Tomography/Computed Tomography (SPECT/CT) image quantification while maintaining rapid renal clearance, as expected for small molecules. The longer tumor retention of FAP-2286 as compared with FAPI-46 resulted in 12- and 9-fold higher time-integrated activity coefficient and absorbed dose delivered to the tumors, respectively, which ultimately lead to greater tumor inhibition.

In a compassionate use setting in Germany, both [68Ga]-FAP-2286 and [177Lu]-FAP-2286 were administered to 11 patients with FAP-expressing solid tumors, including advanced, metastatic adenocarcinoma of the pancreas, breast, rectum, or ovary. Patients received individualized doses, with activities ranging from 2.5 to 9.9 GBq (68–268 mCi). Nine patients received two doses of [177Lu]-FAP-2286 and one patient received a third dose. Results have been presented at several meetings and published by Baum and colleagues.[18] In December 2020, Clovis Oncology activated individual INDs for the imaging and therapeutic agents, [68Ga]-FAP-2286 and [177Lu]-FAP-2286. The first clinical trial of [177Lu]-FAP-2286 is LuMIERE: A Phase 1/2, multicenter, open-label, non-randomized study to investigate the safety and tolerability, pharmacokinetics, dosimetry, and preliminary activity of [177Lu]-FAP-2286 in patients with an advanced solid tumor (Study CO-2286–114, NCT04939610). LuMIERE was initiated in 2021, with the first Phase 1 patient enrolled August of that year. Phase 1 evaluates the safety and tolerability of [177Lu]-FAP-2286 in patients with FAP-expressing solid tumors, as determined by PET/CT with [68Ga]-FAP-2286. Dose escalation follows a Bayesian Optimal Interval design. All dose levels include a flat dose of FAP-2286 peptide with ascending levels of activity, starting at 3.7 GBq (100 mCi) with three possible escalation steps of 50 mCi each, for a maximum possible single dose of 9.25 GBq (250 mCi). [177Lu]-FAP-2286 is administered every 6 weeks, for a maximum of six doses. Organ and tumor dosimetry are evaluated from SPECT/CT images from several time points following each dose.

Phase 2 will begin once a recommended Phase 2 dose (RP2D) is found. The primary endpoint for Phase 2 is the objective response rate (ORR) in each of several tumor-specific cohorts. Clovis Oncology anticipates completing dose escalation and initiating Phase 2 in the second quarter of 2023.

As of December 2022, 17 Phase 1 patients had been enrolled, had PET/CT imaging with [68Ga]-FAP-2286, and received at least one administration of [177Lu]-FAP-2286. Preliminary efficacy signals have been observed, with one confirmed PR of significant duration and several other patients with prolonged SD. Dosimetry findings for kidney and red marrow indicate relatively low exposures, with a mean kidney absorbed dose of ~0.42 Gy/GBq and mean red marrow absorbed dose of ~0.024 Gy/GBq.

There are two investigator-initiated studies of FAP-2286 underway for which Clovis Oncology is collaborator. NCT04621435 is a multi-arm prospective trial that evaluates the ability of novel imaging radiolabeled agents to detect metastatic cancer in participants with solid tumors using a ^{68}Ga- or ^{64}Cu-FAP-2286 tracer for PET/CT imaging. As of December 2022, approximately 60 patients had been enrolled and imaged with a FAP-2286 tracer. NCT05180162 is a single-arm, prospective pilot trial that evaluates the ability of a novel imaging agent, ^{68}Ga-FAP-2286, to identify pathologic fibrosis in the setting of hepatic, cardiac and pulmonary fibrosis. Thomas Hope, MD, of University of California, San Francisco, is the sponsor and primary investigator for both studies.

PNT6555

With the goal of developing new FAP-targeting therapeutic and imaging radiopharmaceuticals, a library of compounds was invented by Professor William Bachovchin, PhD, at Tufts University. POINT Biopharma licensed worldwide rights to the compounds from Bach Biosciences in April 2020 and has advanced the lead clinical candidate, PNT6555, through Investigational New Drug (IND) enabling nonclinical studies, GMP process and method validation and initiation of a first in human clinical trial.

PNT6555 is composed of a DOTA chelator (1,4,7,10-tetraazacyclododecane-1,4,7,10- tetraacetic acid) and an FAP-targeting moiety (Bz-D-Ala-boroPro) connected via an aminomethyl linker (Am). The corresponding [^{68}Ga] ([Ga-68]-DOTA-AmBz-D-Ala-boroPro) and [^{177}Lu] ([Lu-177]-DOTA-AmBz-D-Ala-boroPro) chelates represent the imaging and therapeutic theranostic pair of PNT6555, respectively.

Nonclinical data has shown PNT6555 and its radiometal chelates, to be potent and specific inhibitors of FAP. [Ga-68]-PNT6555 and [Lu-177]-PNT6555 exhibit rapid uptake into FAP expressing tumors, with prolonged tumor retention observed for [Lu-177]-PNT6555, and limited uptake or retention in normal tissues.[19] Unique to boronic acid inhibitors, such as PNT6555, is the ability to form an adduct with the serine of the catalytic site (FAP in this case) through a mechanistic process called "slow binding kinetics." If the sequence of the peptidyl portion of the inhibitor (D-Alanine-Proline for PNT6555) is correctly recognized by the enzyme,

it induces a conformational change to the enzyme-inhibitor complex that is much tighter— and which could explain the enhanced tumor uptake and retention that was observed with PNT6555 relative to other FAP-targeting agents. Further, preclinical therapeutic studies using a single dose of [Lu-177]-PNT6555 or [Ac-225]-PNT6555 showed compelling efficacy in the HEK-mFAP model with several mice experiencing long-term survival greater than 100 days at multiple dose levels tested.

POINT Biopharma's clinical development plan is to investigate the therapeutic benefit and safety of PNT6555 across a variety of FAP-expressing solid tumors. The Phase 1 FRONTIER trial (NCT05432193) commenced dosing in July 2022 and aims to evaluate the safety and tolerability of [Lu-177]-PNT6555 to determine an RP2D. Patients with pancreatic ductal adenocarcinoma, esophageal cancer, colorectal cancer, melanoma skin cancer, and soft tissue sarcoma are being selected for [Lu-177]-PNT6555 therapy using [Ga-68]-PNT6555 PET/CT imaging. Other key endpoints of the study include radiation dosimetry and biodistribution, blood pharmacokinetics, imaging agent characteristics, and preliminary efficacy based on objective response rate and tumor biomarkers.

Diagnostic Trials

Currently, there are 21 clinical studies registered under clinicaltrials.gov using radioligands for diagnostic purpose. In **Fig. 2**, we highlight the products that are under investigation and the breakdown of the phases of each clinical study. As shown, most of these studies use the FAPI family of compounds (^{18}F/^{68}Ga-FAPI-04, ^{68}Ga-FAPI-46, and ^{18}F-FAPI-74), in addition to two studies with ^{68}Ga-FAP-2286. When the data are analyzed based on the phases of clinical studies, we see that 18 of the studies are in early phases of exploration in Phase 0, Not disclosed/NA, or Phase 1. Three studies are in a more advanced clinical development stage in Phase 2 with [^{18}F]FAPI-74 in gastrointestinal cancers and [^{68}Ga]FAPI-46 in pancreatic ductal adenocarcinoma (see **Fig. 2**). Further analysis of the data based on clinical indication and disease area demonstrates that the highest number of studies are conducted in oncology (16 studies) followed by fibrosis composed of three studies and cardiovascular and arthritis each with one study under investigation (**Fig. 3**).

The information highlighted in this section shows that a large number of studies to investigate FAP-targeting ligands for imaging are in clinical trials. However, most of the studies are in early phases

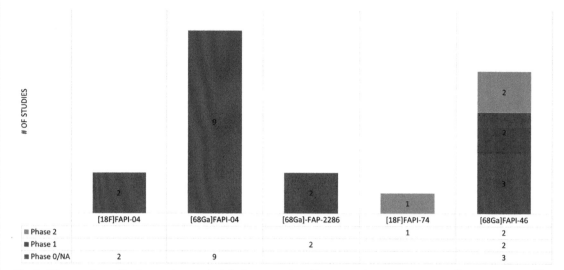

	[18F]FAPI-04	[68Ga]FAPI-04	[68Ga]-FAP-2286	[18F]FAPI-74	[68Ga]FAPI-46
■ Phase 2				1	2
■ Phase 1			2		2
■ Phase 0/NA	2	9			3

Fig. 2. Diagnostic studies by product and trial phase. Depicted here are three studies with [18F]FAPI-74 and [68Ga]FAPI-46 in Phase 2 clinical study stage. Remaining studies are in Phase 0 and Phase 1. NA is "not applicable" designation where a phase of study is not indicated in clinicaltrials.gov. Two imaging studies are with [68Ga]-FAP-2286 and the remaining are conducted with FAPI family of compounds labeled with fluorine-18 or gallium-68.

of development under academic/investigator-initiated studies primarily focused on oncology.

Radioligand Therapy Trials

There are currently three clinical studies registered in clinicaltrials.gov investigating three radioligands for therapy using three products (**Fig. 4**). One product is [177Lu]-EB-FAPI,[20,21] which is Evans blue-modified radiolabeled FAP inhibitor with a β-emitter radionuclide, lutetium-177. Two studies

for this product are in progress, one investigating [177Lu]-EB-FAPI in patients with radioactive iodine refractory thyroid cancer in 20 patients (NCT05410821) and the other examining diagnosis of metastatic tumors with [68Ga]-FAPI-46 PET-CT followed by RLT with [177Lu]-EB-FAPI in 10 patients (NCT05400967). Both studies are in early stages of development examining safety, tolerability, and initial efficacy with start dates of July 15, 2022 and January 1, 2022.

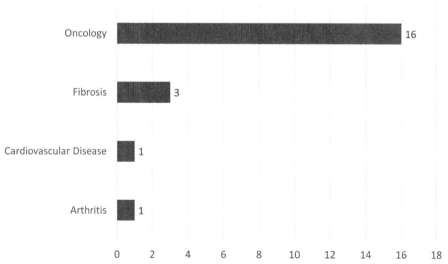

Fig. 3. Diagnostic studies by disease type. Further examination of the 21 diagnostic studies by disease type demonstrated that most of the studies are conducted in oncology, followed by fibrosis, cardiovascular disease, and arthritis.

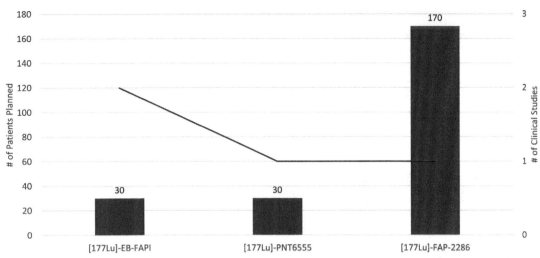

Fig. 4. Radioligand therapeutic studies by product name, patients planned, and number of studies. RLT studies were examined by product name and corresponding patient subjects planned in support of those studies. [^{177}Lu]-EB-FAPI has two studies in progress with a total of 30 patients. [^{177}Lu]-PNT6555 and [^{177}Lu]-FAP-2286 have one study each in progress with 30 and 170 patients planned, respectively.

The second compound by POINT Biopharma leverages a theranostic approach using PNT6555 for both imaging and therapeutic purposes. Named the FRONTIER trial, this is a Phase 1 study with approximately 30 participants to evaluate safety, tolerability, and dosimetry of [^{177}Lu]-PNT6555 for treatment of patients with select solid tumors (NCT05432193). [^{68}Ga]-PNT6555 is used as the imaging agent for patient screening of FAP avid disease. Patients who demonstrate FAP avidity will receive the therapeutic radioligand [^{177}Lu]-PNT6555 at a fixed dose level for up to six doses at an interval of 6 weeks between each dose. The study start date was July 13, 2022.

The third and last product, by Clovis Oncology, is a theranostic approach using FAP-2286 for imaging and therapy purposes. This is a Phase 1/2 multicenter, open-label, non-randomized study to investigate the safety and tolerability, pharmacokinetics, dosimetry, and preliminary activity of [^{177}Lu]-FAP-2286 in patients with an advanced solid tumor. Patients with a positive uptake of the imaging tracer [^{68}Ga]-FAP-2286 will receive the therapeutic radioligand [^{177}Lu]-FAP-2286. Phase 1 of this study features dose escalation to determine the RP2D and schedule in patients with solid tumors and the Phase 2 portion is aimed at a fixed dose of the therapeutic at the RP2D. A total of 170 patients are planned for the study with the trial name LuMIERE and start date of July 30, 2021 (NCT04939610).

Therapeutic/theranostic studies using radioligands for FAP-targeting are still in early stages of development and are currently using a single therapy approach with lutetium-177 as the radioligand of choice. Based on data in clinicaltrials.gov, the anticipated primary completion date for most of these therapeutic studies is between mid-year 2023 and mid-year 2024.

Non-Radioligand Therapy Trials

Based on data available on clinicaltrials.gov, Avacta, Molecular Partners AG, and Roche are three pharmaceutical companies pursuing non-radioligand FAP-targeting therapeutics. Summary information regarding these clinical studies is provided in **Table 2**. The table depicts a total of eight studies, of which five are active, three are completed and four are active and recruiting.

Avacta is pursuing AVA6000[22] in a Phase 1 study (NCT04969835). This product is an FAP-activated prodrug based on the pre|CISION platform, providing a prodrug form of doxorubicin. In its FAP-activated form, the doxorubicin drug moiety is not cell permeable and is an inert agent. In the tumor microenvironment, where the level of the enzyme FAP is substantially higher than elsewhere in the body, the FAP substrate is cleaved, and the active doxorubicin drug is released causing differential targeting of tumor tissue compared with healthy tissue.

Molecular Partners AG is pursuing a Phase 1 study (NCT05098405) with MP0317 (FAP × CD-40)[23] as part of an immune-oncology pipeline. MP0317 includes DARPin domains to bind to

Table 2
Non-radioligand therapies targeting FAP

Sponsor	NCT#	Study Title	Intervention(s)	Trial Phase	Status
Avacta life sciences Ltd	NCT04969835	A study evaluating the safety, pharmacokinetics and early efficacy of AVA6000 in solid tumors	Drug: AVA6000	Phase 1	Recruiting
Molecular partners AG	NCT05098405	First-in-human safety and tolerability of MP0317 in patients with relapsed/refractory advanced solid tumors	Drug: MPO317, a tri-specific fibroblast activation protein (FAP) × CD40 DARPin drug candidate	Phase 1	Recruiting
Hoffmann-La Roche	NCT0385079	A study to evaluate safety and therapeutic activity of RO6874281, in combination with pembrolizumab, in participants with advanced metastatic melanoma	Drug: RO6874281|drug: Pembrolizumab	Phase 1	Completed
Hoffmann-La Roche	NCTO4826003	Study to evaluate safety, pharmacokinetics and pharmacodynamics and preliminary anti-tumor activity of RO7122290, in combination with cibisatamab with obiutuzumab pretreatment	Drug: RO7122290|drug: cibisatamab|drug: obinutuzumab	Phase 1/Phase 2	Recruiting
Hoffmann-La Roche	NCT04857138	A study to evaluate safety, pharmacokinetics and antitumor activity of RO7300490, as a single agent (Part A) or in combination with atezolizumab in participants with advanced solid tumors	Drug: RO7300490|drug: atezolizumab	Phase 1	Recruiting
Hoffmann-La Roche	NCT02627274	A study evaluating safety, pharmacokinetics and therapeutic activity of RO6874281 as a single agent (Part A) or in combination with trastuzumab or cetuximab (Part B or C)	Drug: RO6874281|drug: trastuzumab|drug: cetuximab	Phase 1	Active, not recruiting

(continued on next page)

Table 2
(continued)

Sponsor	NCT#	Study Title	Intervention(s)	Trial Phase	Status
Hoffmann-La Roche	NCT03386721	Basket study to evaluate the therapeutic activity of simlukafusp alfa as a combination therapy in participants with advanced and/or metastatic solid tumors	Drug: simlukafusp alfa| drug: atezolizumab (MPDL3280A), an engineered anti-PD-L1 antibody| drug: gemcitabine| drug: vinorelbine	Phase 2	Completed
Hoffmann-La Roche	NCT02558140	A dose escalation study of RO6874813 in participants with locally advanced or metastatic solid tumors	Biological: RO6874813	Phase 1	Completed

This table demonstrates industry sponsored trials for FAP-targeted non-radioligand therapy. Three industry sites have active non-RLT studies in progress. These include Avacta, Molecular Partners AG, and Roche. Four of the eight studies are currently actively recruiting.

FAP and CD40 molecules. FAP is found in the tumor microenvironment and, by engaging CD40 on immune cells at the same time, clustering occurs that can achieve local activation of immune cells. Based on this model, activation of immune cells only occurs when both targets are simultaneously engaged, resulting in local tumor targeting and avoiding systemic side effects.

Roche has two FAP-targeted antibody and fusion protein products in early phases of clinical development. One is FAP-CD40 (RG6189),[24] a second-generation tumor-targeted CD40 agonist designed to activate antigen-presenting cells to treat cancer in combination with other therapies. The second product is FAP 4-1BBL (RG7827),[25] an agonistic immune modulator and targeted T-cell co-stimulator. RG7827 has an antibody-like structure, with one arm binding to FAP and the other arm carrying the signaling molecule, 4-1BBL. Last, Roche completed studies with a third FAP-targeted compound, Simlukafusp alfa (FAP-IL2v), which has been discontinued.

FUTURE DIRECTIONS

As outlined in this article, the current clinical studies using radioligands for FAP imaging and therapy are in Phase 1 or early Phase 2 stage and hence in early parts of clinical development. We expect that it will take several years before efficacy data for appropriate indications can be obtained in support of new drug application

approvals. In addition to the clinical efforts discussed, several additional radioligands for imaging and therapy are under development and showing promising results in preclinical or first in human studies. The compounds are not registered with clinicaltrials.gov data and thus have not been analyzed in the previous sections. A number of these products are expected to enter the clinical trial process for imaging, therapy or theranostic purpose in the near future. A selection of these prospective radioligands is highlighted below based on information presented at the 2022 ICPO FAP Theranostics Summit.

Ratio Therapeutics (RTX) is using their Trillium technology platform to create proprietary small molecule targeting agents to attack a broad array of cancer targets. The company showed promising preclinical data highlighting the development and optimization of radioligands for theranostic use. These include, but are not limited to, ^{68}Ga-RTX ^{18}F-RTX and ^{67}Cu-RTX radioligands targeting FAP for imaging or therapy. 3B Pharmaceuticals, the originating company behind the theranostic FAP-2286, is developing and optimizing additional products in its FAP pipeline. These include ^{18}F-FAP for imaging, a 3BP-FAP SPECT tracer to meet the needs of regions without access to PET scanners and a new lead FAP ligand for therapeutic use, 3BP-3940. Philogen's platform creates small molecule ligands with antibody-like properties featuring ultra-high affinity to their target antigen and long residence time at the tumor site.

They have developed radiotracers with high affinity for FAP targeting. These radioligands are named "OncoFAP" and are being optimized for imaging and therapy use.[26] Last, homodimers with two squaramide coupled FAPI conjugates [^{177}Lu]Lu-DOTAGA (SA.FAPi)$_2$ show promising preliminary results to treat radioiodine refractory differentiated patients with thyroid cancer in initial studies conducted by Prof Ballal.[27]

SUMMARY

FAP has been an attractive target for therapy and imaging since first identified in the 1980s, with significant growth occurring in FAP targeting, especially in the development of radioligands for imaging and therapeutic use in the recent years. The studies outlined in this article are not meant to be an exhaustive list of all human studies with FAP-targeting ligands, but instead highlight registered studies through clinicaltrials.gov, along with other published and publicly available data on emerging compounds soon entering clinical studies.

Based on the data available, we see significant momentum in FAP imaging with 21 studies in progress. The products at the latest clinical development stage in are [^{18}F]FAPI-74 (gastrointestinal cancers) and [^{68}Ga]FAPI-46 Pancreatic Ductal Adenocarcinoma (PDAC) in phase 2 and most of the remaining imaging studies are investigator-initiated studies in early stages of clinical development. Additional larger prospective studies in key indications are needed to move FAP imaging toward a path for new drug application status.

In FAP targeting for therapy, we currently see studies in early stages of clinical evaluations. In RLT, four clinical studies are in progress using three interventions with ^{177}Lu as the main isotope of choice. Currently, the radioligand studies are monotherapies, and future directions could include combination therapies, with radioligand FAP targeting as one arm of therapy. Further, dosing regiments and use of alpha therapy along with beta therapy options will be interesting areas of development to assess the best therapeutic response in various cancers.

We expect that over the next three years, there will be significant advances in FAP targeting through the availability of data from existing studies, and registration of additional prospective studies that can further result in clinical development of appropriate indications for FAP-targeting ligands in imaging, along with best therapeutic targeting approaches.

CLINICS CARE POINTS

- Investigator initiated studies in Phase 0/1 are critical driving factors for exploring various new clinical indications for new radipharmaceuticals, which have made a great impact on the advancement of FAP interventions. However, moving the promising products through the clinical development pahway and through approvals, requires launch of more prospective clinical studies in key areas of unmet need.

- Activated fibroblasts play a critical role in oncology through CAFs, in addition to their role in non-oncology through activated fibroblast mediated disease (Fibrotic disease, fibroimflammatory disease, cardiovascular disease and more). As a result, distinguishing FAP PET image observations between malignant and non-malignant lesions will be important through establishing optimized FAP imaging protocols and image interpretation guidelines.

DISCLOSURE

S. Mosessian serves as the Chief Scientific Officer at SOFIE, a commercial company with IP rights to the Fibroblast Activation Protein Inhibitor family of compounds for diagnostic and companion diagnostic development. J.D. Jensen serves as the Executive Vice President of Clinical Development at POINT Biopharma, a pre-commercial radiopharmaceutical development company with worldwide rights to a family of Fibroblast Activation Protein Inhibitor compounds invented by Dr William Bachovchin at Tufts University. A. Enke BS serves as a Senior Director of Clinical Development at Clovis Oncology, a publicly traded pharmaceutical development company with US rights to the Fibroblast Activation Protein-targeting peptide, FAP-2286 for diagnostic and therapeutic development.

REFERENCES

1. Rettig WJ, Chesa PG, Beresford HR, et al. Differential expression of cell surface antigens and glial fibrillary acidic protein in human astrocytoma subsets. Cancer Res 1986;46(12 Pt 1):6406–12.
2. Garin-Chesa P, Old LJ, Rettig WJ. Cell surface glycoprotein of reactive stromal fibroblasts as a potential antibody target in human epithelial cancers. Proc Natl Acad Sci U S A 1990;87(18):7235–9.

3. Rettig WJ, Garin-Chesa P, Healey JH, et al. Regulation and heteromeric structure of the fibroblast activation protein in normal and transformed cells of mesenchymal and neuroectodermal origin. Cancer Res 1993;53(14):3327–35.

4. Aoyama A, Chen WT. A 170-kDa membrane-bound protease is associated with the expression of invasiveness by human malignant melanoma cells. Proc Natl Acad Sci U S A 1990;87(21):8296–300.

5. Scanlan MJ, Raj BK, Calvo B, et al. Molecular cloning of fibroblast activation protein alpha, a member of the serine protease family selectively expressed in stromal fibroblasts of epithelial cancers. Proc Natl Acad Sci U S A 1994;91(12):5657–61.

6. Goldstein LA, Ghersi G, Piñeiro-Sánchez ML, et al. Molecular cloning of seprase: a serine integral membrane protease from human melanoma. Biochim Biophys Acta 1997;1361(1):11–9.

7. Piñeiro-Sánchez ML, Goldstein LA, Dodt J, et al. Identification of the 170-kDa melanoma membrane-bound gelatinase (seprase) as a serine integral membrane protease. J Biol Chem 1997;272(12): 7595–601.

8. Gene: FAP ENSG00000078098, Available at: http://uswest.ensembl.org/Homo_sapiens/Gene/ExpressionAtlas?g=ENSG00000078098. Accessed March 19, 2023.

9. The human protein atlas: FAP tissue, Available at: https://www.proteinatlas.org/ENSG00000078098-FA/tissue. Accessed March 19, 2023.

10. Mona CE, Benz MR, Hikmat F, et al. Correlation of 68Ga-FAPi-46 PET biodistribution with FAP expression by immunohistochemistry in patients with solid cancers: interim analysis of a prospective translational exploratory study. J Nucl Med 2022;63(7): 1021–6.

11. Dendl K, Koerber SA, Kratochwil C, et al. FAP and FAPI-PET/CT in malignant and non-malignant diseases: a perfect symbiosis? Cancers 2021;13(19). https://doi.org/10.3390/cancers13194946.

12. Loktev A, Lindner T, Burger EM, et al. Development of fibroblast activation protein-targeted radiotracers with improved tumor retention. J Nucl Med 2019; 60(10):1421–9.

13. Kratochwil C, Flechsig P, Lindner T, et al. Ga-FAPI PET/CT: tracer uptake in 28 different kinds of cancer. J Nucl Med 2019;60(6):801–5.

14. Meyer C, Dahlbom M, Lindner T, et al. Radiation dosimetry and biodistribution of. J Nucl Med 2020; 61(8):1171–7.

15. Fendler WP, Pabst KM, Kessler L, et al. Safety and efficacy of 90Y-FAPI-46 radioligand therapy in patients with advanced sarcoma and other cancer entities. Clin Cancer Res 2022;28(19):4346–53.

16. Giesel FL, Adeberg S, Syed M, et al. FAPI-74 PET/CT using either. J Nucl Med 2021;62(2):201–7.

17. Zboralski D, Hoehne A, Bredenbeck A, et al. Preclinical evaluation of FAP-2286 for fibroblast activation protein targeted radionuclide imaging and therapy. Eur J Nucl Med Mol Imag 2022;49(11):3651–67.

18. Baum RP, Schuchardt C, Singh A, et al. Feasibility, biodistribution, and preliminary dosimetry in peptide-targeted radionuclide therapy of diverse adenocarcinomas using. J Nucl Med 2022;63(3): 415–23.

19. Hallett RM, Poplawski SE, Dornan MH, et al. Pre-clinical characterization of the novel FAP targeting ligand PNT6555 for imaging and therapy of cancer. Cancer Res, 82 (12_Supplement), 2022, 3303.

20. Wen X, Xu P, Shi M, et al. Evans blue-modified radiolabeled fibroblast activation protein inhibitor as long-acting cancer therapeutics. Theranostics 2022; 12(1):422–33.

21. Treatment Using 177Lu-DOTA-EB-FAPI in Patients With Radioactive Iodine Refractory Thyroid Cancer. Available at: https://clinicaltrials.gov/ct2/show/NCT05410821. Accessed March 19, 2023.

22. McLaughlin F., Poplawski S.E. and Sanford D.G., Abstract 1815: AVA6000, a novel Precision medicine, targeted to the tumor microenvironment via Fibroblast Activation Protein (FAP) mediated cleavage, Cancer Res, 2022;82(12_supplement):1815.

23. Ioannou K, Ragusa S, Roquette J. Abstract 1733: MP0317, a CD40xFAP targeting multi-specific DARPin® therapeutic, drives immune activation and reverts myeloid-mediated T-cell suppression in vitro and ex vivo, Cancer Res, 2021;81(13_Supplement):1733.

24. Sum E, Rapp M, Fröbel P, et al. Fibroblast activation protein α-targeted CD40 agonism abrogates systemic toxicity and enables administration of high doses to induce effective antitumor immunity. Clin Cancer Res 2021;27(14):4036–53.

25. Trüb M, Uhlenbrock F, Claus C, et al. Fibroblast activation protein-targeted-4-1BB ligand agonist amplifies effector functions of intratumoral T cells in human cancer. J Immunother Cancer 2020;8(2). https://doi.org/10.1136/jitc-2019-000238.

26. Bartoli F, Elsinga P, Nazario LR, et al. Automated radiosynthesis, preliminary in vitro/in vivo characterization of OncoFAP-based radiopharmaceuticals for cancer imaging and therapy. Pharmaceuticals 2022;15(8). https://doi.org/10.3390/ph15080958.

27. Ballal S, Yadav MP, Moon ES, et al. Novel fibroblast activation protein inhibitor-based targeted theranostics for radioiodine-refractory differentiated thyroid cancer patients: a pilot study. Thyroid 2022;32(1): 65–77. https://doi.org/10.1089/thy.2021.0412.

Moving?

Make sure your subscription moves with you!

To notify us of your new address, find your **Clinics Account Number** (located on your mailing label above your name), and contact customer service at:

Email: journalscustomerservice-usa@elsevier.com

800-654-2452 (subscribers in the U.S. & Canada)
314-447-8871 (subscribers outside of the U.S. & Canada)

Fax number: 314-447-8029

Elsevier Health Sciences Division
Subscription Customer Service
3251 Riverport Lane
Maryland Heights, MO 63043

Printed and bound by CPI Group (UK) Ltd, Croydon, CR0 4YY

03/10/2024

01040365-0015